THE YEAR IN
GASTROENTEROLOGY AND HEPATOLOGY

VOLUME 2

THE YEAR IN GASTROENTEROLOGY AND HEPATOLOGY

VOLUME 2

EDITED BY

NIZAR ZEIN, BRET LASHNER

CLINICAL PUBLISHING
OXFORD

Clinical Publishing

an imprint of Atlas Medical Publishing Ltd

Oxford Centre for Innovation
Mill Street, Oxford OX2 0JX, UK

Tel: +44 1865 811116
Fax: +44 1865 251550
E mail: info@clinicalpublishing.co.uk
Web: www.clinicalpublishing.co.uk

Distributed in USA and Canada by:

Clinical Publishing
30 Amberwood Parkway
Ashland, Ohio 44805, USA
Tel: 800 247 6553
Fax: 419 281 6883
E mail: orders@bookmasters.com

Distributed in UK and Rest of World by:

Marston Book Services Ltd
PO Box 269
Abingdon
Oxon OX14 4YN, UK
Tel: +44 1235 465500
Fax: +44 1235 465555
E mail: trade.orders@marston.co.uk

First published 2007

A catalogue record for this book is available from the British Library

ISBN-13 978 1 904392 81 1
ISBN-10 1 904392 81 4
ISSN 1745-8498

Project Manager: Rosemary Osmond, Helimetrics Ltd, Chipping Norton, Oxon, UK
Typeset by Hope Services (Abingdon) Ltd, Abingdon, Oxon, UK
Printed by T G Hostench SA, Barcelona, Spain

Contents

Part III

Gastrointestinal endoscopy

Part IV

Hepatology and liver transplantation

Editors

Bret A Lashner, MD
Professor of Medicine, Cleveland Clinic Lerner College of Medicine; Director, Center for Inflammatory Bowel Disease, Department of Gastroenterology and Hepatology, Cleveland Clinic, Cleveland, Ohio, USA

Nizar N Zein, MD
Director of Clinical Hepatology, Department of Gastroenterology and Hepatology, Cleveland Clinic, Cleveland, Ohio, USA

Contributors

Edgar Achkar, MD
Vice Chairman, Department of Gastroenterology and Hepatology, Cleveland Clinic, Cleveland, Ohio, USA

Jean-Paul Achkar, MD
Staff Gastroenterologist, Center for Inflammatory Bowel Disease, Department of Gastroenterology and Hepatology, Cleveland Clinic, Cleveland, Ohio, USA

David S Barnes, MD
Acting Head, Section of Hepatology, Department of Gastroenterology and Hepatology; Medical Director of Liver Transplantation, Transplant Center, Cleveland Clinic, Cleveland, Ohio, USA

Laura Bianchi, MD
Chief Fellow, Department of Gastroenterology and Hepatology, Cleveland Clinic, Cleveland, Ohio, USA

Aaron Brzezinski, MD, FRCP(C)
Staff, Center for Inflammatory Bowel Disease, Department of Gastroenterology and Hepatology, Cleveland Clinic, Cleveland, Ohio, USA

Carol A Burke, MD, FACG, FACP
Director, Center for Colon Polyp and Cancer Prevention, Department of Gastroenterology and Hepatology, Cleveland Clinic, Cleveland, Ohio, USA

William D Carey, MD, MACG
Professor of Medicine, Cleveland Clinic Lerner College of Medicine; Department of Gastroenterology and Hepatology, Cleveland Clinic, Cleveland; Professor of Medicine, Ohio State University, Ohio, USA

John A Dumot, MD
Section Head, Gastroenterology Regional Medical Practice, Department of Gastroenterology and Hepatology, Cleveland Clinic, Cleveland, Ohio, USA

Bijan Eghtesad, MD
Staff Surgeon, Department of General Surgery, Section of Liver Transplantation, Cleveland Clinic, Cleveland, Ohio, USA

Ariel E Feldstein, MD
Staff, Department of Pediatric Gastroenterology and Cell Biology, Cleveland Clinic, Cleveland, Ohio, USA

John J Fung, MD, PhD
Chairman, Department of General Surgery; Chief, Transplantation Surgery, Cleveland Clinic, Cleveland, Ohio, USA

Marsha Kay, MD
Staff Physician, Department of Pediatric Gastroenterology and Nutrition, Cleveland Clinic, Cleveland, Ohio, USA

Margaret F Kinnard, MD
Assistant Professor of Medicine, Case Western Reserve University School of Medicine, Cleveland Veterans Affairs Medical Center; Chief, GI Section, Louis Stokes Cleveland VA Medical Center, Cleveland, Ohio, USA

Bret A Lashner, MD
Professor of Medicine, Cleveland Clinic Lerner College of Medicine; Director, Center for Inflammatory Bowel Disease, Department of Gastroenterology and Hepatology, Cleveland Clinic, Cleveland, Ohio, USA

Brent D Lemberg, MD
Chief Fellow, Department of Gastroenterology and Hepatology, Cleveland Clinic, Cleveland, Ohio, USA

Ilche Nonevski, MD
Department of Gastroenterology and Hepatology, Cleveland Clinic, Cleveland, Ohio, USA

Ioannis Oikonomou, MD
Fellow, Department of Gastroenterology and Hepatology, Cleveland Clinic, Cleveland, Ohio, USA

Robert S O'Shea, MD, MScE
Assistant Professor of Medicine, Cleveland Clinic Lerner College of Medicine, Case Western Reserve University; Department of Gastroenterology and Hepatology, Cleveland Clinic, Cleveland, Ohio, USA

Woosuk Park, MD
Department of Gastroenterology and Hepatology, Cleveland Clinic, Cleveland, Ohio, USA

Mark Pimentel, MD
Director, GI Motility Program, Division of Gastroenterology and Hepatology, Cedars-Sinai Medical Center, Los Angeles, California, USA

Kadakkal Radhakrishnan, MD
Staff, Department of Pediatric Gastroenterology, Cleveland Clinic, Cleveland, Ohio, USA

Steven S Shay, MD
Staff Gastroenterologist, Department of Gastroenterology and Hepatology, Cleveland Clinic, Cleveland, Ohio, USA

Bo Shen, MD, FACG
Staff, Department of Gastroenterology and Hepatology, Cleveland Clinic, Cleveland, Ohio, USA

Edy E Soffer, MD, FACG
Co-Director, GI Motility Program, Division of Gastroenterology and Hepatology, Cedars-Sinai Medical Center, Los Angeles, California, USA

John J Vargo, MD, MPG
Staff, Section of Therapeutic and Pancreaticobiliary Endoscopy, Department of Gastroenterology and Hepatology, Cleveland Clinic, Cleveland, Ohio, USA

Jamilé Wakim-Fleming, MD
Assistant Professor, Case Western Reserve University, Cleveland Ohio; Department of Gastroenterology and Hepatology, Cleveland Clinic, Cleveland, Ohio, USA

Anna Wieckowska, MD
Department of Gastroenterology and Hepatology, Cleveland Clinic, Cleveland, Ohio, USA

Robert Wyllie, MD
Chairman, Division of Pediatrics, Physician-in-Chief, The Children's Hospital, Cleveland Clinic, Cleveland, Ohio, USA

Nizar N Zein, MD
Director, Center for Inflammatory Bowel Disease, Department of Gastroenterology and Hepatology, Cleveland Clinic, Cleveland, Ohio, USA

Preface

BRET A LASHNER, MD
Professor of Medicine
Cleveland Clinic Lerner College of Medicine
Director, Center for Inflammatory Bowel Disease

NIZAR N ZEIN, MD
Director of Clinical Hepatology

Department of Gastroenterology and Hepatology
Cleveland Clinic
Cleveland, Ohio, USA

As gastroenterologists, our patients expect us to offer them the latest treatments for their diseases. Indeed, that is the crux of the referral to a specialist. However, the gastroenterology and hepatology literature advances at such a rapid rate that it is impossible for any of us to be 'caught up' with our reading.

We are very happy to offer you this volume of the most important studies published in the last eighteen months. Each article is presented and critiqued by true experts in the field. Oesophageal motility disorders, gastrointestinal cancer, inflammatory bowel disease, irritable bowel syndrome, endoscopic ultrasound, biliary endoscopy, viral hepatitis, cholestasis, fatty liver, portal hypertension, and liver transplantation are some of the areas covered. We must thank our colleagues for writing such outstanding reviews and insightful criticism. It has been a true privilege working with them.

So, try to 'catch up' by sitting back and reading this book cover-to-cover. We think you will agree with us that this was a very good year.

Part I

Diseases of the upper GI tract

1

Oesophageal motility disorders

STEVEN SHAY

Introduction

Oesophageal motility disorders (EMD) are sought in patients with dysphagia and/or chest pain of non-cardiac origin. Classification schemes for the EMD have been proposed (Table 1.1). Only achalasia has well-defined physiological and clinical consequences. The other named disorders in Table 1.1 have no aetiology, lack definite pathophysiologies and do not predictably respond to therapy (even if the motility abnormality resolves).

The development of new technologies is necessary to address the issues discussed above. This review will focus on the advances in technology in the last year. However, some articles are reviewed on achalasia, the only universally accepted EMD.

Table 1.1 Criteria for diagnosing oesophageal motility abnormalities

Function defect	Diagnosis	Manometric findings
Aperistalsis	Achalasia	Absent distal peristalsis Increased LES pressure (>45 mmHg) Incomplete LES relaxation
Uncoordinated activity	DES	≥20% simultaneous contractions Repetitive contractions (>3 peaks) Prolonged duration contractions Incomplete LES relaxation
Hypercontractile	Nutcracker Oesophagus	Increased amplitude (>180 mmHg) Increased peristaltic duration
	Hypertensive LES	Resting LES pressure >45 mmHg Incomplete LES relaxation
Hypocontractile	IEM	>30% non-transmitted peristalsis Peristaltic amplitude <30 mmHg
	Hypotensive LES	Resting LES pressure <10 mmHg

DES, diffuse oesophageal spasm; LES, lower oesophageal sphincter; IEM, ineffective oesophageal motility.

High-resolution manometry (HRM) predicts the success of oesophageal bolus transport and identifies clinically important abnormalities not detected by conventional manometry

Fox M, Hebbard G, Janiak P, *et al. Neurogastroenterol Motil* 2004; **16**: 533–42

BACKGROUND. Bolus transit is complex, as it depends on a normal swallowing act (relaxation of the upper oesophageal sphincter and pharyngeal contraction) to present the bolus to the oesophageal body, normal oesophageal body mechanics (peristalsis and an effective contraction) and timely LES relaxation to allow bolus transport from the pharynx to the stomach. Standard oesophageal manometry catheters are ill equipped to do all the above, because they have only five to eight pressure sites, usually with 5 cm between pressure sites, and most/all pressure sites are unidirectional. As a result, a proportion of symptomatic patients with dysphagia and/or chest pain due to a disorder in a short segment of the tubular oesophagus will be missed by the standard oesophageal manometry catheter. The aim of this multicentre study was to compare high-resolution manometry (HRM) perfusion catheters having 21 and 32 unidirectional pressure sites with standard manometry. Bolus transit was assessed simultaneously by the gold standard, the video-oesophagram. Standard manometry was not performed at a separate time. Instead, sites were chosen from the HRM catheter to simulate standard oesophageal manometry catheters with eight, seven and five channels.

INTERPRETATION. Receiver operating characteristic (ROC) analysis (Fig. 1.1) showed that HRM predicted the presence of abnormal bolus transit more accurately than standard manometry (Fig 1.1). Furthermore, HRM identified clinically important motor dysfunction not detected by manometry and oesophagram, such as localized disturbances of peristalsis and abnormal movement of the LES during oesophageal spasm. The authors conclude that HRM is an important advance in the assessment of oesophageal function and is likely to bring benefits in clinical practice.

Comment

In this study, ten normal subjects and nine with endoscopy-negative dysphagia were given ten swallows of 5 ml water and then at least five swallows of barium at intervals of 30 s or longer. The method allowed findings of HRM to be simultaneously correlated to bolus transit by video-oesophagrametry.

First, HRM was more accurate than conventional manometry in predicting disturbed bolus transport at mild to moderate levels of transit abnormality. Normal bolus transit and complete failure of bolus transit were identified accurately by both methods. Thus, HRM will be of benefit in some, but not all, symptomatic patients.

Secondly, HRM reclassified the findings with some swallows. Swallows classified as hypomotility or oesophageal spasms by HRM were often classified as normal or non-specific oesophageal motor disorder by conventional manometry. Identifying

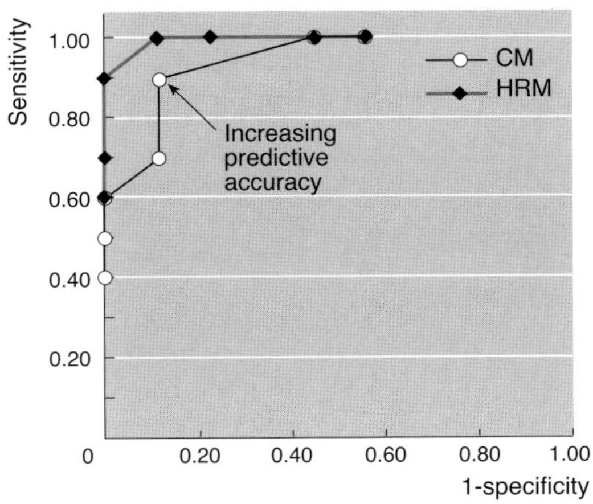

Fig. 1.1 Receiver operating characteristic (ROC) analysis. Both conventional manometry (CM) and high-resolution manometry (HRM) were accurate in predicting both complete success and failure of bolus transport. HRM was more accurate than CM in predicting disturbed bolus transport at mild to moderate levels of transit abnormality. The sensitivity and specificity of HRM were equal to or greater than those of CM at every level. The larger area under the ROC curve indicates that HRM predicts bolus transport more accurately than CM. Source: Fox *et al.* (2004).

more patients with manometric abnormalities may be useful. For example, patients who will develop dysphagia after fundoplication may be identified, because conventional manometry has not been found to be consistently helpful |**1**|.

The authors of this report have been using HRM for 5 years in clinical practice for patients with no oesophagitis and dysphagia. They have found that about 10% of patients had a definite diagnosis made by HRM when conventional manometry was non-diagnostic. In 212 unselected patients, Clouse *et al.* found manometry disagreement in 12% and diagnostic disagreement in 5% between HRM and conventional manometry |**2**|.

The improved diagnostic accuracy of HRM over conventional manometry and the successful prediction of bolus transport are strong arguments for HRM becoming the state-of-the-art method for assessing oesophageal motor function. Furthermore, software allows data from all pressure sites to be presented as a spatiotemporal plot (STP; Fig. 1.2). Experienced users find it easier to interpret STP plots than to analyse separate line tracings, though line tracings are also available for review if the reader of the data prefers.

There are other benefits in using HRM. First, HRM is a shorter study as there is no need for a pull-through to measure LES pressure. Secondly, there is an accurate swallow marker (both pharyngeal pressure and upper oesophageal sphincter relaxation are measured), and separate swallow and respiratory signals are not

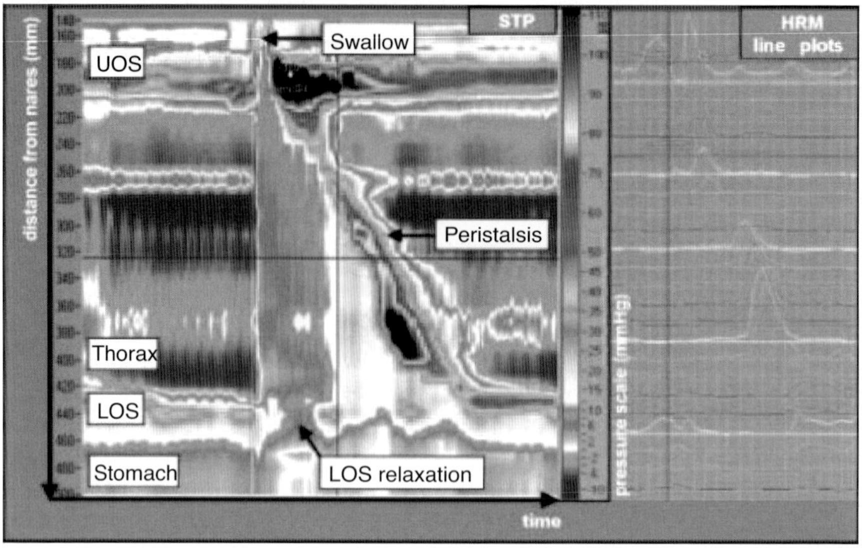

Fig. 1.2 Normal 32-channel high-resolution manometry (HRM) of 10 ml water swallows. The HRM spatiotemporal plot (STP) depicts the direction and force of pressure activity in the oesophagus from the pharynx to the stomach. Time is on the x-axis and distance from the nares is on the y-axis. Each pressure is assigned a colour. Source: Fox *et al.* (2004).

necessary. Thirdly, intragastric pressure is available at all times, so the gastro-oesophageal pressure gradient can be measured, and movement and coughing artefact can be identified accurately. Fourthly, LES relaxation is better measured as discussed in the next article (Bredenoord *et al.*, 2005).

There are disadvantages of HRM that must be considered, as described by Bredenoord *et al.* below. First, this more sophisticated equipment is more expensive; secondly, the additional signals make interpretation more challenging.

A solid-state HRM catheter is now commercially available (Sierra Scientific Instruments, Los Angeles, CA, USA). The catheter has 36 circumferential pressure sensors 1 cm apart from the pharynx to the stomach, and the spatiotemporal plot is derived by analysing all 36 pressure sites.

Sleeve sensor versus high-resolution manometry (HRM) for the detection of transient lower esophageal sphincter relaxations (TLESR)

Bredenoord J, Weuste B, Timmer R, Smout A. *Am J Physiol Gastrointest Liver Physiol* 2005; **288**: G1190–4

BACKGROUND. In conventional manometry, a single perfused side-hole or miniature pressure transducer is positioned in the lumen of the LES. Axial movement of the distal oesophagus relative to the catheter occurs with a swallow. Complete LES relaxation has been reported to occur in 30% of achalasia patients [3] but may be a measurement artefact from axial movement. The sleeve sensor was developed to address this problem, and is traditionally accepted as the best method of measuring LES relaxation. The aim of this study was to compare the sleeve sensor with HRM in detecting transient LES relaxations.

INTERPRETATION. High-resolution manometry is at least as accurate as the sleeve sensor in detecting transient relaxations of the lower oesophageal sphincter. These findings should also apply to swallow-associated relaxations of the lower oesophageal sphincter, which were not assessed in this study.

Comment

LES relaxation was examined in twelve gastro-oesophageal reflux disease (GERD) patients 30 min before and 90 min after a meal. LES was assessed by HRM (seven perfused sites 1 cm apart) with at least the most distal pressure site in the stomach, and a sleeve sensor straddling the LES. Impedance detected gas and/or liquid reflux and pH monitoring acid reflux to correlate with transient lower oesophageal sphincter relaxations (TLESRs).

Of 145 TLESRs identified by either method, the sleeve sensor detected 75% and HRM 81% (Fig. 1.3). Median TLESR duration and the proportion of TLESRs associated with reflux were not significantly different for TLESRs diagnosed by HRM compared with the sleeve sensor. However, there was a higher proportion of TLESRs diagnosed only by HRM than by the sleeve sensor. This suggests the sleeve sensor may have occasional false-positive TLESRs. The authors did not assess swallow-associated LESRs. However, since HRM has sites at intervals of 1 cm from the stomach to the distal oesophagus, it is reasonable to assume that the accuracy is similar for swallow-associated LESRs and TLESRs despite axial oesophageal movement with the former.

The importance of this article, when taken in conjunction with the previous article (Fox *et al.*, 2004), is the value of HRM in assessing LES function in addition to oesophageal body function. The limitation of a single side-hole at the LES and gaps between pressure sites of 5 cm in most commercial conventional catheters are simultaneously addressed.

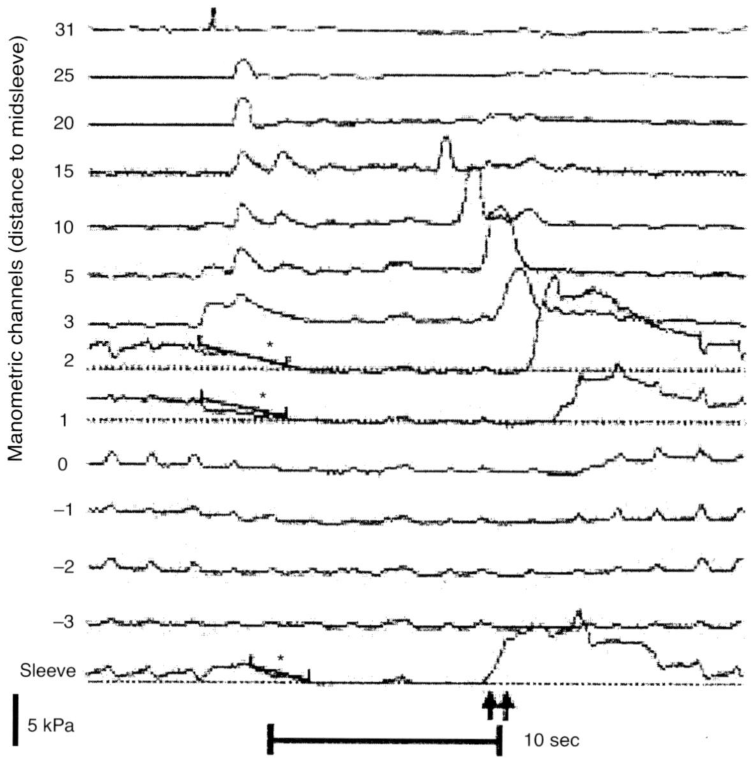

Fig. 1.3 Transient LES relaxation (TLESR). Channels 1 and 2 and the sleeve show relaxation to gastric pressure (*) followed by secondary peristalsis. The increase in pressure in the proximal end of the sleeve (arrows) induced by the peristaltic contraction makes the relaxation last shorter in the sleeve sensor. The dotted line indicates gastric pressure. Source: Bredenoord *et al.* (2005).

Assessment of oesophageal motor function using combined perfusion manometry and multichannel intraluminal impedance measurement in normal subjects

Nguyen J, Rigda R, Tipper M, Concillo J, Smout A, Holloway R. *Neurogastroenterol Motil* 2005; **17**: 458–65

BACKGROUND. Manometry findings can only infer or predict bolus transport efficacy. Video-oesophagram is the gold standard for the assessment of bolus transit. However, oesophageal impedance monitoring (EIM) has been developed recently to assess bolus entry and bolus clearance from the oesophagus (Fig. 1.4). This was supported by a study this year showing excellent correlation of bolus transit when

barium oesophagrametry and impedance monitoring were done simultaneously. However, only normal subjects were studied |4|. The aim of this study was to establish normal values for simultaneous impedance monitoring and manometry using perfusion catheters.

Interpretation. Using impedance criteria, normal oesophageal bolus clearance is defined when an individual completely clears at least 70% of liquid responses and 60% of viscous responses. Normal values are now available for application in the research and clinical settings.

Comment

The methods used in this multicentre study from Europe and Australia added impedance electrode pairs to perfusion catheters. The main clinical finding is that normal bolus transit with 70% of liquid swallows and 60% of viscous swallows defines the normal limit. These are the same normal values as those reported in a multicentre study from the USA with a solid-state catheter |**5**|. Moreover, these values were the same despite the studies being done in different postures and the catheters having different impedance/manometry sites in the two reports.

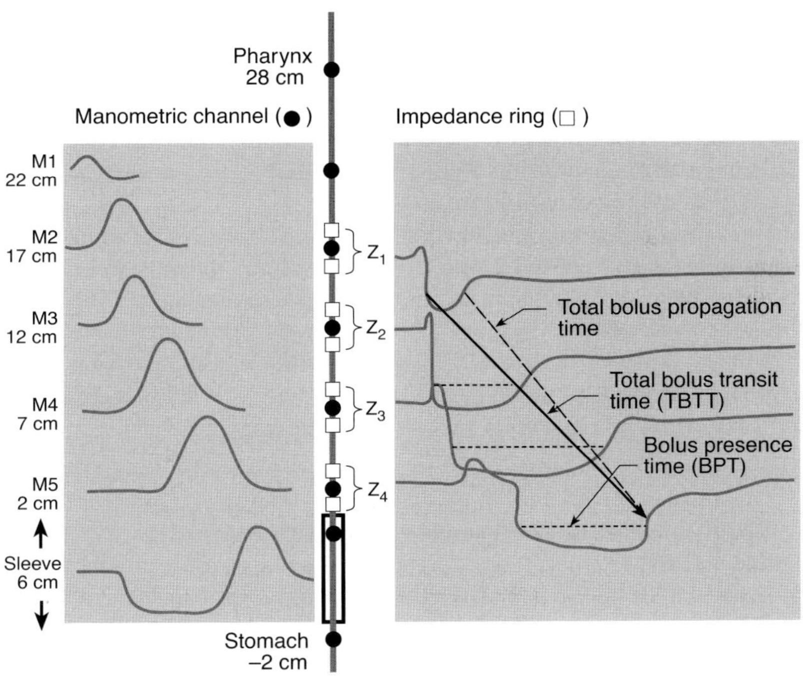

Fig. 1.4 Schematic depiction of the combined perfusion manometry and impedance recording assembly and important impedance variables. Source: Nguyen *et al.* (2005).

There were additional findings in this study. First, liquid swallows followed by normal peristalsis were rarely associated with an abnormal total bolus transit time (2%) as defined in Fig. 1.4, though an abnormal bolus presence time (Fig. 1.4) at one or more sites was present in 13%. Importantly, hypotensive and simultaneous contractions were usually associated with both normal liquid total bolus transit time (83 and 88% respectively) and normal bolus presence time (72 and 75%). These findings are similar to those of the previous study [5], and highlight the importance of simultaneously assessing bolus clearance with abnormal manometric findings.

In contrast to hypotensive and simultaneous contractions, failed swallows (wave amplitude <10 mmHg at any of four sites) were usually associated with both abnormal liquid total bolus transit time (62%) and bolus presence time (65%). This suggests that failed swallows are a more severe manometric finding.

Furthermore, the area of abnormality was important. Most non-peristaltic responses with normal clearance had proximal (12 and 17 cm above LES) oesophageal motor abnormalities. In contrast, even focal failure in the distal oesophagus was associated with impaired clearance.

Finally, viscous boluses were more likely to exhibit failed clearance than liquid boluses. This suggests that the viscous medium may provide a more sensitive and discriminating bolus in the detection of abnormal oesophageal motor function.

Studies comparing HRM and pressure-impedance monitoring have not yet been done. Possibly the increased pressure sites in HRM will consistently predict bolus transit successfully, as shown by Fox *et al.* (reviewed above). On the other hand, some abnormalities found with HRM may not cause abnormal bolus transit, since the current study with pressure sites 5 cm apart commonly found normal bolus transit in the face of manometry abnormalities.

Oesophageal impedance monitoring has limitations. Like HRM, impedance monitoring requires experience in interpretation. In addition, the impedance baseline may be low because of oesophagitis, Barrett's oesophagus or stasis. EIM has not been reported in these settings. Validation with barium oesophagram has been done only in normal subjects to date. Finally, though EIM has confirmed abnormal bolus transit with oesophageal motility disorders, characteristic abnormal impedance patterns for the various disorders have not been reported.

Esophageal manometry: assessment of interpreter consistency

Nayar D, Khandwala F, Achkar E, *et al. Clin Gastroenterol Hepatol* 2005; **3**: 218–24

BACKGROUND. The diagnosis of oesophageal motility disorders by manometry is based on predefined criteria (Table 1.1). Some have well-defined therapeutic options (e.g. achalasia), though others are of uncertain clinical significance (e.g. nutcracker oesophagus). The diagnosis of these disorders is dependent on the physician's

accuracy and consistency in interpreting manometry tracings. The aim of this prospective, multiobserver, randomized, double-blind study was to assess the reliability of interpretation of oesophageal manometry by highly experienced (*n* = 3), moderately experienced (*n* = 3) and inexperienced (*n* = 2) interpreters. They all interpreted the same 72 tracings selected from archives at a large tertiary referral centre without knowledge of the original diagnosis or the diagnosis by the other observers. An equal number of tracings with seven diagnoses (normal or one of the six motility disorders listed in Table 1.1) was selected randomly.

INTERPRETATION. Interobserver agreement for achalasia and normal manometry data was good. However, there was only fair agreement for the other disorders (nutcracker, DES, IEM, hypotensive and hypertensive LES). The authors conclude that poor interobserver consistency and uncertain clinical implications for these other disorders should lead to their redefinition or elimination from practice.

Comment

The authors investigated why there was diagnostic inconsistency in this study. They found three reasons. Poor adherence to established manometric criteria was the most common cause, and was felt to be responsible for about 50% of errors. For example, the normal cut-off level for LES pressure and oesophageal body amplitude was not consistently followed. In my opinion, the difficulty in precise determination of mid-expiratory pressure may be partially responsible. In addition, DES patients were frequently diagnosed as IEM and *vice versa*. This was primarily due to some interpreters assigning simultaneous oesophageal contractions with normal or decreased contraction amplitude to DES and other interpreters assigning it to IEM. Though not stated in the criteria of Table 1.1, simultaneous contractions of increased amplitude should be categorized as simultaneous, while a simultaneous contraction with decreased amplitude should be categorized as ineffective.

Misinterpretation of intrabolus pressure was felt to be responsible for 30% of errors. In my opinion, it is occasionally impossible to discriminate intrabolus pressure from the take-off point for peristalsis, especially in patients with early achalasia. Hopefully, HRM or impedance-pressure manometry will be shown to be effective in this difficult situation. A technically inadequate study was felt to be responsible for 20% of errors.

There were other findings. Intra-observer agreement was good. Moreover, interobserver agreement improved with increasing experience from low experience (k = 0.30, fair) to moderate experience (k = 0.39, fair) and highly experienced (k = 0.44, moderate).

The authors comment that patients with difficult manometry tracings to interpret should have a barium swallow, as these studies are complementary. Simultaneous video-oesophagram and manometry has shown that radiography is insensitive to contractions in the oesophageal segments devoid of bolus, while manometry was insensitive to contractions that were non-occlusive **|6|**.

High-resolution manometry or impedance-pressure monitoring, already discussed, may not only improve the accuracy of interpretation but may also be used to assess the importance of correctly interpreted findings on bolus transit. A categorization of oesophageal motility disorders based on both pressure and bolus transit findings may be better than one based on manometric findings only, and one scheme has recently been suggested in a study using impedance-pressure monitoring in 350 consecutive patients |**7**|.

Motor and sensory function of the esophagus: revelations through ultrasound imaging

Mittal R. *J Clin Gastroenterol* 2005; **39**: S42–8

BACKGROUND. This is a review article discussing endoscopic ultrasonography in the assessment of motor and sensory function of the oesophagus. Although it reviews the state of the art, its focus is on the ability of oesophageal ultrasonography to determine the role of the longitudinal muscle layer of the oesophagus. Although half of the oesophageal muscle mass is longitudinal muscle, its function has been poorly understood until now. Thus, the aim of this review was to assess the role of longitudinal muscle in normal oesophageal motility and bolus transit, oesophageal motility disorders, and symptoms.

INTERPRETATION. There is synchrony in the timing as well as the amplitude of contraction between the longitudinal and circular muscle layers of the oesophagus in normal patients, and asynchrony for both timing and contraction amplitude of the two muscle layers during contractions in patients with spastic motor disorders. Hypertrophy of increasing severity of longitudinal and circular muscle has been described in patients with nutcracker oesophagus, DES and achalasia. Sustained contractions of longitudinal muscle have been temporally associated with chest pain and heartburn.

Comment

High-resolution manometry and oesophageal impedance monitoring assess oesophageal function. In contrast, ultrasonography assesses detailed oesophageal structure. Simultaneous ultrasonography and oesophageal motility testing has been described recently. Not only can this method correlate structural changes by ultrasonography with oesophageal contractions, but it can also determine whether symptoms have corresponding anatomical and/or pressure changes. Targets for therapy may be identified by ultrasonography. The author of the paper believes that oesophageal ultrasound has the potential to become a useful clinical tool for assessing oesophageal function with improved technology.

Several concepts are reviewed in this article. First, the change in oesophageal cross-sectional area is a marker for longitudinal muscle contraction, while oesophageal pressure is the marker for circular muscle contraction. The ability to measure both muscles simultaneously allows abnormalities to be identified in patients with spastic motor disorders compared with normal subjects, as shown in Fig. 1.5.

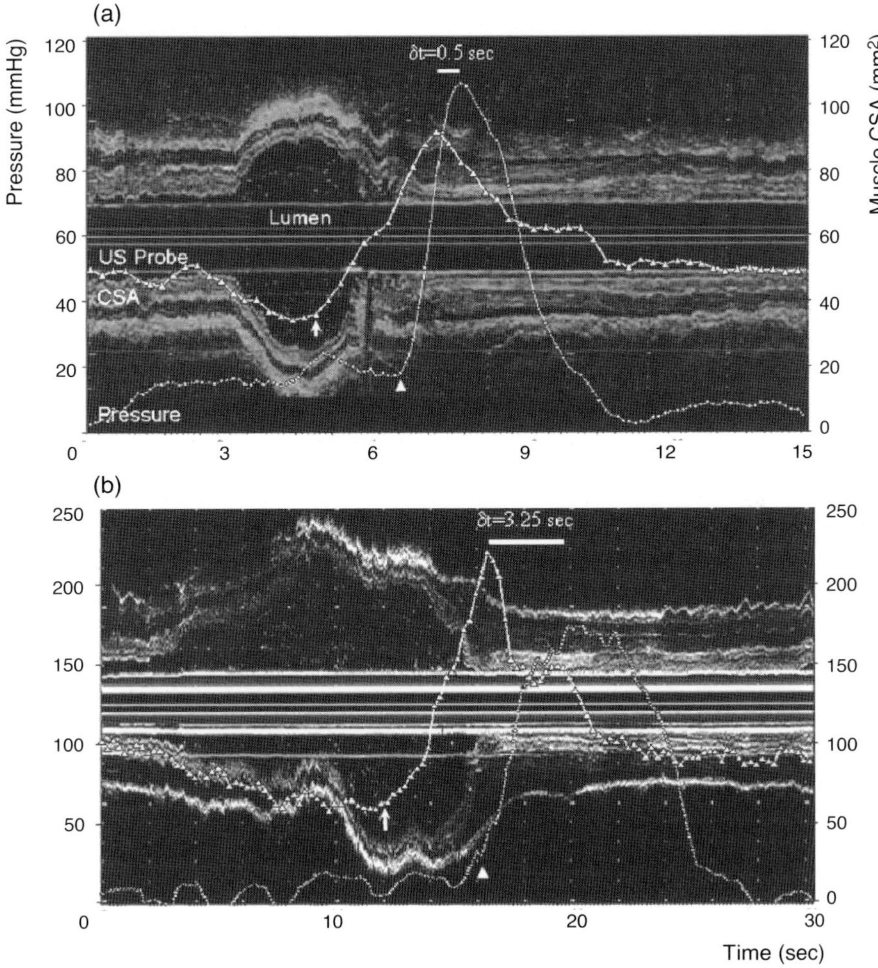

Fig. 1.5 (a) Relationship between M-mode ultrasound images, muscle cross-sectional area (CSA) and the pressure wave in a normal subject. Note that the onset of lumen collapse occurs at the same time as the onset of muscle CSA. The pressure wave occurs at the same time as the first complete collapse of the lumen on the manometric probe. The peak of manometric contraction and the peak CSA occurred with delta-t ≤0.5. (b) An example of dissociation between circular (CM) and longitudinal (LM) muscle contraction in a patient with nutcracker oesophagus. These recordings were obtained 2 cm above the LES. Note the disassociation between the peak pressure and peak muscle CSA. Source: Mittal (2005).

Secondly, differences in muscle thickness have been identified in spastic motor disorders. Graded increases in thickness have been seen from normal to achalasia, as described above. Novel insights into the pathogenesis of the spastic motor disorders may be derived from this method.

Thirdly, simultaneous pH, pressure and ultrasound monitoring has shown sustained longitudinal muscle contraction with 67% of chest pain episodes. Importantly, these episodes of pain occurred while pH was above 4 and no dysmotility was seen. Prolonged motility and pH studies have failed to show significant relationships between oesophageal contractions and pH with symptoms [8]. Thus, measuring longitudinal muscle contraction may be of value in assessing symptoms of unknown origin.

Long-term outcome of pneumatic dilation in the treatment of achalasia

Karamanolis G, Sgouros S, Karatzias G, *et al. Am J Gastroenterol* 2005; **100**: 270–4

BACKGROUND. There are limited data on the long-term outcome after pneumatic dilation for achalasia. The aim of this study from a single centre in Greece was to review retrospectively the long-term outcome of a large series of patients with achalasia treated with pneumatic dilation done by a single investigator.

INTERPRETATION. Although 51% of patients continued to be in clinical remission more than 15 years after the initial pneumatic dilation, the long-term success rate of pneumatic dilation drops progressively with time.

Comment

This study reviews the long-term results of 260 pneumatic dilations in 153 patients. There were good or excellent results initially in 90% of patients. Good or excellent results were 76% in those followed for 5 years and 51% in those followed for at least 15 years. There was only one perforation in these 260 pneumatic dilations, and LES decreased from a mean of 29 to 12 mmHg. There are several aspects that warrant further comment.

Importantly, survivor analysis showed that 50% of patients developed symptoms after 10.92 years (Fig. 1.6). Thus, the longer the follow-up after pneumatic dilation, the lower the success rate.

The pneumatic dilator used was a handmade dilator before 1994 and a Rigiflex dilator thereafter. There was a higher success rate with Rigiflex balloons (81.6 vs 71.9%), which are the pneumatic dilators used in most centres today.

Not only was there symptom follow-up every 1–2 years, but also the maximal diameter of the oesophageal body was determined upright after a barium oesophagram. In patients who responded, an immediate and sustained reduction in oesophageal diameter occurred with a mean (SD) of 3.7 (1.2) cm at 5 years and

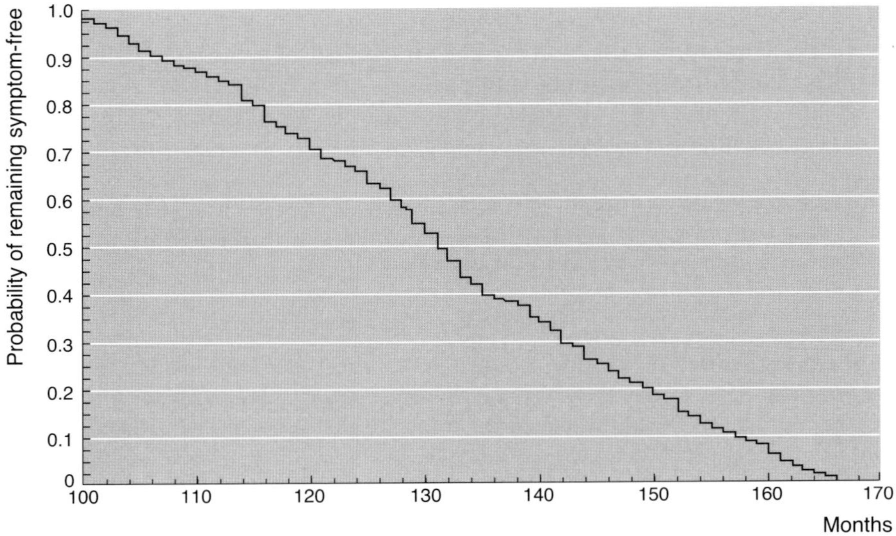

Fig. 1.6 Kaplan–Meier survival analysis estimating the probability of remaining symptom-free. Source: Karamanolis *et al.* (2005).

3.9 (0.8) cm at 15 years. Furthermore, the success rate differed according to previous oesophageal diameter. More patients with mild to moderate oesophageal dilation (5–8 cm; 72/82) were in clinical remission than those with a diameter <5 cm (41/62) or >8 cm (3/9).

This study supports the role of pneumatic dilation as an effective primary treatment option along with laparoscopic Heller myotomy for the initial treatment of achalasia. A large study of pneumatic dilation and Heller myotomy in achalasia found a similar short-term efficacy – 86% with pneumatic dilation and 89% with Heller myotomy – in improving symptoms, and 54 vs 45% in improving oesophageal emptying more than 80% with a timed barium swallow |**9**|. These results are similar to the initial results of pneumatic dilation in the present study. There is also a review this year of the surgical therapy of achalasia |**10**| in which controversies are discussed, such as how long the myotomy should be extended, and whether partial fundoplication (or whether Dor or Toupet) should be included to prevent symptomatic gastro-oesphageal reflux (GER), which occurs in 10–20% of patients.

Pneumatic dilation for the treatment of achalasia in untreated patients and patients with failed Heller myotomy

Guardino J, Vela M, Connor J, Richter J. *J Clin Gastroenterol* 2004; **38**: 855–60

BACKGROUND. Some patients with achalasia who choose to have Heller myotomy fail to have their symptoms adequately relieved. Unfortunately, there is little information on pneumatic dilation after failed Heller myotomy. The aim of this study was to assess the efficacy and safety of graded pneumatic dilation with Rigiflex pneumatic dilation in patients with achalasia after Heller myotomy.

INTERPRETATION. The risk of perforation is not higher after pneumatic dilation in patients after Heller myotomy than after pneumatic dilation in untreated patients with achalasia. However, patients with pneumatic dilation after Heller myotomy did not have as good an outcome as untreated patients with achalasia. In the patients symptomatic after Heller myotomy, better outcomes after pneumatic dilation were found in those who were older and had a higher LES pressure.

Comment

In this retrospective study, twelve patients with persistent symptoms after Heller myotomy who underwent a total of 22 pneumatic dilations were compared with 96 untreated patients with achalasia treated with 117 pneumatic dilations as their initial therapy. A highly experienced gastroenterologist performed all the pneumatic dilations, and the overall perforation rate with pneumatic dilation was 2% with both perforations in the 108 patients in the untreated achalasia group. It is important to note that none of the Heller myotomy patients had fundoplication as part of their surgery.

Unfortunately, though pneumatic dilation was safe in the Heller myotomy patients, persistent symptoms occurred in 50% and physiological success (80% emptying of barium with a timed barium swallow) in only 10%. This was substantially less than the 74% with a symptomatic response and 52% physiological success in the previously untreated patients. Mean follow-up for all patients was 10 months. The subgroup of Heller myotomy patients who did have symptomatic improvement (5/12) were older, and they had a higher LES pressure, suggesting they had an incomplete Heller myotomy.

Achalasia presenting after operative and non-operative trauma

Shah R, Izanec J, Friedel D, Axelrod P, Parkman H, Fisher R. *Dig Dis Sci* 2004; **49**: 1818–24

BACKGROUND. The pathophysiology of primary achalasia is incompletely understood. Secondary achalasia from malignancy, infiltrative disorders and infection (*Trypanasoma cruzi.*) probably occurs as a result of vagal nerve damage. A few case reports have implicated vagal nerve injury after surgery as a cause of achalasia [11]. However, non-operative trauma has not been implicated as a cause of achalasia. The aim of this study was to review retrospectively the records of 64 patients with achalasia on oesophageal manometry, and compare them with 73 patients who had similar symptoms but normal oesophageal manometry.

INTERPRETATION. Significantly more patients with achalasia had a preceding history of trauma than patients with similar symptoms and normal oesophageal manometry. In fact, 25% of patients diagnosed with achalasia had a history of operative or non-operative trauma to the chest or upper gastrointestinal tract.

Comment.

This retrospective study did show a significant difference if there was a preceding history of trauma in patients with achalasia (P <0.016; odds ratio 3.1). However, there was only a trend for each of the two trauma types: non-operative trauma events ($P = 0.098$), all of which were chest trauma in a motor vehicle accident; and operative trauma ($P = 0.06$). In addition, selection bias may have occurred since only 64 patients out of 125 diagnosed with achalasia over the 6-year study period had records complete enough for review. Therefore, the association of non-operative trauma with achalasia is intriguing, but a larger, optimally prospective study will be needed to confirm or refute this observation.

In the operative group who subsequently developed achalasia, there were six patients with previous upper gastrointestinal surgery (two with bariatric surgery; one with Billroth II with vagotomy; two with repair of an oesophageal fistula/perforation; one with a tetralogy of Fallot repair). The authors suggest that vagal disruption leading to neuropathic dysfunction may be responsible for the development of achalasia in these patients.

The symptoms were different in post-traumatic achalasia patients compared with the other achalasia patients. They were more likely to complain of chest pain ($P = 0.012$) and less likely to have regurgitation ($P = 0.01$). However, the main symptom in all achalasia patients was dysphagia, and there was no difference in manometric findings between the two achalasia groups.

Impaired bolus transit across the esophagogastric junction in post-fundoplication dysphagia

Scheffer R, Sansom M, Haverkamp A, Oors T, Hebbard G, Gooszen H. *Am J Gastroenterol* 2005; **100**: 1677–84

BACKGROUND. Dysphagia is a common symptom after fundoplication. The effect of antireflux surgery on transit through the oesophagogastric junction after fundoplication has not been examined prospectively. The aim of this study was to determine the effect of a successful laparoscopic fundoplication on oesophagogastric junction transit efficacy for both liquids and solids, oesophagogastric junction opening mechanics, and the relationship between oesophagogastric junction transit parameters and dysphagia. Eleven patients were studied by simultaneous HRM of the oesophagogastric junction and video-oesophagram both before and after a fundoplication.

INTERPRETATION. Fundoplication patients exhibit restricted hiatal opening and incomplete deglutative oesophagogastric junction relaxation (Fig. 1.7). To facilitate oesophagogastric junction transit despite these altered oesophagogastric junction dynamics, a higher intrabolus pressure is created by augmented bolus compression. Fundoplication increased oesophagogastric junction transit times of liquids from a mean of 6.9 to 9.8 s, and of solids from 2.8 to 5.8 s.

Comment

This study used HRM to assess the oesophagogastric junction, with eleven pressure sites 1 cm apart over the oesophagogastric junction. It shows how HRM allows detailed assessment of the oesophagogastric junction compared with conventional manometry, especially when presented in the topographic format (Fig. 1.7). The combination of HRM with video-oesophagrametry elegantly shows the impact of fundoplication on bolus transit. Several aspects of this study deserve additional comment.

This study was done upright, which simulates the normal ingestion of a liquid and solid meal. However, this posture does not eliminate the effect of gravity on oesophageal emptying. Furthermore, this study was done twice, once with a catheter across the oesophagogastric junction and on a second occasion with the catheter above the oesophagogastric junction. Since the results were no different in the two studies, this provides the important information that a catheter across the oesophagogastric junction does not influence either bolus transit or manometric findings. Finally, solid radio-opaque boluses (1 cm^3) made of gelatin mixed with barium were assessed in addition to 10 ml liquid barium boluses. Curiously, bolus transit of the solid was faster than liquid transit.

Interestingly, although oesophagogastric junction transit time was increased after fundoplication, this was entirely the result of an increased time from bolus arrival at the oesophagogastric junction until the opening of the oesophagogastric

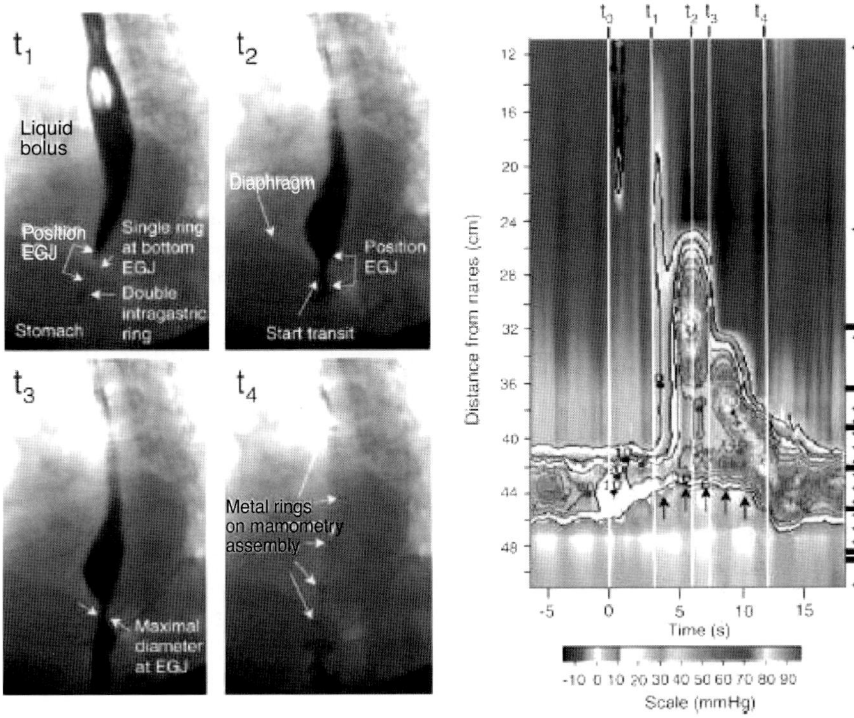

Fig. 1.7 Fluoroscopic and manometric data on emptying across the oesophagogastric junction in a representative post-fundoplication patient. Note that relaxation of the junction is incomplete (*arrows*), the intrabolus pressure is increased, and that a narrowed and elongated outflow tract is associated with reduced axial bolus length measured after fundoplication. Source: Scheffer *et al.* (2005).

junction and the start of bolus entry. Once bolus entry into the oesophagogastric junction began, as a result of increased intrabolus pressure, the time the oesophagogastric junction was open was the same as with prefundoplication.

The degree of dysphagia correlated with oesophagogastric junction transit duration, as determined by video-oesophagram, but not with any manometric parameter. Thus, video-oesophagram findings may be a useful marker in symptomatic patients, and this shows the importance of bolus transit studies done in addition to even detailed manometric data. Possibly patients with more severe symptoms, especially those being considered for reoperation, may have abnormal manometry findings not identified in this study. Additional studies using similar methods in patients with more severe symptoms should clarify this question.

Does diffuse esophageal spasm progress to achalasia? A prospective cohort study

Khatami S, Khandwala F, Shay S, Vaezi M. *Dig Dis Sci* 2005; **50**: 1605–10

BACKGROUND. DES and achalasia share both clinical and manometric characteristics. Some reports have described progression of DES to achalasia, but these are primarily case reports. The aim of this study was to assess prospectively the rate of progression of DES to achalasia by performing repeat oesophageal motility and symptom assessment in twelve patients with DES.

INTERPRETATION. Progression from DES to achalasia is uncommon (8%), though 58% of patients continued to have DES by manometry. Interestingly, 25% had normal oesophageal manometry. Since changes in manometric findings over time occurred in 42% of patients with an original diagnosis of DES, there is doubt about the specific nature of such a diagnosis.

Comment

This is the first prospective cohort study of DES patients to assess manometric change over time. DES was diagnosed only when two oesophageal experts agreed on the diagnosis after reviewing the manometry tracings. Thirty-two patients were diagnosed with DES over an 11-year period at a tertiary referral centre (1992–2003). However, only twelve agreed to participate, though there were no demographic, symptomatic or manometric differences compared with the 20 patients who were not included for a variety of reasons.

Though symptom type (primarily dysphagia and chest pain) did not change over time, symptom intensity was significantly less in the years between oesophageal motility measurements (mean 4.8 years, SD 3.4). In addition, although one may expect the number of simultaneous contractions or the degree of LES relaxation to play a role in predicting future worsening of oesophageal function and possible progression to achalasia, this was not supported by the data. The limitations of this study are that only twelve patients were in the cohort, and that the length of follow-up was variable.

Conclusion

The major advance in EMD in 2005 was the further development of new technologies. The article by Nayar *et al.* showed the limitations in standard oesophageal motility, the gold standard for the diagnosis of EMD for many years. They found only fair agreement among experienced readers for the diagnosis of DES, IEM, nutcracker oesophagus, and hypertensive and hypotensive LES. Not only do these disorders have uncertain clinical implications, but up to 50% of patients with dysphagia and/or chest pain have a normal study. Problems with conventional manometry in differentiating increased intrabolus pressure from the take-off of an oesophageal contraction and consistency in lower oesophageal sphincter pressure (LESP) determination were identified. For these reasons, better methods to assess patients with suspected EMD are needed.

The new methods discussed in this review address two aspects of oesophageal testing: bolus transit and functional anatomy. First, tests predicting or measuring bolus transit are reviewed. Simultaneous manometry and video-oesophagram is the gold standard for this approach. Scheffer *et al.* show how fundoplication restricts hiatal opening and results in prolonged liquid and solid bolus transit. Though X-ray exposure limits the use of fluoroscopy as a diagnostic test, it is a useful gold standard in the comparison of candidate methods for their ability to assess bolus transit.

High-resolution manometry was evaluated by Fox *et al.* Simultaneous video-oesophagram and HRM showed that HRM predicted abnormal bolus transit more accurately than conventional manometry. Furthermore, Bredenoord *et al.* found that HRM is at least as accurate as a sleeve sensor for detecting TLESRs. Thus, HRM simultaneously addresses two limitations of conventional manometry: a single side-hole at the LES and 5 cm gaps between pressure sites. The additional advantages of a shorter test, an accurate swallow marker and constant monitoring of intragastric pressure make HRM a strong candidate for the new gold standard.

Secondly, detailed oesophageal anatomy by ultrasonography is reviewed by Mittal. The ability to simultaneously measure longitudinal and circular muscle, peristalsis and pH has identified patients with chest pain and heartburn associated with sustained longitudinal muscle contractions, but normal motility and pH. This method should offer novel insights into the pathogenesis of the spastic motor disorders, and may identify the cause of symptoms when pressure, bolus transit and pH are normal.

This review also includes articles related to the aetiology of achalasia and its treatment with pneumatic dilation. Shah *et al.* show an increased incidence of achalasia after chest trauma, and suggest that this may be due to vagal disruption. Khatami *et al.* show that DES uncommonly progresses to achalasia. Karamanolis *et al.* found that 51% of 153 patients remained in remission 15 years after initial pneumatic dilation, but that long-term success decreased progressively with time. Finally, Guardino *et al.* show that patients with Heller myotomy (and no fundoplication) did not have an increased risk of perforation after pneumatic dilation, but that the outcome was not as good as in untreated patients with achalasia.

What should we expect in 2006? Further experience with HRM and impedance manometry – especially a head-to-head comparison – is eagerly awaited. Eventually, their roles will be defined by outcome studies. Hopefully, new technologies will lead to advances in the pathogenesis of the EMD, a new classification of EMD based on bolus transit and/or anatomical derangements in addition to manometric findings, more consistent correlation of symptoms with observed findings, and better results from specific therapies.

References

1. Fibbe C, Layer P, Keller J. Esophageal motility in reflux disease before and after fundoplication: a prospective, randomized, clinical, and manometric study. *Gastroenterology* 2001; **121**: 514–20.
2. Clouse R, Staiano A, Alrakawi A, Harioan L. Application of topographical methods to clinical esophageal manometry. *Am J Gastroenterol* 2000; **95**: 2720–30.
3. Katz P, Richter J, Cowan R, Castell D. Apparent complete lower esophageal sphincter relaxation in achalasia. *Gastroenterology* 1986; **90**: 978–87.
4. Imam H, Shay S, Ali A, Baker M. Bolus transit patterns in healthy subjects: a study using simultaneous impedance monitoring, videoesophagram, and esophageal manometry. *Am J Physiol Gastrointest Liver Physiol* 2005; **288**: G1000–6.
5. Tutuian R, Vela M, Balaji N, Wise J, Murray J, Peters J, Shay S, Castell D. Esophageal function testing with combined multichannel intraluminal impedance and manometry: multicenter study in healthy volunteers. *Clin Gastroenterol Hepatol* 2003; **1**: 174–82.
6. Massey B, Dodds W, Hogan W. Abnormal esophageal motility. An analysis of concurrent radiographic and manometric findings. *Gastroenterology* 1991; **101**: 334–54.
7. Tutuian R, Castell D. Combined multichannel intraluminal impedance and manometry clarifies esophageal function abnormalities: a study in 350 patients. *Am J Gastroenterol* 2004; **99**: 1011–19.
8. Peters L, Maas L, Petty D. Spontaneous non-cardiac chest pain: evaluation by 24-hour ambulatory esophageal motility and pH monitoring. *Gastroenterology* 1988; **94**: 878–86.
9. Vela M, Richter J, Wachsberger D, Connor J, Rice T. Complexities of managing achalasia at a tertiary referral center: use of pneumatic dilatation, Heller myotomy, and Botulinum toxin injection. *Am J Gastroenterol* 2004; **99**: 1029–36.
10. Woltman T, Pellegrini C, Oelschlager B. Achalasia. *Surg Clin N Am* 2005; **85**: 483–93.
11. Dauntemann T, Dresner D. Achalasia-like syndrome presenting after highly selective vagotomy. *Dig Dis Sci* 1995; **40**: 2081–3.

2

Acid disorders of the oesophagus

EDGAR ACHKAR, WOOSUK PARK, ILCHE NONEVSKI

Introduction

Since the introduction of proton pump inhibitors (PPIs), the treatment of acid-related disorders has altered significantly. Ulcer surgery for pain is almost unheard of and perforation from peptic ulcers has become very rare. A significant proportion of duodenal ulcers and about half of all gastric ulcers are managed by eradication of *Helicobacter pylori.* Aspirin and non-steroidal anti-inflammatory agents account for the majority of the remaining gastric ulcers. In the oesophagus, however, acid reflux is a widespread problem. Heartburn affects as many as 40% of adults and complications such as peptic strictures and Barrett's oesophagus are encountered regularly in medical practice. Barrett's oesophagus affects only a small percentage of patients with gastro-oesophageal reflux disease (GERD) but its cancer potential has led to a search for improved screening and surveillance methods.

We have assembled a group of articles dealing with some of the diagnostic methods for acid reflux and Barrett's oesophagus, such as the wireless pH test, capsule endoscopy and chromoendoscopy. One article addresses the issue of night-time heartburn and another reports the results of PPI use during pregnancy. Two new methods for the endoscopic treatment of reflux are reviewed, and there is a study on the management of rings by periodic dilatations and another on the role of intralesional steroid injection. We review an important observation on the prevalence of Barrett's oesophagus, and finally a paper on the role of crystal violet chromoendoscopy in the diagnosis of dysplasia in Barrett's oesophagus. Anti-inflammatory agents account for significant morbidity and mortality, particularly in the elderly. PPIs have a protective effect and should be used prophylactically in patients taking non-steroidal anti-inflammatory drugs (NSAIDs) chronically. Besides their ulcerogenic effect, these drugs, including cyclooxygenase 2 (COX-2) inhibitors, are also known to cause heartburn, abdominal pain and nausea.

Value of extended recording time with wireless pH monitoring in evaluating gastroesophageal reflux disease

Prakash C, Clouse RE. *Clin Gastroenterol Hepatol* 2005; **3**: 329–34

BACKGROUND. Prolonged ambulatory pH monitoring is an important tool in the evaluation and diagnosis of GERD. The wireless system alleviates patient discomfort and the inconvenience associated with the conventional nasogastric catheter-based pH probe and allows extended monitoring to 48 h, twice the monitoring time of the conventional catheter-based system. The aim of this study was to evaluate the clinical significance of the extended wireless pH monitoring system. Subjects who had at least one reflux symptom, either typical or atypical, were evaluated. Acid exposure time, symptom index and reflux-associated symptom probability at day 1 and day 2 of recording were compared.

INTERPRETATION. A total of 157 subjects underwent wireless pH monitoring. The study was performed off antireflux therapy in 121 subjects (off-therapy group) and on PPI therapy in 36 subjects (on-therapy group). In the off-therapy group, extending the recording time was associated with an increase in the number of recorded symptoms from 115 on day 1 to 121 on day 2 (an increase of 5.2%). The number of symptoms associated with reflux events doubled from 15.2 on day 1 to 31.5 on day 2 (P <0.0001). Similarly, in the on-therapy group, the number of recorded symptoms increased from 12 to 26 (P <0.0001). In this group, number of symptoms associated with the reflux event also increased but the difference was not statistically significant. Overall, 48-h monitoring yielded a 30.1% increase in the detection of a positive symptom index and reflux–symptom association, as well as an elevated acid exposure time, compared with 24-h monitoring.

Comment

Wireless pH monitoring is an attractive alternative to the conventional catheter-based system because it minimizes patient discomfort, allows greater freedom to carry out a normal daily routine and enables monitoring over a longer period of time [1]. Until now, the added benefit of extending the pH monitoring period afforded by the wireless system has been unknown. This study shows that extending the pH monitoring time from the conventional 24 h to 48 h increases the likelihood of detecting more reflux events. Additionally, the association between symptoms and reflux events using the symptom index or reflux-associated symptom probability may be enhanced with a longer monitoring time. Thus, its use is expected to be more widespread in the near future.

A prospective study of the diagnostic accuracy of PillCam Eso esophageal capsule endoscopy versus conventional upper endoscopy in patients with chronic gastroesophageal reflux disease

Eliakim R, Sharma VK, Yassin K, *et al. J Clin Gastroenterol* 2005; **39**: 572–8

BACKGROUND. The PillCam ESO® capsule endoscope is a new device for examining the oesophagus in an office setting without sedation or the discomfort of conventional upper endoscopy (oesophagogastroduodenoscopy [EGD]). Hence, capsule endoscopy may have better patient acceptance and cost less than EGD. However, the test characteristics of capsule endoscopy in comparison with EGD are unknown. The aim of this study was to establish the test characteristics of capsule endoscopy using EGD as the gold standard and to assess the safety profile.

INTERPRETATION. In this multicentre cohort study, 106 subjects with either symptoms of GERD ($n = 93$) or Barrett's oesophagus ($n = 13$) were enrolled. Each subject underwent capsule endoscopy followed by EGD. Using intention-to-treat analysis, in patients with Barrett's oesophagus, capsule endoscopy had a sensitivity of 92%, a specificity of 99%, a negative predictive value of 96% and a positive predictive value of 97%. In patients with oesophagitis, capsule endoscopy had a sensitivity of 85%, a specificity of 99%, a negative predictive value of 92% and a positive predictive value of 92%. Most patients tolerated capsule endoscopy well and no adverse events were reported.

Comment

EGD is frequently performed for various reasons, including the evaluation of chronic GERD symptoms and screening for Barrett's oesophagus. The disadvantages of EGD are the associated cost and risks. Capsule endoscopy appears to be a safe and cost-effective approach in comparison with EGD. It is convenient and easily tolerated. In this study, capsule endoscopy was shown to be highly accurate in screening for Barrett's oesophagus and the detection of oesophagitis. However, it has lower sensitivity than EGD and therefore its role in screening for oesophagitis is debatable. Furthermore, the diagnosis of Barrett's oesophagus requires histological examination. Consequently, EGD may not be avoidable in many patients with questionable Barrett's oesophagus on capsule endoscopy. Similarly, patients with strictures will need EGD for further evaluation and therapy. In conclusion, capsule endoscopy appears to be a useful tool for examining the oesophagus in place of EGD. However, the indications and patient selection for this test should be further evaluated and defined. In patients with a high level of suspicion of Barrett's oesophagus or strictures, EGD should be the test of choice.

The safety of proton pump inhibitors in pregnancy: a multicentre prospective controlled study

Diav-Citrin O, Arnon J, Shechtman S, *et al. Aliment Pharmacol Ther* 2005; **21**: 269–75

BACKGROUND. Heartburn is a common symptom during pregnancy, affecting 30–50% of all women. The aetiology of GERD in pregnancy is multifactorial, but the greatest contributing factor appears to be the reduction in lower oesophageal sphincter pressure seen with increases in plasma progesterone [2]. While many women achieve symptomatic relief with over-the-counter antacids or H_2 receptor antagonists, symptoms of GERD persist in a considerable number. Several case reports and cohort studies have suggested that omeprazole appears safe during pregnancy. This study evaluated prospectively the rate of major congenital anomalies in women who were taking PPIs (omeprazole, lansoprazole or pantoprazole) during pregnancy compared with a control population obtained from an international teratogen database.

INTERPRETATION. The study involved 410 pregnancies with exposure to PPIs and 868 control pregnancies. The primary end-point was the rate of major congenital anomalies, and secondary end-points included pregnancy outcome, birth weight and gestational age at delivery. After controlling for several variables, including maternal age, pregnancy order, parity, past miscarriages and elective termination of pregnancy, information on pregnancy outcomes was obtained by the use of self-reported questionnaires and post-partum maternal interviews. The study was powered to find a 2.72-fold increase in the overall rate of major anomalies after exposure to omeprazole. The median duration of treatment was 14–22 days, with greater than 85% of PPI use occurring in the first trimester. Major anomalies were found in 3.6% of the omeprazole group compared with 3.8% in the control group ($P = 0.9$). Similar insignificant rates of major teratogenic anomalies were seen in the lansoprazole and pantoprazole groups. Of the secondary end-points, only a 60-g difference in birth weight between the omeprazole group and controls was significant. There was a higher rate of elective termination of pregnancy in the omeprazole and lansoprazole groups compared with controls. The authors relate this finding to a possible increase in the effect of fear of medication on pregnancy.

Comment

This multicentre study adds to the growing body of literature suggesting that PPI use, even during the first trimester, does not increase the risk of teratogenicity. The authors recognized the limitations of the study, including reliance on maternal questionnaires and interviews for information on abnormal pregnancy, but contend that applying the same protocol to both treatment and control arms minimized potential biases. The median duration of treatment was 14 days, and the most common indications were treatment for *H. pylori*-associated peptic ulcers, peptic ulcer disease and reflux oesophagitis. However, in practice the predominant indications for the use of PPIs during pregnancy are GERD and dyspepsia, and both require prolonged treatment. Further studies of PPI use during pregnancy should take into account the potential need for prolonged treatment.

Effect of esomeprazole on night-time heartburn and sleep quality in patients with GERD: a randomized, placebo-controlled trial

Johnson DA, Orr WC, Crawley JA, *et al. Am J Gastroenterol* 2005; **100**: 1914–22

BACKGROUND. Heartburn affects a large number of people and accounts for a large proportion of health expenditure. Night-time heartburn and acid regurgitation are reported by 75% of patients with heartburn, and the same proportion reports sleep disturbances. Night symptoms are rarely addressed separately as they are considered to be part of the GERD complex. This study attempted to evaluate the effect of esomeprazole on night symptoms and work productivity.

INTERPRETATION. Adult patients with a history of heartburn or acid regurgitation for more than 3 months were entered in the study after a screening period. They were randomized to receive esomeprazole 40 mg, esomeprazole 20 mg or placebo. The primary outcome of the study was the relief of night-time heartburn during the last 7 days of a 4-week trial, as recorded on diary cards. Other outcomes included relief or complete resolution of sleep disturbances, improvement on a sleep quality index, and complete resolution of daytime and 24-h heartburn. Night-time heartburn was relieved in only 50% of patients with both 20 and 40 mg of esomeprazole, compared with a 12.7% placebo rate. Sleep disturbances improved in 73% of patients with either dose compared with 41% with placebo. The effects on work hours and regular activity were also significantly improved with the medication.

Comment

Acid suppression with esomeprazole in patients complaining of heartburn and acid regurgitation is indeed effective in reducing night-time heartburn and in improving the quality of sleep. The assessment of sleep in this study was subjective, however, and there were no pH studies to link the improvement to the effect on acid secretion. While only 50% of patients reported relief of night-time heartburn, as many as 74% reported resolution of sleep disturbances. This difference implies that sleep improvement may not be entirely related to the resolution of night-time heartburn. It is interesting to note also that 41% of patients on placebo reported resolution of sleep disturbances and 55% some improvement in sleeping.

The choice of the last 7 days of a 4-week trial as the time to assess treatment results appears somewhat arbitrary. We do not know the long-term effects of treatment on night-time heartburn. It is also surprising that while all study patients had moderate to severe heartburn only 50% reported relief at night as well as during the day, and the figures for complete resolution were even lower. This may reflect the fact that patients were selected only on the basis of symptoms and were not representative of patients who have acid reflux on the basis of objective tests. It is hoped that the results would be even more impressive in such patients.

One may conclude that esomeprazole is helpful in relieving night symptoms effectively, but it is abundantly clear that more than half the patients continue to complain of the same symptoms. The question, unanswered by this study, is whether higher doses would achieve better results.

Endoscopic full-thickness plication for the treatment of GERD: 12-month follow-up for the North American open-label trial

Pleskow D, Rothstein R, Lo S, *et al.* *Gastrointest Endosc* 2005; **61**: 643–9

Long-term outcomes of endoluminal gastroplication: a US multicenter trial

Chen YK, Raijman I, Ben-Menachem T, *et al.* *Gastrointest Endosc* 2005; **61**: 659–67

BACKGROUND. Endoscopic therapy for GERD is a novel approach in the management of acid reflux. These two articles report the outcomes of two full-thickness plication techniques: the Endoscopic Plication System® (EPS) and Endocinch®.

INTERPRETATION. The study by Pleskow *et al.* assessed a 12-month safety and efficacy of the EPS®. Sixty-four patients with chronic GERD received a single endoscopic full-thickness plication in the gastric cardia 1 cm distal to the gastro-oesophageal junction. At the 12-month follow-up, 40 of 57 patients who completed the study (70%) were off PPI therapy. Additionally, the GERD health-related quality of life score improved compared with baseline (median 19.0 vs 5.0; $P < 0.0001$) and improvement in pH monitoring was observed in 40 of 51 (80%) patients. Three serious adverse events occurred acutely (one case of pneumothorax and two cases of pneumoperitoneum) and no new adverse events occurred during the extended 12-month follow-up.

The study by Chen *et al.* was a multicentre trial assessing the Endocinch® device in 85 patients. They found a significant reduction in heartburn scores compared with baseline ($P < 0.0001$) at the 1- and 2-year follow-ups. Additionally, complete heartburn symptom resolution was achieved in 59% at 1 year and in 52% at the 2-year follow-up ($P < 0.0001$ vs baseline). Similarly, resolution of regurgitation symptoms was found in 83% at 1 year and 77% at 2 years ($P < 0.0001$ vs baseline). Adverse events occurred in seven patients, including gastrointestinal bleeding, bronchospasm and dysphagia.

Comment

The two studies show improvement in reflux symptom scores and a decrease in PPI use with endoscopic plication. However, these studies are limited by the lack of controls. The data on the efficacy of these novel techniques are inconsistent. For example, a recent sham-controlled study, reported in abstract form, showed no difference between the Endocinch and sham control groups (Park *et al.*, DDW 2005) [3]. Furthermore, a failure rate of 80% has been reported for the Endocinch at 18 months of follow-up [4]. Some of these therapy failures were attributed to the loss of sutures over time. Given these conflicting findings, further randomized, controlled studies are warranted to assess the long-term efficacy and safety of these devices. In recent years, numerous approaches to endoscopic therapy for GERD have been introduced, but many were withdrawn from the market because of safety concerns. For example, Enteryx® (Boston Scientific) was withdrawn in 2005 because of associated morbidity and mortality, including one confirmed death related to this procedure. Thus, caution is warranted when using these new therapies in patients with a benign disease such as GERD.

Long-term acid suppressive therapy may prevent the relapse of lower esophageal (Schatzki's) rings: a prospective, randomized, placebo-controlled study

Sgouros SN, Vlachogiannakos J, Karamanolis G, *et al. Am J Gastroenterol* 2005; **100**: 1929–34

BACKGROUND. Lower oesophageal (Schatzki's) ring is frequently found in patients with intermittent solid food dysphagia. It is thought to occur as a result of inflammatory insult, primarily from GERD. Schatzki's ring is usually treated with oesophageal dilatation in conjunction with acid suppression therapy with PPI to minimize the risk of recurrence. However, the efficacy of antireflux therapy has not been studied. Therefore, the aim of this prospective, randomized, double-blind, placebo-controlled study was to evaluate the effect of long-term PPI therapy on the relapse rate of lower oesophageal rings after oesophageal dilatation with Savary dilators.

INTERPRETATION. A total of 44 patients with symptomatic Schatzki's ring underwent oesophageal dilatation. Of these patients, 14 had documented GERD by EGD or 24-h ambulatory pH monitoring and were treated with open-label omeprazole 20 mg daily. The remaining 30 patients were randomized to receive either omeprazole 20 mg daily or a placebo. The group with documented GERD ($n = 14$) had a mean follow-up period of about 44 months and had no recurrence of Shatzki's ring. The treatment group ($n = 15$) had a mean follow-up of 37 months and one patient relapsed after 13 months of follow-up. In the placebo group ($n = 15$), seven patients relapsed after a mean follow-up of about 20 months. Kaplan–Meier analysis showed that the treatment group was less likely to have a relapse compared with the control group ($P = 0.0008$) (Fig. 2.1).

Comment

The causal relationship between GERD and Schatzki's ring is not well established. In this study, only 14 out of 44 patients (32%) with Schatzki's ring had either

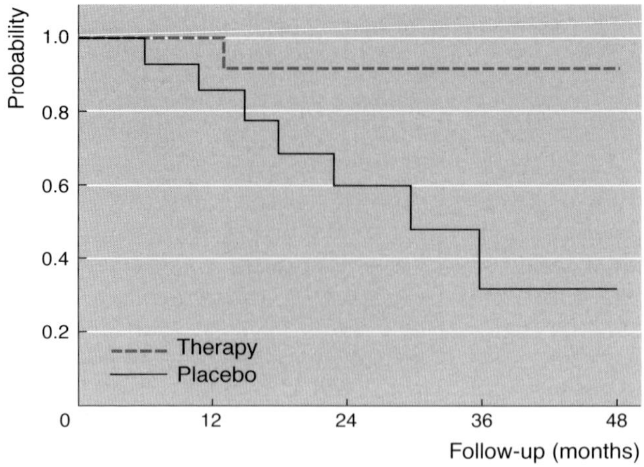

Fig. 2.1 Probability of remaining free from relapse of Schatzki's ring after successful endoscopic treatment. Source: Sgouros *et al.* (2005).

abnormal pH monitoring or EGD to suggest GERD as the cause. In the group with documented GERD, daily PPI therapy was shown to be highly effective in preventing relapses. What is interesting, however, is that even in the absence of evidence for GERD, empirical PPI therapy was shown to decrease the recurrence of Shatzki's ring significantly. These results suggest that patients with symptomatic Schatzki's ring should be treated with PPIs after bougienage regardless of the presence or absence of symptoms suggesting GERD. Unfortunately, the duration of therapy was not addressed in this study. Therefore, further studies on the dose and duration of therapy would be helpful.

A prospective randomized, double-blind, placebo-controlled trial of endoscopic steroid injection for recalcitrant esophageal peptic strictures

Ramage JI Jr, Rumalla A, Baron TH, *et al. Am J Gastroenterol* 2005; **100**: 2419–25

BACKGROUND. Peptic oesophageal strictures and associated dysphagia cause significant symptoms and decreased quality of life. Approximately 50% of patients will require dilatation and subsequent repeat procedures |5–7|. The use of PPIs has substantially reduced the rate of stricture recurrence to 30% over a 1-year period |8|. However, many of these patients still require dilatation. Several uncontrolled studies have suggested that intralesional corticosteroid injection during dilatation may delay or prevent stricture recurrence.

INTERPRETATION. This was a carefully performed, randomized, double-blind, placebo-controlled study that enrolled 30 patients with documented peptic stricture and previous dilatation to receive a sham injection and subsequent dilatation versus injection of the strictured area with triamcinolone followed by dilatation. Patients were stratified according to the number of dilatations, the severity of stricture, the presence of dysphagia, and previous therapy with PPIs. Body mass index was higher in the steroid-treated group (28.9 kg/m^2) than in the sham group (25.1 kg/m^2). All patients received a standardized PPI regimen, which served as an additional control. The need for repeat injection and dilatation was assessed periodically over a 1-year period using a modified dysphagia severity questionnaire. One patient in each group died of unrelated causes. Two patients in each group underwent fundoplication. The study found that 13% of patients in the steroid-treated group required repeat dilatation, compared with 60% in the sham group ($P = 0.011$). Furthermore, the time to first dilatation was significantly longer for the steroid-treated group than for the sham group. (Fig. 2.2) The difference in dysphagia frequency and dietary tolerance between the groups did not reach statistical significance during the study period.

Comment

This study confirms prospectively what had been observed in various retrospective studies: patients receiving intralesional steroid injection for recurrent peptic oesophageal strictures require repeat dilatation less frequently. The mechanism

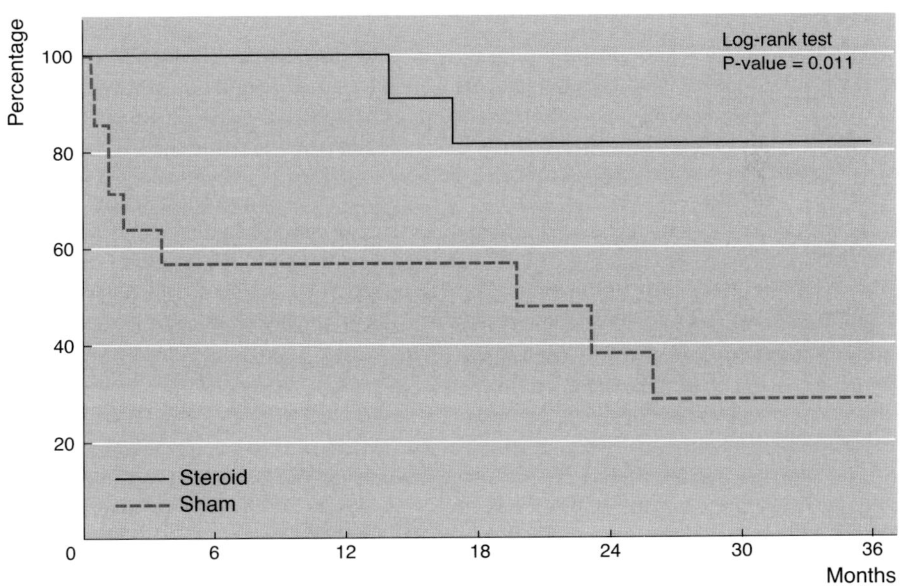

Fig. 2.2 Time to first repeat dilatation. Source: Ramage *et al.* (2005).

proposed is that corticosteroids inhibit wound healing and thereby delay the development of the scarring and wound contraction that leads to stricture formation. As acid reflux is the offending agent in the development of strictures, this study attempted to minimize the contribution of acid suppression by maintaining both the study and control subjects on PPIs throughout the 1-year period. While the low incidence of recalcitrant peptic stricture patients did not allow a larger sample size, there was still a significant difference in the interval to repeat dilatation therapy in the triamcinolone group. However, there was no difference in dysphagia and dietary tolerance between the two groups. While intralesional steroid injection is not advocated as routine practice, the results of this study should generate further interest in treating both peptic and non-peptic oesophageal strictures with similar endoscopic modalities.

Prevalence of Barrett's esophagus in the general population: an endoscopic study

Ronkainen J, Aro P, Storskrubb T, *et al.* *Gastroenterology* 2005; **29**: 1825–31

Background. Barrett's oesophagus is a significant public health problem because of the associated increased risk of developing oesophageal adenocarcinoma. The reported prevalence of Barrett's oesophagus in patients with reflux symptoms ranges from 0.4% to 8.3%. However, the prevalence of Barrett's oesophagus in the general population unrelated to reflux symptoms has not been established.

Interpretation. In this study, 3000 randomly selected adults from two municipalities with an adult population of 21 610 in northern Sweden were contacted by mail for a survey using a validated abdominal symptom questionnaire. Of the responders ($n = 2122$; 71%), a randomly selected 1000 adults underwent upper endoscopy. Of the 1000 subjects who underwent endoscopy, 40% had reflux symptoms and 15.5% had oesophagitis. Endoscopic findings suggestive of Barrett's oesophagus, such as mucosal tongue or proximally displaced oesophagogastric junction, were found in 103 (10.3%) subjects. A histological diagnosis of Barrett's oesophagus was made in 16 subjects (1.6%): eleven (1.1%) with short-segment and five (0.5%) with long-segment Barrett's oesophagus (Table 2.1). The prevalence of Barrett's oesophagus was 2.3% in those with reflux symptoms and 1.2% in those without. Additionally, Barrett's oesophagus was found in 2.6% of those with oesophagitis and 1.4% of those without oesophagitis. Alcohol ($P = 0.04$) and smoking ($P = 0.047$) were independent risk factors for Barrett's oesophagus.

Comment

This study is the first to assess the prevalence of Barrett's oesophagus in the general population irrespective of reflux symptoms. In this study, the overall prevalence of Barrett's oesophagus in northern Sweden was 1.6% and about half of the Barrett's oesophagus cases had no associated reflux symptoms. This finding suggests that the

Table 2.1 Prevalence of Barrett's oesophagus

	Barrett's oesophagus	Long-segment Barrett's oesophagus	Short-segment Barrett's oesophagus	No Barrett's oesophagus
No. of cases (%)	16 (1.6)	5 (0.5)	11 (1.1)	984 (98.4)
With GERD symptoms (%)	56.3	80	45.5	39.7
With oesophagitis (%)	25.0	60.0	9.1	15.4

GERD, gastro-oesophageal reflux disease.
Source: Ronkainen *et al.* (2005).

current screening guidelines based on the presence of chronic reflux symptoms may be inadequate and that screening in the asymptomatic population may be necessary. It has been reported that about 40% of patients with oesophageal adenocarcinoma have no reflux symptoms, further supporting the need for general screening for Barrett's oesophagus [9]. With the advent of office-based, sedationless, ultrathin endoscopy and oesophageal capsule endoscopy, mass screening for Barrett's oesophagus is feasible. However, before such mass screening is implemented, further studies showing the morbidity and mortality benefit and its cost-effectiveness are needed. Until then, screening for Barrett's oesophagus remains controversial.

Crystal violet chromoendoscopy with mucosal pit pattern diagnosis is useful for surveillance of short-segment Barrett's esophagus

Amano Y, Kushiyama Y, Ishihara S, *et al. Am J Gastroenterol* 2005; **100**: 21–6

BACKGROUND. Current practice guidelines recommend endoscopic surveillance for dysplasia in patients with Barrett's oesophagus. This involves four quadrant biopsies at intervals of 1–2 cm along the entire Barrett's segment. This approach has various limitations, such as sampling error and poor cost-effectiveness. Methylene blue chromoendoscopy selectively stains non-dysplastic Barrett's mucosa. However, its use may be limited to long-segment Barrett's oesophagus because of low sensitivity and specificity in short-segment Barrett's oesophagus [10]. On the other hand, crystal violet chromoendoscopy, which has been used in screening for dysplasia in the colon, has shown promise in surveillance for Barrett's oesophagus [11]. Thus, the aim of this study was to evaluate methylene blue and crystal violet chromoendoscopy in surveillance for dysplasia in short-segment Barrett's oesophagus. In this study, 400 patients with suspected short-segment Barrett's oesophagus on endoscopy were randomly assigned to undergo chromoendoscopy with 0.05% crystal violet, 0.1% crystal violet, 0.05% methylene blue or 0.1% methylene blue. During chromoendoscopy, biopsies were taken from both stained and unstained columnar-appearing epithelium.

Interpretation. Of the 400 patients in the study, 230 were diagnosed as having Barrett's oesophagus, defined by the presence of goblet cell metaplasia. In this group with Barrett's oesophagus, nine patients had low-grade dysplasia, five had high-grade dysplasia and four had adenocarcinoma. Both methylene blue and crystal violet stained Barrett's epithelium more effectively than non-Barrett's epithelium. Furthermore, 0.05% crystal violet was found to be the most effective and had the highest sensitivity (89.2%), specificity (85.7%), and diagnostic accuracy (88.0%) for detecting Barrett's epithelium compared with 0.1% crystal violet or methylene blue. Additionally, chromoendoscopy with 0.05% crystal violet was shown to yield the best pit pattern identification, which aids in the detection of dysplastic Barrett's epithelium.

Comment

This study shows that chromoendoscopy using 0.05% crystal violet may enhance screening and surveillance for Barrett's oesophagus. The current guideline for surveillance for Barrett's dysplasia recommends four quadrant biopsies every 1–2 cm, which can be time-consuming. Furthermore, dysplastic lesions can easily be missed because of sampling error. In this study, 0.05% crystal violet was shown to stain Barrett's epithelium effectively and to allow pit pattern identification. Since pit pattern identification may facilitate targeted biopsies in surveillance for dysplasia, chromoendoscopy appears promising in improving the effectiveness of surveillance for dysplasia. However, staining can be tedious and may prolong the procedure time, and may not be reproducible among different endoscopists. Because of these limitations and the lack of guidelines regarding the use of chromoendoscopy in surveillance for Barrett's oesophagus, chromoendoscopy should be considered a promising tool that requires further study.

Improvements with esomeprazole in patients with upper gastrointestinal symptoms taking non-steroidal anti-inflammatory drugs, including selective COX-2 inhibitors

Hawkey C, Talley NJ, Yeomans ND, *et al.*; NASA1 SPACE1 Study Group. *Am J Gastroenterol* 2005; **100**: 1028–36

Background. PPIs are effective in reducing acid-related conditions caused by NSAIDs and COX-2 inhibitors. However, these agents are also known to cause upper gastrointestinal symptoms such as dyspepsia, heartburn and abdominal pain. It is not clear that dyspeptic symptoms are necessarily acid-related. The authors evaluated the effect of esomeprazole on upper gastrointestinal symptoms in a group of patients with medical conditions requiring chronic intake of anti-inflammatory agents.

Interpretation. This is a multicentre, multinational, randomized, double-blind placebo-controlled study. Patients with chronic conditions requiring the chronic use of NSAIDs or COX-2 inhibitors were included after patients with ulcer disease by endoscopy had been eliminated. Patients were randomized to receive esomeprazole 20 or 40 mg or placebo. They had all taken NSAIDs or COX-2 inhibitors for 7 months or longer. Gastrointestinal symptoms and health-related quality of life were assessed at baseline and after 4 weeks of treatment. Esomeprazole 20 and 40 mg daily were significantly superior to placebo in reducing symptoms and improving quality-of-life scores (Fig. 2.3). Similar results were observed in the two trials.

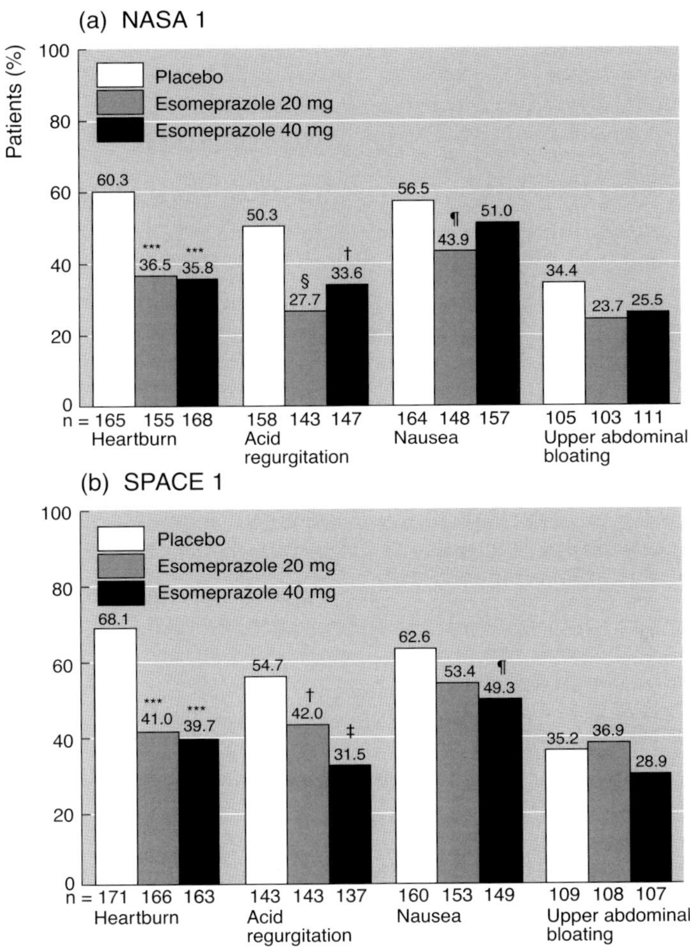

Fig. 2.3 Percentage of patients with upper gastrointestinal symptoms after 4 weeks of therapy as a proportion of those who had the symptom at baseline. (a) ***P <0.0001; §P = 0.0001; †P = 0.0044; ¶P = 0.0269. (b) ***P <0.0001; †P = 0.0404; ‡P = 0.0002; ¶P = 0.0256. Source: Hawkey *et al.* (2005).

Comment

The significant improvement in upper gastrointestinal symptoms with esomeprazole even in patients who were taking COX-2 inhibitors suggests that these symptoms are acid-related whether the patient is taking NSAIDs or a COX-2 inhibitor, even though the study did not include pH testing. While the two doses of esomeprazole had equivalent effects in reducing symptoms, it should be noted that the investigators' assessment of symptoms showed significant improvement of heartburn and acid regurgitation but not of nausea or bloating. In addition, the number of patients continuing to complain of heartburn and acid regurgitation after 4 weeks of treatment was reduced by half or less.

The rate of improvement with placebo, 30–40%, is not surprising, as shown by previous studies involving patients with dyspepsia.

The studies suffer from selection bias because the patients who were included had sought medical attention precisely because of the presence of upper gastrointestinal symptoms and may have been more willing to participate in the study. Therefore this patient population does not represent the entire population of chronic NSAID users.

It is difficult to ascertain the exact contribution of NSAIDs or COX-2 inhibitors to the quality of life, since the patients had chronic conditions known to affect quality-of-life parameters. Nevertheless, esomeprazole showed an overall positive effect.

We may conclude that a dose of 20 mg of esomeprazole is indicated and effective in patients taking NSAIDs or COX-2 inhibitors regularly. Such a low dose, however, may not be sufficient to prevent ulcers or bleeding. Whether all patients taking anti-inflammatory agents chronically should receive a PPI or whether the drug should be reserved for selective groups remains unanswered.

Conclusion

This review highlights some of the most important developments in the past year in the diagnosis and management of acid-related disorders.

While the symptom complex of GERD is easy to identify in most cases and empirical treatment is reasonable, objective measurement of acid reflux is often needed. The wireless pH probe is certainly much better tolerated by patients and appears quite accurate, providing prolonged pH monitoring. The role of capsule endoscopy in the diagnosis of oesophagitis is ill-defined but it may be a quick and safe screening method for Barrett's oesophagus, provided that such screening is beneficial in the long run. The effects of various medications during pregnancy do not usually receive much attention in the gastroenterology literature. According to the study we reviewed, PPIs appear safe during pregnancy, although the authors looked only at short-term use. More observations are needed before we can safely say that pregnant women can take PPIs throughout their pregnancy with impunity.

A large proportion of patients with GERD report night-time heartburn and sleep disturbances. Esomeprazole appears to affect night-time symptoms favourably but the effect is far from being universal. New endoscopic methods for treating GERD are reported, although this past year saw the withdrawal of one agent, Enteryx®, because of serious side effects. The clinical observation that patients with Schatzki's rings benefit from periodic dilatations and treatment with PPIs is vindicated by a small but well-designed study. Local injection of steroids in some forms of peptic strictures also appears to be beneficial. An important epidemiological study revealed that the presence of Barrett's oesophagus in the general population is unrelated to reflux symptoms, and crystal violet chromoendoscopy may be a useful method of improving screening for Barrett's oesophagus. Finally, while we know that PPIs protect from ulcers induced by NSAIDs, it appears that esomeprazole is effective in relieving dyspeptic symptoms in patients taking NSAIDs as well as in those taking COX-2 inhibitors, suggesting that these symptoms may also be acid-related.

References

1. Pandolfino JE, Richter JE, Ours T, Guardino JM, Chapman J, Kahrilas PJ. Ambulatory esophageal pH monitoring using a wireless system. *Am J Gastroenterol* 2003; **98**: 740–9.
2. Richter JE. Gastroesophageal reflux disease during pregnancy. *Gastroenterol Clin North Am* 2003; **32**: 235–61.
3. Park PO, Hall-Angeras M, Ohlin B, *et al.* A prospective, multicenter, randomized, single-blind, parallel group study on the comparison between endoscopic cardia suturing and sham operation as a treatment of patients with gastroesophageal reflux symptoms. *Gastroenterology* 2005; **128**(4 Suppl 2): A95.
4. Schiefke I, Zabel-Langhennig A, Neumann S, Feisthammel J, Moessner J, Caca K. Long-term failure of endoscopic gastroplication (EndoCinch). *Gut* 2005; **54**: 752–8.
5. Patterson DJ, Graham DY, Smith JL, Schwartz JT, Alpert E, Lanza FL, Cain GD. Natural history of benign esophageal stricture treated by dilatation. *Gastroenterology* 1983; **85**: 346–50.
6. Ogilvie AL, Ferguson R, Atkinson M. Outlook with conservative treatment of peptic oesophageal stricture. *Gut* 1980; **21**: 23–5.
7. Hands LJ, Papavramidis S, Bishop H, Dennison AR, McIntyre RL, Kettlewell MG. The natural history of peptic oesophageal strictures treated by dilatation and antireflux therapy alone. *Ann R Coll Surg Engl* 1989; **71**: 306–9.
8. Smith PM, Kerr GD, Cockel R, Ross BA, Bate CM, Brown P, Dronfield MW, Green JR, Hislop WS, Theodossi A, *et al.* A comparison of omeprazole and ranitidine in the

prevention of recurrence of benign esophageal stricture. *Gastroenterology* 1994; **107**: 1312–18.

9. Lagergren J, Bergstrom R, Lindgren A, Nyren O. Symptomatic gastroesophageal reflux as a risk factor for esophageal adenocarcinoma. *N Engl J Med* 1999; **340**: 825–31.

10. Sharma P, Topalovski M, Mayo MS, Weston AP. Methylene blue chromoendoscopy for detection of short-segment Barrett's esophagus. *Gastrointest Endosc* 2001; **54**: 289–93.

11. Amano Y, Komazawa Y, Ishimura N, Ohara S, Aimi M, Fujishiro H, Ishihara S, Adachi K, Kinoshita Y. Two cases of superficial cancer in Barrett's esophagus detected by chromoendoscopy with crystal violet. *Gastrointest Endosc* 2004; **59**: 143–6.

Part II

Diseases of the lower GI tract

3

Colorectal neoplasia

LAURA BIANCHI, CAROL BURKE

Introduction

Many governmental agencies have made the prevention of colorectal cancer one of their top priorities. The adenoma–carcinoma sequence is a suitable biologic paradigm for the prevention and early detection of disease. We have chosen a series of articles that address multiple areas in colorectal neoplasia prevention. Four of the articles provide the latest data on the chemoprevention of colorectal neoplasia. These include studies on primary prevention with dietary fibre and the use of 3-hydroxy-3 methylglutaryl coenzyme A (HMG-CoA) reductase inhibitors, i.e. the statins. Cyclooxygenase 2 (COX-2) inhibitors have been shown to decrease the risk of colorectal neoplasia.

Two long awaited, long-term adenoma prevention trials have been completed. While the efficacy data have not been published, the safety data are available from one trial utilizing rofecoxib and another one using celecoxib. Colorectal cancer screening is recommended by all major gastrointestinal societies. Options for average risk individuals include annual faecal occult blood testing (FOBT), flexible sigmoidoscopy (FS) every 5 years, air contrast barium enema (ACBE) every 5 years or colonoscopy every 10 years beginning at the age of 50 years. One article elucidates the risks and benefits of screening in the elderly population. Since no guidelines recommend the time to cease screening, data from this study can help us guide our patients to make informed decisions about screening. New colorectal cancer screening technologies are being developed. One of the newest technologies, computed tomographic colonoscopy (CTC), is emerging as a promising screening modality. However, the accuracy of CTC has been found to vary widely in published studies. One article, a meta-analysis, attempts to determine the true accuracy of CTC and the reasons for the wide heterogeneity in its reported sensitivity. Another study compares the accuracy of colonoscopy, CTC and ACBE and provides support for colonoscopy as the preferred screening modality. When clinicians recommend colorectal screening and surveillance strategies to patients, those with the highest risk of cancer are usually recommended the most aggressive surveillance. An interesting international study elaborates the differing risks of colorectal and extra-colonic cancers in families meeting the Amsterdam criteria who harbour mismatch repair (MMR) mutations compared to those families that have no evidence of

MMR mutations. The findings are likely to change cancer surveillance based on the genetic cause of hereditary non-polyposis colorectal cancer. Our last study compares the short-term outcomes of conventional versus laparoscopic-assisted surgery in patients with colorectal cancer.

Dietary fiber intake and risk of colorectal cancer: a pooled analysis of prospective cohort studies

Park Y, Hunter D, Spiegelman D, *et al.* *JAMA* 2005; **294**: 2849–57

BACKGROUND. Dietary fibre has been hypothesized to reduce the risk of colorectal cancer. Data regarding the association between fibre and the prevention of colorectal diseases including colorectal cancer are conflicting. Several epidemiologic and case–control studies have shown an inverse relationship between dietary fibre intake and risk of colorectal cancer while other prospective studies, including randomized controlled intervention trials, have found no association. A recent European study found a significantly decreased risk of colorectal cancer or adenoma in patients with substantial dietary fibre intake.

INTERPRETATION. The Pooling Project of Prospective Studies of Diet and Cancer was established to summarize the association between dietary factors and risk of cancers. In an effort to analyse the association between dietary fibre intake and risk of colorectal cancer, the Pooling Project authors identified 13 cohort studies which met pre-specified criteria. Each study utilized a food frequency questionnaire and energy-adjusted intakes were calculated. During follow-up times of 6 to 20 years, 7 328 414 person-years were accumulated and 8081 incident colorectal cancer cases were identified. The median energy-adjusted dietary fibre intake ranged from 14 to 28 g/day in men and from 13 to 24 g/day in women. Cereals were the major contributor to dietary fibre in Europe while fruits and vegetables were the main fibre sources in North American studies. The age-adjusted model revealed a significant inverse association between the highest versus lowest quintile of dietary fibre intake and a risk of colorectal cancer (relative risk [RR] 0.84; 95% confidence interval [CI] 0.77–0.92). However, when multivariate analysis was performed to account for other colorectal cancer risk factors, including non-dietary risk factors, multivitamin use, total energy intake, intake of folate, alcohol, and red meat, this association was no longer statistically significant (RR 0.94; 95% CI 0.86–1.03) (Fig. 3.1).

Comment

This study performed a systematic analysis of the association between dietary fibre intake and risk of colorectal cancer in 13 prospective cohort studies. The pooled data from these homogeneous studies revealed a significant inverse association between dietary fibre intake and risk of colorectal cancer in an age-adjusted model. However, in the multivariate analysis, after adjustment for other colorectal cancer risk factors, no benefit of fibre was seen. Therefore, high reported dietary fibre intake was not shown to be associated with a reduced risk of colorectal cancer. Based on this evidence, high dietary fibre is not proven to prevent colorectal

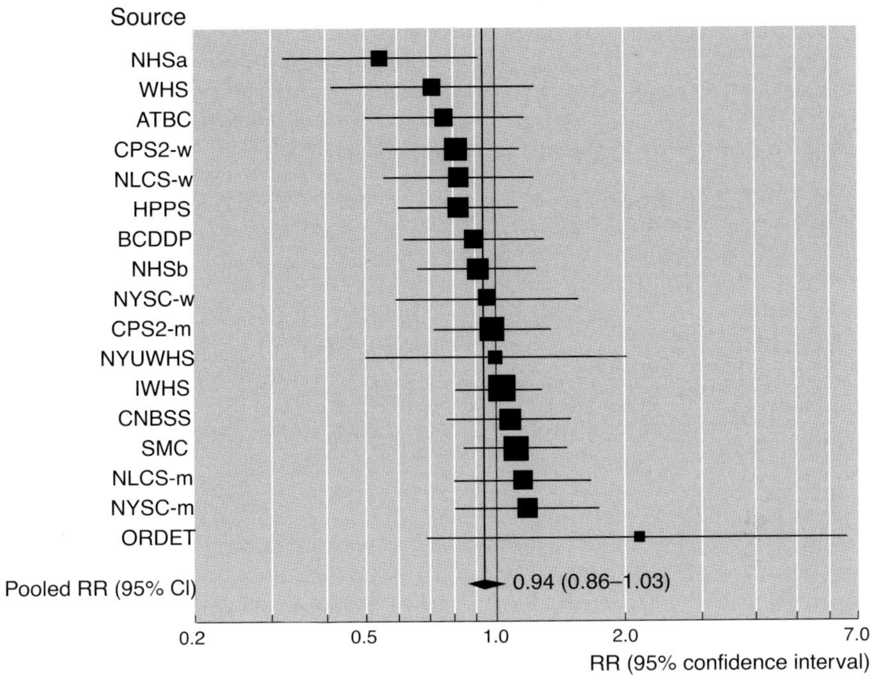

Fig. 3.1 Study-specific and pooled multivariate relative risks (RRs) of colorectal cancer comparing the highest versus the lowest quintile of dietary fibre intake. The *squares* and *horizontal lines* correspond with the multivariate study-specific RRs and 95% CIs for the highest quintile of dietary fibre intake compared with the lowest. The size of a *square* reflects the study-specific weight (inverse of the variance), and the *diamond* represents the pooled RR and 95% CI. The vertical *dotted line* represents the pooled RR. Source: Park *et al.* (2005).

neoplasia. Of note, this study utilized data regarding baseline fibre intake and did not assess lifelong fibre intake or intake earlier in life. While there may be a role of fibre in general gastrointestinal health and lower risks of heart disease and diabetes, this study adds to the mounting evidence that a high fibre diet is not associated with a decreased risk of colonic cancer.

Colonoscopic screening of average-risk women for colorectal neoplasia

Schoenfeld P, Cash B, Flood A, *et al.*; CONCeRN Study Investigators. *N Engl J Med* 2005; **352**: 2061–8

Background. A recent study showed that a significant portion of advanced colonic neoplasms would be missed with the use of flexible sigmoidoscopy in men.

Women have been shown to have a lower prevalence of colorectal neoplasia than men and it has been suggested that 'lower risk' individuals, i.e. women under the age of 60, undergo colorectal cancer screening with flexible sigmoidoscopy. Unfortunately, limiting colorectal cancer screening to an investigation of the distal colon may lead to missed proximal advanced lesions. The predictive value of flexible sigmoidoscopy to detect women with advanced proximal neoplasia is unknown.

Interpretation. In this multicentre study, asymptomatic women referred for colorectal cancer screening underwent colonoscopy. The findings in the distal colon visualized on colonoscopy were used as a surrogate for the yield of flexible sigmoidoscopy. Lesions were considered detectable by flexible sigmoidoscopy if they were in the distal colon or they were in the proximal colon in subjects who had concurrent adenomas in the distal colon. The participants included average risk women aged 50–79 and women aged 40–79 with a family history of colorectal cancer in a first-degree relative. Colonoscopy was completed in 1463 (98.7%) of the eligible participants. A total of 446 neoplasms were identified in 299 women (20.4%). Of these women, 72 (4.9%) had advanced neoplasms (>1 cm adenoma, villous adenoma, adenoma with high grade dysplasia, or invasive colorectal cancer) detected on colonoscopy. The diagnostic yield of flexible sigmoidoscopy for advanced neoplasia was 34.7% (25 of 72 cases detected) (Fig. 3.2). Advanced neoplasia would have been identified in 1.7% of women and missed in 3.2% based upon the distal findings. There was no significant difference in the diagnostic yield of flexible sigmoidoscopy when women with and without a family history of colon cancer were compared or when age-adjusted stratification was performed. 93.5% of women had no neoplasia in the distal colon (defined as rectum and sigmoid). The prevalence of proximal advanced neoplasia was not different in women with no distal colorectal neoplasms (3.4%) compared to women with distal colorectal neoplasia (3.2%). If the distal colon findings were the trigger for colonoscopy, 94% of cases of advanced neoplasia in the proximal colon would have been missed.

When the prevalence of advanced neoplasia in asymptomatic men with negative faecal occult blood test and no family history of colon cancer were compared with age-matched women, men were more likely to have advanced neoplasia than women (8.6 % men vs 4.5% women; $P = 0.002$). Additionally, flexible sigmoidoscopy had a significantly greater yield for detection of advanced neoplasms in men (66.3% men vs 35.2% women; $P < 0.001$).

Comment

The diagnostic yield of flexible sigmoidoscopy for the detection of advanced neoplasia in women is 34.7% and is much lower than the yield in men at 66.3%. Advanced neoplasia would be missed in nearly two-thirds of women undergoing flexible sigmoidoscopy. This study used colonoscopic findings in the distal colon as a surrogate for flexible sigmoidoscopy, therefore the true yield of flexible sigmoidoscopy is not known. Since flexible sigmoidosocopy is typically done without sedation, by endoscopists of variable proficiency, and with a more limited preparation, this study may have overestimated the yield of flexible sigmoidoscopy. Published guidelines recommend either flexible sigmoidoscopy every 5 years with annual faecal occult blood testing or colonoscopy every 10 years for colorectal cancer

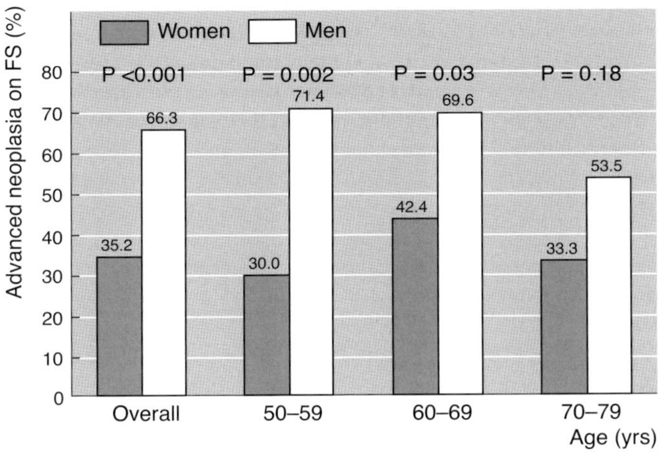

Fig. 3.2 Yield of flexible sigmoidoscopy (FS) for advanced colorectal neoplasia anywhere in the colon in men and women, according to age. The yield of FS was defined as the proportion of patients with advanced colorectal neoplasia who were found to have advanced lesions in the distal colon or advanced lesions in the proximal colon along with small adenomas in the distal colon, which would have triggered the performance of colonoscopy. The women were from the current study, and the men were from VA Cooperative Study 380. Source: Schoenfeld *et al.* (2005).

screening in asymptomatic patients. This study presents strong evidence to support the use of colonoscopy for colorectal cancer screening in average risk women in view of the fact that flexible sigmoidoscopy alone would have missed the vast majority of advanced neoplasms in women.

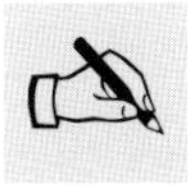

Analysis of air contrast barium enema, computed tomographic colonography, and colonoscopy: prospective comparison

Rockey DC, Paulson E, Niedzwiecki D, *et al.* *Lancet* 2005; **365**: 305–11

Background. Air contrast barium enemas (ACBE) and colonoscopy have been the mainstays of colonic imaging. Computed tomographic colonography (CTC) is a relatively new technique, and the sensitivity of CTC for the detection of colorectal polyps and cancer is variable. The investigators of this study intended to compare the sensitivity of these three imaging modalities in a cohort of patients with an increased risk of colorectal neoplasia.

Interpretation. This multicentre study was performed between 2000 and 2004. Subjects were eligible if they had either a positive faecal occult blood test, haematochezia, iron-deficiency anaemia, or a family history of colorectal neoplasia.

ACBE was performed first, after standard preparation. Within 2 weeks CTC was performed after bowel preparation using a four- or eight-slice multidetector scanner with a 2.5 mm slice thickness. Image interpretation was primarily two-dimensional with three-dimensional reading for problem solving. Colonoscopy was done the same day as CTC in the standard fashion. The mean duration of experience for ACBE readers was 19 years. Approximately half the CTC readers had read more than 50 cases and those that had not read 50 cases completed a CTC training module. The imaging findings were revealed during colonoscopy by 'segmental unblinding' to reconcile discrepancies regarding lesions. Size and location (caecum, ascending, transverse, descending, sigmoid, rectum) of lesions detected during each imaging modality were recorded. The reference standard in this study was the combined dataset for all three imaging studies. The sensitivity of each imaging study was calculated on a per-patient, per-lesion and per-histology basis. Of 775 subjects, 614 (79%) completed all three diagnostic studies. The per-patient sensitivity of colonoscopy for lesions ≥10 mm was 0.984 (95% CI 0.91–1.00) while it was 0.48 for ACBE (95% CI 0.35–0.61), and 0.59 for CTC (95% CI 0.45–0.71) (Table 3.1). The results were similar for lesions 6–9 mm and lesions ≥6 mm. Colonoscopy had the highest specificity for lesions ≥10 mm (0.996; 95% CI 0.99–1.00) and 6–9 mm (0.996; 95% CI 0.98–1.00). The quality of preparation did not significantly alter the sensitivity of any of the imaging studies and reader experience was inversely proportional to the number of lesions detected on CTC. The authors report that no serious procedure-related adverse events occurred.

Comment

In this multicentre study, colonoscopy had the highest sensitivity and specificity for the detection of colonic lesions greater than 6 mm. While ACBE and CTC proved to be highly specific for lesions greater than 1 cm in size, neither test exhibited the high degree of sensitivity seen with colonoscopy which is needed before widespread use of CTC can be considered. Although CTC reader inexperience may be presumed to limit the study's accuracy, this study found that increased reader experience is not associated with greater diagnostic accuracy. In fact the less experienced interpreters detected more colonic lesions ≥10 mm than the more seasoned interpreters (70% vs 47%; $P = 0.0775$). All three studies appeared to be equally safe as no procedure-related adverse events were documented. Colonoscopy is more sensitive and specific than either ACBE or CTC for detection of colonic lesions greater than 6 mm in size. This study confirms the limited role of ACBE and the unacceptable accuracy of CTC for the detection of colonic neoplasms. CTC is a rapidly evolving field, and comparisons between colonoscopy and future CTC technology may yield different results.

Until evidence suggests otherwise, colonoscopy should remain the test of choice for the detection of colorectal neoplasms.

Table 3.1 Colon imaging test sensitivity

	Sensitivity (95% CI)					
	Per patient	***P***	**Per lesion**	***P***	**Per histology**	***P***
Lesion size ≥10 mm						
Number	63		76		55	
ACBE	0.48 (0.35–0.61)	0.1083	0.45 (0.33–0.57)	0.2008	0.55 (0.40–0.68)	0.2253
CTC	0.59 (0.45–0.71)	<0.0001	0.53 (0.41–0.64)	<0.0001	0.64 (0.49–0.77)	<0.0001
Colonoscopy	0.984 (0.91–1.00)		0.987 (0.93–1.00)		0.982 (0.90–1.00)	
Lesion size 6–9 mm						
Number	116		158		97	
ACBE	0.35 (0.27–0.45)	0.0080	0.30 (0.23–0.38)	0.0005	0.31 (0.22–0.41)	<0.0001
CTC	0.51 (0.41–0.60)	<0.0001	0.47 (0.39–0.56)	<0.0001	0.60 (0.49–0.70)	<0.0001
Colonoscopy	0.99 (0.95–1.00)		0.987 (0.96–1.00)		1.00 (0.96–1.00)	
Lesion size ≥6 mm						
Number	155		234		152	
ACBE	0.41 (0.33–0.49)	0.0033	0.35 (0.29–0.41)	0.0002	0.39 (0.32–0.48)	<0.0001
CTC	0.55 (0.47–0.63)	<0.0001	0.49 (0.43–0.56)	<0.0001	0.61 (0.53–0.69)	<0.0001
Colonoscopy	0.987 (0.95–1.00)		0.987 (0.96–1.00)		0.993 (0.96–1.00)	

Sensitivity is based on lesion size and method of analysis, i.e. whether per patient, per lesion, or per histology (adenoma or cancer). *P*-values associated with ACBE are for ACBE vs CTC. *P*-values associated with CTC are for CTC vs colonoscopy. *P*-values are not shown for ACBE vs colonoscopy, but all were $P < 0.0001$.
Source: Rockey *et al.* (2005).

Meta-analysis: computed tomographic colonography

Mulhall B, Veerappan G, Jackson J. *Ann Intern Med* 2005; **142**: 635–50

Background. CTC is an imaging technique with rapidly evolving technology. Proponents of CTC suggest it may be better tolerated by patients than colonoscopy and may improve patient adherence with colorectal cancer screening. Studies of the test characteristics of CTC have had mixed results with only one study showing a sensitivity of CTC similar to colonoscopy. The source of the discrepancy of the accuracy of CTC among these studies is unclear. A systematic review of the literature and meta-analysis was undertaken to determine the source of the discrepant results.

Interpretation. The investigators identified prospective studies of adults undergoing CTC with colonoscopy or surgery as the gold standard. Pooled sensitivities and specificities per patient overall and for the detection of polyps <6mm, 6–9 mm and >9 mm were abstracted. Technical characteristics of the CTC scanner and mode of image interpretation were analysed. Thirty-three prospective studies met the inclusion criteria involving 6393 subjects. The sensitivity of CTC increased progressively as polyp size increased; 48% (95% CI 14–86%) for polyps <6mm, to 70% (95% CI 55–84%) for polyps 6–9 mm, to 85% (95% CI 79–81%) for polyps >9mm (Fig. 3.3). The analyses were heterogeneous (P <0.001) and most of the variance was due to between-study heterogeneity. The sources for some of the heterogeneity were identified. Every 1 mm increase in collimation width decreased the sensitivity by 4.9%. Multidetector scanners had homogeneously higher sensitivity (95% CI 92–99%) when compared with single-detector scanners (82% CI 76–92%), although the latter results were heterogeneous. Studies using two-dimensional imaging with confirmation by three-dimensional imaging when necessary yielded a sensitivity of 81.9% (CI 71–91%) versus studies using fly-through technology where the pooled sensitivity was 99% (CI 95–100%). The per-patient specificity was 93% (95% CI 91–95%) for polyps 6–9 mm and 97% (95% CI 96–97%) for polyps >9 mm.

Comment

CTC appears to be highly specific, but with widely variable sensitivities. These authors determined some, but not all, of the factors that account for the wide range of sensitivities. Higher sensitivities were linked to thinner collimation slices, multi-detector scanners, and mode of image interpretation. It is likely that reader expertise, stool tagging, electronic cleansing of the colon and other technological factors will enhance the accuracy of CTC for the detection of colorectal neoplasia. Until widespread and consistently high sensitivity of CTC is attained, colonoscopy is still the 'gold standard' for the detection of colorectal neoplasia.

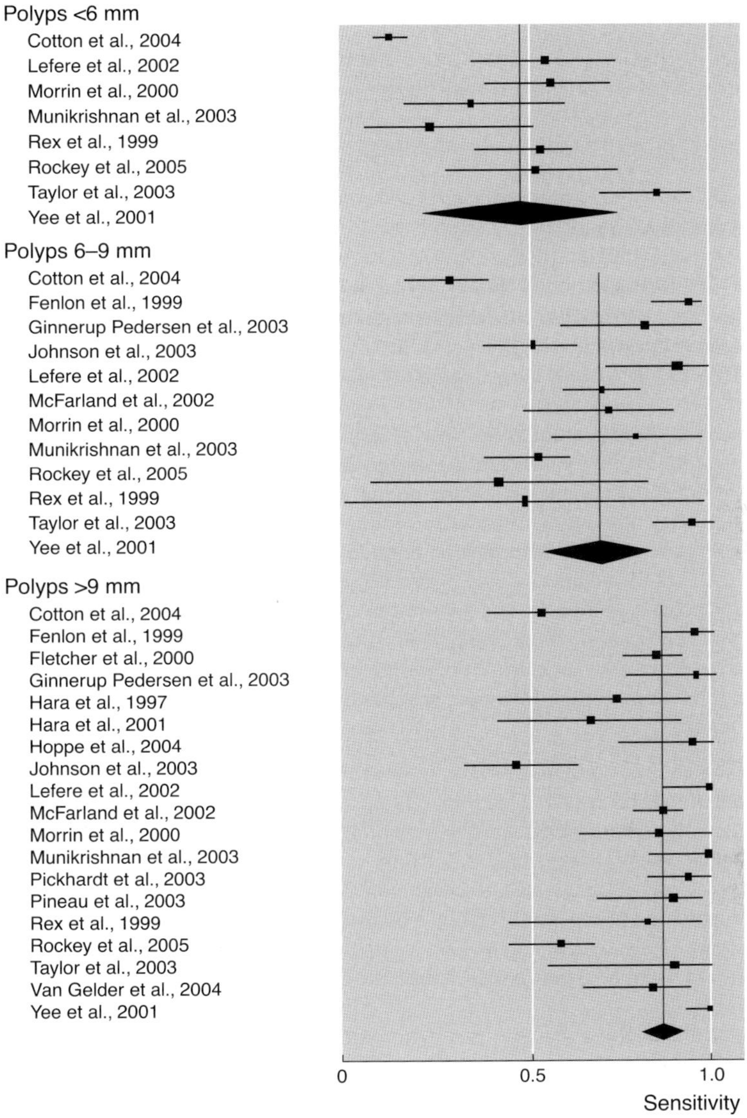

Fig. 3.3 Reported per-patient sensitivities in the included studies, by polyp size. Summary statistics: for polyps <6 mm, 0.48 (95% CI 0.25–0.70); for polyps 6–9 mm, 0.70 (CI 0.55–0.84); for polyps >9 mm, 0.85 (CI 0.79–0.91). Source: Mulhall *et al.* (2005).

Cardiovascular events associated with rofecoxib in a colorectal adenoma chemoprevention trial

Bresalier R, Sandler R, Quan H, *et al.*; Adenomatous Polyp Prevention on Vioxx (APPROVe) Trial Investigators. *N Engl J Med* 2005; **352**: 1092–102

Cardiovascular risk associated with celecoxib in a clinical trial for colorectal adenoma prevention

Solomon S, McMurray J, Pfeffer M, *et al.*; Adenoma Prevention with Celecoxib (APC) Study Investigators. *N Engl J Med* 2005; **352**: 1071–80

Background. COX-2 is expressed at sites of inflammation and benign and malignant neoplasms. COX-2 inhibition reduces the development of colorectal neoplasia in colorectal cancer cells lines and animal models. Celecoxib, a COX-2 inhibitor, has been shown in a 6-month trial to reduce the size and number of colorectal adenomas in patients with familial adenomatous polyposis (FAP). Celecoxib is approved by the FDA for adjunctive use in the management of FAP patients. The effectiveness of COX-2 inhibitors for the prevention of adenomas in individuals with a lesser risk of colorectal cancer is unknown. Cohort and case–control studies have suggested an adverse cardiovascular safety profile of COX-2 inhibitors and other non-steroidal anti-inflammatories. However, prospective data on the safety of COX-2 inhibitors are lacking.

Interpretation. These two multicentre, international studies were designed to assess the effect of long-term COX-2 inhibitor use on the risk of recurrent neoplastic polyps of the colon in patients with a history of colorectal adenomas. Due to their large size and prospective nature, the adverse event data were utilized to determine the cardiovascular safety of rofecoxib and celecoxib in individuals with a history of colorectal adenomas. Both studies utilized a data safety monitoring board and a cardiovascular safety committee which developed cardiovascular end-point definitions as guidelines for adjudication. Both trials were terminated prematurely on the basis of the cardiovascular risks.

The rofecoxib study randomized 2586 patients to either rofecoxib 25 mg per day or placebo for three years. Randomization was concealed and the study was double-blinded. Follow-up of patients occurred at regular intervals throughout the three-year study and adverse events were reported and confirmed by an adjudication committee. Forty-six patients (1.50 events per 100 patient-years) in the rofecoxib group had thrombotic events compared with 26 patients (0.78 events per 100 patient-years) in the placebo group (RR 1.92; 95% CI 1.19–3.11) (Table 3.2). The increased relative risk became apparent after 18 months of treatment. The difference between the two groups was predominantly due to the increased number of myocardial infarctions and strokes in the rofecoxib group. In addition, other investigator-reported cardiovascular events, including hypertension, oedema, and congestive heart failure, were reported more

Table 3.2 Incidence of adjudicated thrombotic adverse events*

Adverse event	**Rofecoxib group (*n* = 1287)**		**Placebo group (*n* = 1299)**		**Hazard ratio (95% CI)**
	No. of patients (%)	**Rate/100 patient-yr**	**No. of patients (%)**	**Rate/100 patient-yr**	
Total	46 (3.6)	1.50	26 (2.0)	0.78	1.92 (1.19–3.11)
Cardiac events	31 (2.4)	1.01	12 (0.9)	0.36	2.80 (1.44–5.45)
Myocardial infarction	21		9		
Fatal myocardial infarction	2		3		
Sudden death from cardiac causes	3		1		
Unstable angina pectoris	7		4		
Cerebrovascular events	15 (1.2)	0.49	7 (0.5)	0.21	2.32 (0.89–6.74)
Fatal ischaemic stroke	1		0		
Ischaemic stroke	11		6		
Transient ischaemic attack	5		2		
Peripheral vascular events	3 (0.2)	0.10	7 (0.5)	0.21	0.46 (0.08–2.03)
Peripheral arterial thrombosis	1		1		
Peripheral venous thrombosis	2		4		
Pulmonary embolism	0		2		

*The total duration of follow-up was 3059 patient-years in the rofecoxib group and 3327 patient-years in the placebo group. Although a patient may have had two or more clinical adverse events, the patient was counted once within a category. The same patient may appear in different categories. CI, confidence interval.
Source: Bresalier *et al.* (2005).

frequently in the rofecoxib group when compared to controls (Table 3.3). Overall and cardiovascular mortality were similar in the two groups.

The celecoxib trial investigators randomized 2035 patients to 200 mg celecoxib twice daily, 400 mg celecoxib twice daily, or placebo. The incidence of pre-specified composite cardiovascular end-point (death from cardiovascular causes, non-fatal myocardial infarction, stroke and heart failure) were compared. A mid-study analysis revealed a dose-related increase in the composite end-point in patients taking celecoxib. This included 16 subjects (2.3%) of the group given 200 mg of celecoxib twice daily (hazard ratio 2.3; 95% CI 0.9–5.5), 23 subjects (3.4%) receiving 400 mg of celecoxib twice daily (hazard ratio 3.4; 95% CI 1.4–7.8) versus 7 subjects (1.0%) in the placebo group. The hazard ratio associated with celecoxib was not significantly affected by baseline characteristics of the subjects including history of cardiovascular events, age, gender, diabetes, smoking, use of lipid-lowering agents or aspirin use.

Table 3.3 Incidence of individual cardiovascular and fatal events

End-point	Placebo (n = 679)	Celecoxib, 200 mg twice daily (n = 685)	Celecoxib, 400 mg twice daily (n = 671)	Both celecoxib groups (n = 1356)
	No. of patients (%)			
Death from any cause	6 (0.9)	6 (0.9)	9 (1.3)	15 (1.1)
Death from cardiovascular causes	1 (0.1)	3 (0.4)	6 (0.9)	9 (0.7)
Death from non-cardiovascular causes	5 (0.7)	3 (0.4)	3 (0.4)	6 (0.4)
Non-fatal cardiovascular events				
Myocardial infarction	3 (0.4)	9 (1.3)	9 (1.3)	18 (1.3)
Stroke	3 (0.4)	3 (0.4)	5 (0.7)	8 (0.6)
Heart failure	2 (0.3)	1 (0.1)	4 (0.6)	5 (0.4)
Thromoembolic event	1 (0.1)	3 (0.4)	4 (0.6)	7 (0.5)
Resuscitation after sudden cardiac arrest	0	0	1 (0.1)	1 (0.1)
Hospitalization for unstable angina	5 (0.7)	4 (0.6)	2 (0.3)	6 (0.4)
Arrhythmia	9 (1.3)	4 (0.6)	7 (1.0)	11 (0.8)
Cardiovascular procedure	7 (1.0)	9 (1.3)	6 (0.9)	15 (1.1)
Other	9 (1.3)	11 (1.6)	14 (2.1)	25 (1.8)

Source: Solomon *et al.* (2005).

Comment

These two, prospective polyp prevention trials have demonstrated an increased cardiovascular risk in patients using daily rofecoxib and celecoxib. The increase in adverse events was noted after long-term exposure: 12 months in the celecoxib trial and 18 months in the rofecoxib study. There appeared to be a dose effect with the use of celecoxib. Unfortunately no baseline characteristics were associated with the increased hazard ratio of cardiovascular events which makes it difficult to predict who is most likely to have serious side effects from celebrex. The mechanisms for the increased cardiovascular complications in patients taking COX-2 inhibitors are unknown, but may be related to promotion of thrombosis due to sustained prostacyclin inhibition, increasing blood pressure, decreasing angiogenesis and perhaps destabilization of atherosclerotic plaques. The cardiovascular risks of COX-2 inhibitors appear to outweigh any potential chemopreventive benefit and they should not be considered for the prevention of colorectal neoplasia in patients with sporadic colorectal adenomas.

Statins in the risk of colorectal cancer

Poynter J, Gruber S, Higgins P, *et al.* *N Engl J Med* 2005; **352**: 2184–92

BACKGROUND. HMG-CoA reductase has been shown to be over-expressed in colorectal cancer cells. Statins inhibit HMG-CoA reductase, and have been shown to inhibit the growth of colon cancer cell lines and reduce the risk of colorectal cancer in some, but not all, cardiovascular clinical trials. The Molecular Epidemiology of Colorectal Cancer study is a population-based case–control study of patients who received a diagnosis of colorectal cancer. These investigators sought to establish whether statin use was associated with a decreased risk of colorectal cancer.

INTERPRETATION. This is a case–control study of the incident colorectal cancers in a northern Israeli population. A total of 3181 patients given a diagnosis of colorectal cancer between 31 May 1998 and 31 March 2004 were identified from the northern Israeli Clalit Heath Services (CHS) database. Of these patients, 2146 were alive and completed an interview. The response rate of eligible participants was 67.5%. Cases were confirmed by pathologic review. Two thousand and fifteen controls were identified from the same database and matched for birth year, sex, ethnicity (Jewish or non-Jewish) and site of primary care clinic. From these subjects, 1651 matched pairs were identified. Patient demographics and an extensive medical and family history were obtained by interview and questionnaire. Patients were asked to recall all medications they used for 5 or more years, including statins, aspirin, and other non-steroidal anti-inflammatory drugs (NSAIDs). Statin use was validated in some patients by matching patients' reports of statin use with database prescription records. There were significantly more Ashkenazi Jews among the cases ($P < 0.001$), significantly more controls than patients reported hypercholesterolaemia ($P < 0.001$), and more controls than patients used statins for at least 5 years (11.6% vs 6.1%). Statin use of 5 or more years was associated with a significant reduction in the unadjusted risk of colorectal cancer (odds ratio [OR] 0.50; 95% CI 0.40–0.63) that persisted after adjusting for NSAID use, dietary factors and family history (OR 0.57; 95% CI 0.44–0.73). In order to determine if the association between statin use and reduced risk of colorectal cancer was due to the specific action of the statins or to the lowering of cholesterol, the investigators looked for an association between the non-statin cholesterol-lowering medication bezafibrate and risk of colorectal cancer; no association was detected (OR 1.08; 95% CI 0.59–2.01). Additionally, the study questioned whether ASA (aspirin) or NSAID use in conjunction with statin therapy modified the effect of the statins, and they found no evidence of effect modification ($P = 0.36$). Statins were also shown to be equally protective in patients with and without a family history of colorectal cancer (OR 0.41; 95% CI 0.19–0.93). In order to evaluate for indication bias, the authors compared statin use among patients with a history of hypercholesterolaemia and ischaemic heart disease. Statins were protective with regard to colorectal cancer in both groups.

Comment

This study detected a strong inverse association between the use of statins for at least 5 years and risk of colorectal cancer. A 47% reduction in relative risk was seen in long-term users versus non-users of statins. While there were some significant variations in the two populations (family history of colorectal cancer, participation in sports, vegetable consumption, personal diagnosis of hypercholesterolaemia), adjusting for these and other confounders did not alter the significant inverse association between long-term statin use and risk of colon and rectal cancer. These data do not provide us with information on dose or frequency of statin use and thus a dose response cannot be determined. Since this study was performed in a genetically homogenous population it is not known if these results are generalizable to other populations. Statins are commonly prescribed and are associated with an acceptable adverse-effect profile. Additional studies on the chemopreventive benefits of statins should be performed in other populations to determine their benefit and cost-effectiveness, and safety data need to be gathered before this medication can be recommended purely for its chemopreventive effects.

Colorectal cancer in patients under close colonoscopic surveillance

Robertson DJ, Greenberg ER, Beach M, *et al. Gastroenterology* 2005; **129**: 34–41

BACKGROUND. Colorectal adenomas are the precursor to colorectal cancer. Individuals with adenomatous polyps are considered to be at higher risk of colorectal cancer compared to the average risk population. Large case–control and cohort trials have suggested that colonoscopy with polypectomy is associated with decrease in colorectal cancer incidence. Methodological differences in these studies prevent certainty of the estimate of efficacy of polypectomy and colonoscopic surveillance.

INTERPRETATION. Robertson *et al.* determined the incidence of colorectal cancer in 2915 subjects who were under colonoscopic surveillance after complete clearing of adenomas from their colorectum. The subjects were drawn from three multicentre, randomized, adenoma chemoprevention trials. Nineteen cases (0.9%) of colorectal cancer occurred over a mean follow-up of 3.7 years. The overall incidence of colorectal cancer was 1.74/1000 person-years. However the incidence was 3.79 (95% CI 1.63–7.47) per 1000 person-years through the first year of follow-up colonoscopy and 0.96 (95% CI 0.31–2.24) for the interval between the one- and up to 4-year colonoscopy ($P = 0.01$). Fifteen cancer cases were found on the surveillance exam and four cases were discovered on an exam done due to symptoms. Eleven cases were Stage III or worse and two subjects died of colorectal carcinoma. The rate of cancer development was higher in men and in subjects with a prior history of adenoma. Overall, the incidence of cancer was similar to that expected from Surveillance, Epidemiology, and End Results (SEER) data (standardized incidence ratio 0.98; 95% CI 0.63–1.54).

Comment

Colorectal cancer occurs more frequently after colonoscopy than is generally expected. The rate of cancer observed in this study is similar to other clinical trials involving colonoscopic follow-up of subjects with resected colorectal adenomas. However, these results contrast with the benefit of polypectomy reported from the National Polyp Study (NPS) which is widely cited as representing the effectiveness of colonoscopy. NPS investigators reported a risk reduction of 76% compared to SEER data with an incidence of 0.6 cancers/1000 person-years. No apparent benefit from polypectomy was seen in Robertson *et al.*'s study. The authors propose a few possibilities that could account for cancer soon after complete colonoscopy. These include missing prevalent neoplasia on baseline colonoscopy or incomplete excision of adenomas. Five invasive cancers were diagnosed in a colonic segment where a large adenoma had been removed on the prior colonoscopy. The third possibility is that some lesions transition quickly to cancer or are *de novo* cancers. The implications of this study highlight the potential for missed lesions on colonoscopy or development of interval cancers. Both of these issues should be acknowledged as potential risks of colonoscopy to patients during the informed consent process. Careful diagnostic and therapeutic techniques should always be utilized by endoscopists to enhance the quality and efficacy of colonoscopy.

Comparing risks and benefits of colorectal cancer screening in elderly patients

Ko CW, Sonnenberg A. *Gastroenterology* 2005; **129**: 1163–70

BACKGROUND. Current guidelines recommend that colorectal cancer screening begins at age 50, but there is a paucity of data regarding the benefits of continued screening in the elderly. An older population with comorbid medical conditions may be at greater risk for procedural complications and receive less benefit from screening. Evidence regarding the risks and benefits of screening in the elderly and the effect of comorbid illnesses on these outcomes are needed to guide informed decisions.

INTERPRETATION. The investigators utilized complex modelling to examine the probability of colorectal cancer screening-related benefit and harm in patients aged 70–94 years with varying health status. They estimated the risk of dying from colorectal cancer and the potential reduction in mortality with different methods of colorectal cancer screening, including annual faecal occult blood testing, flexible sigmoidoscopy every 5 years, and colonoscopy every 10 years.

A sensitivity analysis was performed to examine the effect of uncertainty from the true benefits and risk of colonoscopy. Age- and sex-specific estimates of median life expectancy were gathered, and similar information with respect to colorectal cancer-related mortality rates was collected from the SEER program. The benefit, or number needed to screen to prevent one cancer-related death (NNS), and harm, or number needed to encounter one screening-related complication (NNC), related to colorectal cancer screening were calculated. Overall, the NNS with colonoscopy was significantly

Table 3.4 Expected colorectal cancer mortality and NNS in men

			NNS†		
Age group (y)	**Life expectancy (y)***	**Risk of colorectal cancer death (%)**	**Faecal occult blood test**	**Flexible sigmoidoscopy**	**Colonoscopy**
50–54	36	4.1	138 (116–166)	62 (50–83)	33 (28–42)
	28.5	2.3	255 (219–306)	115 (92–153)	61 (51–77)
	19.6	1.0	629 (539–754)	283 (226–377)	151 (126–189)
70–74	18	3.8	177 (152–212)	80 (75–106)	42 (35–53)
	12.4	2.1	380 (326–456)	171 (137–228)	91 (76–114)
	6.7	0.9	1877 (1609–2252)	845 (676–1126)	450 (375–563)
75–79	14.2	3.6	207 (177–248)	93 (75–124)	50 (41–62)
	9.3	1.9	525 (450–630)	236 (189–315)	126 (105–157)
	4.9	0.9	–	–	–
80–84	10.8	3.2	277 (237–332)	125 (100–166)	66 (55–83)
	6.7	1.8	945 (810–1134)	425 (340–567)	227 (189–283)
	3.3	0.8	–	–	–
85–89	7.9	2.7	554 (475–665)	249 (199–332)	133 (111–166)
	4.7	1.6	–	–	–
	2.2	0.8	–	–	–
90 or older	5.8	2.0	2008 (1721–2409)	903 (723–1205)	482 (402–602)
	3.2	1.1	–	–	–
	1.5	0.5	–	–	–

*Life expectancy was estimated from US life tables and represents the 75th, 50th and 25th percentiles for given age- and sex-specific groups. Patients with good health would have greater anticipated life expectancy (75th percentile), and patients with poor health would have lower anticipated life expectancy (25th percentile).
†The numbers in parentheses represent sensitivity analyses for the estimated range of efficacy for faecal occult blood testing (15–21%), flexible sigmoidoscopy (30–50%), and colonoscopy (60–90%), respectively. The higher NNS is estimated from the lower estimate of efficacy, and the lower NNS is estimated from the higher estimate of efficacy.
Source: Ko and Sonnenberg (2005).

Table 3.5 Expected colorectal cancer mortality and NNS in women

			NNS†		
Age group (y)	**Life expectancy (y)***	**Risk of colorectal cancer death (%)**	**Faecal occult blood test**	**Flexible sigmoidoscopy**	**Colonoscopy**
50–54	40	3.8	147 (126–176)	66 (53–88)	35 (29–44)
	33	2.2	263 (226–316)	119 (95–158)	63 (53–79)
	24.5	1.0	577 (495–693)	260 (208–346)	139 (115–173)
70–74	21.3	3.5	178 (153–214)	80 (64–107)	43 (36–53)
	15.7	2.0	340 (291–408)	153 (122–204)	82 (68–102)
	9.5	0.9	1046 (897–1255)	471 (377–628)	251 (209–314)
75–79	17	3.3	204 (175–245)	92 (74–123)	49 (41–61)
	11.9	2.0	408 (349–489)	183 (147–245)	98 (82–122)
	6.8	0.9	1797 (1540–2156)	808 (647–1078)	431 (359–539)
80–84	13	3.0	262 (224–314)	118 (94–157)	63 (52–78)
	8.6	1.8	581 (498–698)	262 (209–249)	140 (116–174)
	4.6	0.8	–	–	–
85–89	9.6	2.5	455 (390–456)	205 (164–273)	109 (91–137)
	5.9	1.6	2326 (1994–2791)	1047 (837–1396)	558 (465–698)
	2.9	0.8	–	–	–
90 or older	6.8	1.8	1163 (997–1396)	523 (419–698)	279 (23–349)
	3.9	1.0	–	–	–
	1.5	0.4	–	–	–

*Life expectancy was estimated from US life tables and represents the 75th, 50th and 25th percentiles for given age- and sex-specific groups. Patients with good health would have greater anticipated life expectancy (75th percentile), and patients with poor health would have lower anticipated life expectancy (25th percentile).
†The numbers in parentheses represent sensitivity analyses for the estimated range of efficacy for faecal occult blood testing (15–21%), flexible sigmoidoscopy (30–50%), and colonoscopy (60–90%), respectively. The higher NNS is estimated from the lower estimate of efficacy, and the lower NNS is estimated from the higher estimate of efficacy.
Source: Ko and Sonnenberg (2005).

Table 3.6 NNC in men

		NNC		
Age group (y)	**Life expectancy (y)***	**FOBT**	**FS**	**Colon**
50–54	36	352 (211–1057)	159 (95–476)	68 (41–204)
	28.5	375 (225–1126)	222 (133–667)	93 (87–435)
	19.6	**447** (268–1340)	370 (222–1111)	**145** (87–435)
70–74	18	462 (277–1385)	370 (222–1111)	145 (87–435)
	12.4	643 (386–1928)	556 (333–1667)	256 (154–769)
	6.7	1996 (1197–5987)	1111 (667–3333)	**333** (200–1000)
75–79	14.2	556 (334–1669)	556 (333–1667)	256 (154–769)
	9.3	909 (545–2727)	1111 (667–3333)	333 (200–1000)
	4.9	–	–	–
80–84	10.8	790 (474–2369)	556 (333–1667)	256 (154–769)
	6.7	1996 (1197–5987)	1111 (667–3333)	333 (200–1000)
	3.3	–	–	–
85–89	7.9	1390 (834–4171)	1111 (667–3333)	333 (200–1000)
	4.7	–	–	–
	2.2	–	–	–
90–94	5.8	3817 (2290–1145)	1111 (667–3333)	**333** (200–1000)
	3.2	–	–	–
	1.5	–	–	–

FOBT, faecal occult bood testing annually; FS, flexible sigmoidoscopy every 5 years; colon, colonoscopy every 10 years. Estimates that exceed the number of cases needed to avoid one cancer-related death are shown in bold.
Source: Ko and Sonnenberg (2005).

lower than FS or FOBT while the NNC was higher in FS and FOBT groups (Tables 3.4, 3.5, 3.6, 3.7). For most age, gender and life expectancy groups, the benefits of colonoscopy outweighed the risks. The populations that would have more screening-related complications than benefits from screening included: women aged 80–89 with poor health, women over 90 years of age with average or poor health, men aged 75–84 with poor health, and men over 85 years of age with average or poor health.

Comment

Published guidelines recommend initiation of colorectal cancer screening at age 50 in average risk patients. The age to cease screening is unknown and should be based, in part, on the health status of the individual as well as their life expectancy. This study determined that the potential benefit from colorectal cancer screening varied widely with age, life expectancy and screening modality. Colonoscopy had the greatest benefit and the highest complications. The potential reduction in mortality from screening outweighed the risk of colonoscopy-related death at all ages and life expectancies with the exception of: women aged 75–79 in poor health; women aged 85–89 in average health; men aged 70–74 in poor health; and men aged 90–94 in

Table 3.7 NNC in women

Age group (y)	Life expectancy (y)*	NNC		
		FOBT	FS	Colon
50–54	40	346 (209–1039)	139 (83–417)	64 (28–192)
	33	359 (215–1076)	185 (111–556)	85 (51–256)
	24.5	**397** (238–1192)	278 (167–833)	**128** (77–385)
70–74	21.3	423 (254–1268)	278 (167–833)	128 (77–385)
	15.7	26 (315–1577)	370 (222–1111)	145 (87–435)
	9.5	**909** (545–2727)	1111 (667–3333)	333 (200–1000)
75–79	17	480 (288–1439)	370 (222–1111)	145 (87–435)
	11.9	705 (423–2116)	556 (333–1667)	256 (154–769)
	6.8	996 (1197–5987)	1111 (667–3333)	**333** (200–1000)
80–84	13	95 (357–1784)	556 (333–1667)	256 (154–769)
	8.6	1089 (653–3266)	1111 (667–3333)	333 (200–1000)
	4.6	–	–	–
85–89	9.6	909 (545–2727)	1111 (667–3333)	333 (200–1000)
	5.9	3917 (2290–11451)	1111 (667–3333)	**333** (200–1000)
	2.9	–	–	–
90–94	6.8	1996 (1197–5987)	1111 (667–3333)	333 (200–1000)
	3.9	–	–	–
	1.5	–	–	–

FOBT, fecal occult bood testing annually; FS, flexible sigmoidoscopy every 5 years; colon, colonoscopy every 10 years. Estimates that exceed the number of cases needed to avoid one cancer-related death are shown in outline format.
Source: Ko and Sonnenberg (2005).

good health. These data can help guide clinicians in their discussion of colorectal cancer screening options with elderly patients.

Lower cancer incidence in Amsterdam-I criteria families without mismatch repair deficiency: familial colorectal cancer type X

Lindor N, Rabe K, Peterson G, *et al*. *JAMA* 2005; **293**: 1979–85

Background. Hereditary non-polyposis colorectal cancer (HNPCC) is a dominantly inherited cancer syndrome which is associated with an increased risk of colorectal cancer as well as cancer of the endometrium, small intestine, stomach, kidney, ovary, and hepatobiliary system. A germline alteration in one of the MMR genes is present in about 60% of families that meet the Amsterdam-I criteria (AC-I) for HNPCC: at least three relatives with histologically verified colorectal cancer—one a first-degree relative of the other two; at least two successive generations should be affected; one of the relatives' colorectal cancers should be diagnosed prior to age 50. The risk of cancer for individuals in AC-1 families without evidence of a heritable DNA MMR

defect is unknown. It is in this subset of patients that cancer risk and screening recommendations are uncertain.

INTERPRETATION. These authors compared the cancer risks in relatives in AC-1 families with no apparent deficiency in DNA MMR to those with DNA MMR abnormalities. One hundred and seventy-three families who met Amsterdam-I criteria were identified. The majority of families were drawn from the National Cancer Institute supported Colon Cooperative Family Registry and a few other sites in the United States and Germany. Colorectal tumour blocks were tested for microsatellite instability (MSI) using 10 microsatellite loci. Tumours were classified as MSI-high (MSI-H) if more than 3 of the loci demonstrated instability, MSI-low (MSI-L) if 3 or fewer of the loci were unstable and microsatellite stable (MSS) if no loci demonstrated instability. If MSI status was not available, deleterious mutations of *hMLH1* or *hMSH2* genes, or the absence of expression of *hMLH1* or *hMSH2* by immunohistochemistry in tumour blocks were used as surrogates implying DNA MMR deficiency. Using these data, the families were divided into two groups: Group A included families with MSI-H and surrogates implying DNA MMR deficiency, and Group B included the families with MSI-L and MSS corresponding to intact DNA MMR capability. Standard incidence ratios (SIR) for various cancers in relatives were calculated by comparing the observed number of cancer cases in each group to the expected number of cancer cases as determined from the SEER database. All analyses were stratified by MSI status, method of ascertainment (population and clinic base groups), and primary (first zone relatives [50% risk of being a carrier]) and secondary (second-degree relatives [25% risk of being a carrier]) zone relatives. Group A relatives had a significantly increased risk of colorectal, uterine, stomach, urinary (kidney/ureter), ovarian, and small bowel carcinoma (Table 3.8). Group B had only an increased risk of colorectal cancer and the SIR was less than half of that seen in Group A. Group A secondary zone relatives had an increased risk of colorectal cancer but this was not true of Group B subjects. Both Group A and B subjects develop colorectal cancer at a younger age than the general population but the age of onset in Group A is younger (mean 48.7 years) than Group B relatives (mean 60.7 years).

Comment

This study found that the risk of colorectal cancer in families who meet AC-I criteria but do not have hereditary MMR deficiency is only modestly increased compared to the general US population and is significantly lower than those families with evidence of MMR deficiency. No increase in the incidence of extra-colonic tumours was seen in Group B families. Given this study's data, families without documented MMR deficiency do not warrant screening for extra-colonic tumours. In addition, the later age of onset for colon cancer in families without MMR deficiency calls into question the need to start screening for colon cancer between the ages of 20–25 years of age. This study's authors suggest that better characterization of these families is required to help guide screening recommendations for these heterogeneous and genetically distinct groups.

Table 3.8 Standardized incidence ratios comparing first- and second-degree relatives of Group A vs Group B

	Group A (MSI-H) (n = 1855)*		Group B (MSI-L/MSS) (n = 1567)*		
Tumour site	**No. of tumours (men/women)**	**SIR (95% CI)†**	**No. of tumours (men/women)**	**SIR (95% CI)†**	***P*-value‡**
Colorectum	182 (94/88)	6.1 (5.2–7.2)§	55 (23/32)	2.3 (1.7–3.0)§	<0.001
Uterus	41 (0/41)	4.1 (2.9–5.6)§	6 (0/6)	0.8 (0.3–1.6)	<0.001
Stomach	21 (14/7)	4.6 (2.7–6.6)§	5 (1/4)	1.4 (0.3–2.8)	0.008
Breast	21 (0/21)	0.5 (0.3–0.7)	13 (0/13)	0.4 (0.2–0.6)	0.59
Kidney	15 (6/9)	2.6 (1.4–4.0)§	4 (2/2)	0.9 (0.2–1.8)	0.04
Lung	12 (9/3)	0.3 (0.2–0.5)	7 (3/4)	0.2 (0.1–0.4)	0.55
Ovary	12 (0/12)	2.0 (1.0–3.2)§	7 (0/7)	1.5 (0.4–2.9)	0.60
Haematopoietic	11 (5/6)	0.5 (0.2–0.8)	5 (3/2)	0.3 (0.1–0.6)	0.29
Pancreas	10 (6/4)	1.7 (0.7–2.8)	2 (1/1)	0.4 (0.0–1.2)	0.05
Prostate	10 (10/0)	0.3 (0.1–0.6)	9 (9/0)	0.4 (0.1–0.6)	0.79
Small intestine	6 (3/3)	7.6 (2.5–13.9)§	1 (0/1)	1.6 (0.0–5.1)	0.10
Cervix	6 (0/6)	0.3 (0.1–0.5)	5 (0/5)	0.3 (0.1–0.6)	0.96
Bladder	5 (2/3)	0.4 (0.1–0.9)	1 (1/0)	0.1 (0.0–0.3)	0.17
Liver	4 (0/4)	2.4 (0.6–5.0)	1 (1/0)	0.8 (0.0–2.3)	0.28
Ureter	4 (2/2)	9.0 (2.0–18.3)§	1 (1/0)	2.9 (0.0–9.2)	0.29
Brain	3 (0/3)	0.7 (0.0–1.7)	2 (2/0)	0.6 (0.0–1.4)	0.84
Head/neck	3 (3/0)	0.3 (0.0–0.6)	3 (2/1)	0.3 (0.0–0.8)	0.79
Melanoma	2 (0/2)	0.2 (0.0–0.4)	1 (1/0)	0.1 (0.0–0.3)	0.71

CI, confidence interval; MSI-H, microsatellite instability-high; MSI-L, microsatellite instability-low; MSS, microsatellite stable; SIR, standardized incidence ratio.
*Number of first- and second-degree relatives of triad members fulfilling Amsterdam-I criteria.
†SIRs and bootstrapped 95% CIs of specific cancers, by DNA mismatch repair status, combining population- and clinic-based families.
‡Computed by comparing the SIR of the DNA mismatch repair groups (Group A vs Group B).
§Statistically significant estimate compared with the Surveillance, Epidemiology, and End Results population.
Source: Lindor *et al.* (2005).

Short-term end-points of conventional versus laparoscopic-assisted surgery in patients with colorectal cancer (MRC CLASICC trial): multicentre, randomized controlled trial

Guillou P, Quirke P, Thorpe H, *et al.*; MRC CLASICC trial group. *Lancet* 2005; **365**: 1718–26

Background. Early detection of colorectal cancer and advancements in therapy has improved outcomes for patients with colorectal cancer. Surgical resection remains the mainstay of colorectal cancer therapy. Laparoscopic-assisted surgery has become the standard technique for several operations. Minimally invasive surgery may have advantages over conventional surgery for colorectal cancer, including faster recovery, fewer complications and shorter hospitalizations, but convincing data regarding these proposed advantages is lacking.

Interpretation. The MRC CLASSIC trial randomized subjects with colon or rectal cancer from 27 centres in the United Kingdom to laparoscopic-assisted surgery or conventional surgery to compare the short-term outcomes of surgery. Surgeons were required to have undertaken at least 20 laparoscopic-assisted resections and subjects with adenocarcinoma of the transverse colon were excluded. The end-points of the study were tumour and nodal status, tumour at the resection margins, in-hospital mortality, complication rates during surgery and at 30 days and 3 months after surgery, transfusion requirements, and quality of life measurements measured 3 months after surgery. A total of 794 patients were randomized to either laparoscopic or open surgery in a 2:1 ratio. Randomization was concealed and stratified by surgeon, proposed site of operation, presence of liver metastases, and pre-operative radiotherapy. The baseline characteristics of both groups were comparable. The lymph node yield, proportion of Duke's C tumours, in-hospital mortality, post-surgical complication rates, peri-operative transfusion requirements and quality of life scores were similar in the two treatment groups. Positive resection margins were similar in the two groups except for subjects undergoing laparoscopic anterior resection for rectal cancer where positive circumferential margins were noted in 12% vs 6% for the open, anterior resection group. Twenty-nine per cent of patients in the laparoscopic group underwent intra-operative conversion to open surgery because of excessive tumour fixity, uncertain tumour clearance, inaccessibility of tumour, and obesity. Conversion rates were higher for patients undergoing laparoscopic rectal excision. Converted subjects had a higher death rate than open or laparoscopic subjects (9% vs 5% vs 1%, respectively; $P = \text{ns}$). Intra-operative complications, including clinically significant haemorrhage, cardiopulmonary insufficiency, and bowel, bladder or vascular injury, were not significantly different between the two groups, although complication rates in the conversion group were higher than either the conventional surgery group or the laparoscopic group ($P = 0.002$). The rate of conversions fell by year of study from 38% in year 1 to 16% in year 6.

Comment

This randomized study has shown laparoscopic-assisted colon cancer surgery to have similar short-term end-points, complication rates and quality of life when compared to conventional surgery except in patients who require conversion. Patient and tumour related factors associated with a need for conversion were identified and clearly the learning curve for laparoscopic colorectal cancer surgery was underestimated in this trial as the conversion rate fell each year of recruitment. Apart from patients' undergoing laparoscopic anterior resection for rectal cancer, rates of positive margins were similar. Laparoscopic-assisted surgery for colon cancer appears to be safe and effective in the short term. Impaired short-term outcomes after laparascopic anterior resection for rectal cancer do not justify its routine use.

Conclusion

This series of articles provides insight into the safety and efficacy of colorectal cancer screening techniques and agents used for chemoprevention of colorectal neoplasia. The Pooling Project demonstrates the lack of effect that high dietary fibre intake has on reducing the risk of colorectal cancer in many different populations. In contrast, a case–control trial has found that exposure to the class of cholesterol lowering agents called statins, which inhibit HMG-CoA reductase, is associated with a significantly lower risk of colorectal cancer. While the trial could not provide any information on the dose effect, randomized, intervention trials should be considered to confirm this benefit in other populations. A big disappointment in the quest for safe and effective chemopreventive agents was uncovered this year. While COX-2 inhibitors showed marked promise in their ability to inhibit colorectal neoplasia with a safe gastrointestinal profile, serious cardiovascular side effects were confirmed in two of the coxib polyp prevention trials. Rofecoxib was removed from the world-wide market and the use of celecoxib has been limited in some countries due to the serious cardiovascular side effects that occurred after 12 to 18 months of use. While the risk benefit profile for the use of celecoxib in patients with FAP may be favorable, these new results cannot justify the use of COX-2 inhibitors in patients with lower risks for colorectal neoplasia. Colonoscopy continues to be the colorectal cancer screening test of choice. Its greater effectiveness than flexible sigmoidoscopy to detect advanced neoplasia in women is demonstrated. Colonoscopy is also the most effective screening modality in elderly subjects, dependant on health status, where the number needed to screen to prevent one colorectal cancer related death outweighs the number of complications incurred. While CTC is an exciting emerging technology it and ACBE have inferior accuracy to colonoscopy to detect polyps ≥6 mm. Reasons for the variable sensitivities of CTC reported in the literature are being elucidated and include technical factors such as the mode of image interpretation, width of collimation, and number of detectors.

Until CTC technology and interpretative factors become standardized, it cannot be endorsed as a colorectal cancer screening choice. Laparoscopic-assisted colorectal cancer surgery is another emerging technique. Data show that the skill of the surgeon is very important in laparoscopic surgery outcomes. Laparoscopy appears to be safe and has comparable short-term outcomes compared to open colon cancer surgery however the acceptance of laparoscopic anterior resection for rectal cancer needs more study before widespread acceptance.

Further reading

1. Lawes DA, Pearson T, Sengupta S, Boulos PB. The role of MLH1, MSH2 and MSH6 in the development of multiple colorectal cancers. *Br J Cancer* 2005; **93**: 472–7.
2. Lieberman DA, Weiss DG. One-time screening for colorectal cancer with combined fecal occult-blood testing and examination of the distal colon. *N Engl J Med* 2001; **345**: 555–60.
3. O'Brien MJ, Winawer SJ, Zauber AG, Bushey MT, Sternberg SS, Gottlieb LS, Bond JH, Waye JD, Schapiro M; National Polyp Study Workgroup. Flat adenomas in the National Polyp Study: is there increased risk for high-grade dysplasia initially or during surveillance. *Clin Gastroenterol Hepatol* 2004; **2**(10): 905–11.
4. Yiu R, Qiu H, Lee SH, Garcia-Aguilar J. Mechanisms of microsatellite instability in colorectal cancer patients in different age groups. *Dis Colon Rectum* 2005; **48**: 2061–9.
5. Winawer SJ, Zauber AG, Ho MN, O'Brien MJ, Gottlieb LS, Sternberg SS, Waye JD, Schapiro M, Bond JH, Panish JF, *et al.* Prevention of colorectal cancer by colonoscopic polypectomy. The National Polyp Study Workgroup. *N Engl J Med* 1993; **329**(27): 1977–81.
6. Pickhardt PJ, Choi JR, Hwang I, Butler JA, Puckett ML, Hildebrandt HA, Wong RK, Nugent PA, Mysliwiec PA, Schindler WR. Computed tomographic virtual colonoscopy to screen for colorectal neoplasia in asymptomatic adults. *N Engl J Med* 2003; **349**(23): 2191–200.

4

Irritable bowel syndrome

EDY SOFFER, MARK PIMENTEL

Introduction

This chapter covers important papers concerned with various aspects of irritable bowel syndrome (IBS). We have selected articles that provide new insight into the pathophysiology of IBS and ones that affect clinical practice. Topics covered include the link between gut infections and IBS, genetic aspects, and treatment modalities that seek to manipulate the bacterial flora of the gut.

Origin of gas retention and symptoms in patients with bloating

Salvioli B, Serra J, Azpiroz F, *et al. Gastroenterology* 2005; **128**: 574–9

BACKGROUND. Bloating is a very common gastrointestinal symptom, affecting up to 30% of the population in community-based studies. However, the pathophysiology is poorly understood and treatment is consequently ineffective. It is not a simple matter of excess gas in the bowel, as studies attempting to quantify gas volume by abdominal X-ray films or computed tomography scans have produced conflicting results. It is not clear whether symptoms correlate with objective documentation of abdominal distension. Recent studies have shown that patients with IBS and functional bloating develop intestinal gas retention and symptoms with volumes of infused jejunal gas that are well tolerated by healthy subjects. The aims of this study were to determine which segment of the gut is responsible for delayed gut transit, and to correlate symptoms with abdominal distension.

INTERPRETATION. Thirty patients fulfilling the Rome II criteria of IBS and functional bloating, with bloating as the predominant symptom, and 22 healthy subjects were studied in two experiments. In the first experiment, a mixture of gas to which radiolabelled xenon had been added was infused into the jejunum. The segmental transit of gas was assessed with a gamma camera. In the second experiment, gas was infused into the jejunum, ileum and caecum of subgroups of patients and healthy subjects and the effluent was collected in a rectal tube. Retention of gas and the effect of infusion on symptoms and abdominal girth were assessed and compared between and within groups.

The first experiment showed that gas transit was significantly delayed in the patients compared with the healthy controls; retention at the end of the study was 589 ± 194 and 72 ± 18 ml respectively (P <0.05). This was associated with a significantly higher symptom score in patients (3.5 ± 0.6 vs 1.3 ± 0.3; P <0.05). The second experiment showed that healthy subjects were able to evacuate gas regardless of the site of infusion. In contrast, patients were able to expel gas adequately when it was infused into the ileum or the caecum but had significantly more gas retention than control subjects when it was infused into the jejunum. This indicates that the small bowel is the site of abnormal retention (Fig. 4.1). Healthy subjects tolerated gas infusion with minimal symptoms, and the score was comparable among the three sites. In patients, jejunal infusion resulted in a symptom score that was significantly higher than that of controls, while scores induced by infusion in the ileum and caecum were not significantly different from those in controls. The effect of infusion on abdominal girth followed a similar pattern. A significant increase was seen in patients compared with controls during jejunal infusion but not during infusion in the ileum or caecum. In patients who complain of bloating, intestinal gas retention and abdominal distension are significantly higher than in healthy subjects. The segment responsible for these abnormalities is the small bowel.

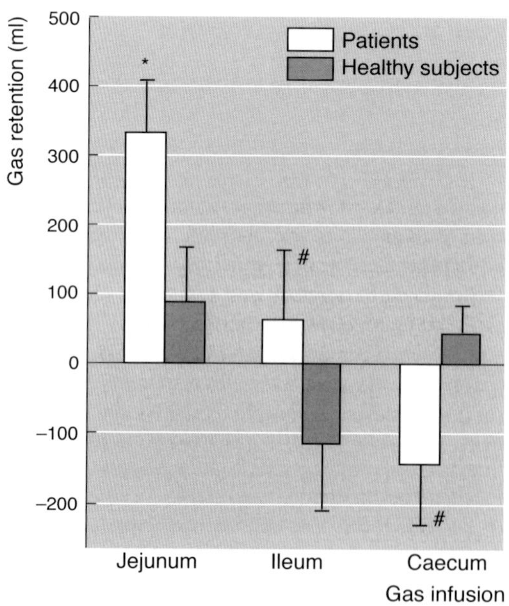

Fig. 4.1 Response to proximal and distal gas infusion. Compared with healthy subjects, patients developed significant gas retention during jejunal (n = 12; *P <0.05 vs healthy subjects) but not during ileal or caecal gas infusion (n = 6 each; #P <0.05 vs jejunal infusion). Source: Salvioli *et al.* (2005).

Comment

There is a large body of information on the transit of solids and liquids in the gut, obtained mainly by the use of scintigraphic techniques. The movement of gas in the bowel has received much less attention. Fortunately, there is growing interest in this area and techniques are being used that can quantify gas dynamics in the bowel, primarily by infusion of gas directly into the intestine, while measuring concomitant evacuation. Using such a technique, the authors found that the source of delayed gas transit is the small bowel, perhaps in contrast to the intuitive assumption that the colon is the culprit. They also showed that objective distension is correlated with symptoms. Although the number of patients in each group was small, given the complexity of the study, the data obtained by the use of these scientific techniques provide an important addition to our understanding of intestinal gas homeostasis. This is particularly intriguing, given the evolving evidence of bacterial overgrowth in the small intestine in patients with IBS, which results in gas production in the small bowel.

Mechanisms underlying the maintenance of muscle hypercontractility in a model of postinfective gut dysfunction

Akiho H, Deng Y, Blennerhassett P, Kanbayashi H, Collins SM.
Gastroenterology 2005; **129**: 131–41

BACKGROUND. A number of groups are examining the role of gut bacteria in IBS. Specifically, there is now a clear link between acute gastroenteritis and the development of IBS. In fact, patients can recall the event heralding their IBS as a bout of acute gastroenteritis. Although data have demonstrated that this so-called post-infectious IBS is real, there is still no understanding of the proportion of IBS that is post-infectious since most patients cannot recall a mild case of gastroenteritis from 10 years earlier. In order to understand how an individual who is a normal host of gut bacteria becomes a patient with IBS induced by acute gastroenteritis, it is important to understand the steps of this evolution and the mechanisms by which these events sustain themselves. One obvious means of sustaining a gut reaction after infection is through an altered immune response. In this study, the authors attempted to identify the mechanism behind altered intestinal muscular hypercontractility in an established model of post-infectious IBS (infection with *Trichinella spiralis*). The authors tested the muscle response to cytokines.

INTERPRETATION. NIH Swiss mice were infected with *T. spiralis*, after which muscle cells were isolated from the longitudinal portion of the jejunal muscle layer and cultured. From this culture was derived mRNA of transforming growth factor β1 (TGF-β1), interleukin (IL)-4 and TGF-β type IIR. These were examined in cultured smooth muscle cells from infected and uninfected mice. Cells were also incubated with or without a cytokine cocktail (IL-4, IL-13 and TGF-β1). Expression of cyclooxygenase 2 (COX-2) was then measured using western blotting with and without the cytokine incubation. Under various cytokine conditions as well as the basal state, muscle contractility was determined using carbachol, by measuring muscle cell length.

In pre-infected mice, the use of carbachol resulted in a 52% increase in muscle contractility. Overnight incubation of muscle cells with IL-4 or IL-13 did not change the muscle response to carbachol. Levels of polymerase chain reaction (PCR) products for TGF-β1 mRNA and protein levels in the muscle at day 10 after infection were higher than in controls. This was consistent up to 35 days after infection. Incubation with IL-4 or IL-13 increased TGF-β1 protein expression in infected mice. COX-2 levels were also inducible by these cytokines. COX-2 inhibitors reduced the effect of incubation with TGF-β1 on the contractile response of smooth muscle to carbachol.

It appears that the hypercontractility of intestinal smooth muscle after infection is dictated by mediators within the muscle cell. The two cytokines may exaggerate the TGF-β1 and COX-2 response of the smooth muscle.

Comment

This article is a major step forward in trying to understand the complex events that take place in post-infectious IBS. The reproduction of these results in humans may provide an argument for the role of infection in the sustained abnormal events in gut responses. Moreover, these results may guide us to therapies that may be of benefit in IBS as a whole.

Rectal mucosal nitric oxide in differentiation of inflammatory bowel disease and irritable bowel syndrome

Reinders CI, Herulf M, Ljung T, *et al. Clin Gastroenterol Hepatol* 2005; **3**: 777–83

BACKGROUND. Nitric oxide (NO) is involved in many functions throughout the gastrointestinal tract in health and disease. In the presence of inflammatory conditions and under the influence of proinflammatory cytokines, NO release is increased as a result of upregulation of the enzyme NO synthase. If luminal levels of NO can be determined, then perhaps NO can serve as a marker of inflammatory conditions in the gut. The authors postulated that NO can distinguish between inflammatory bowel disease (IBD) and IBS, two conditions with overlapping clinical features.

INTERPRETATION. The rectal concentration of NO was evaluated in healthy controls and three groups of patients: patients with IBS; patients with IBD, including ulcerative colitis and Crohn's disease; and patients with collagenous colitis. A subgroup of healthy subjects and patients with ulcerative colitis underwent a repeat study. Nitric oxide was sampled with a rectal balloon inflated with a small amount of room air that contained less than 5 parts per billion (ppb) of NO. The balloon was left in the rectum for 10 min, during which time NO in the rectum would diffuse into the balloon according to the concentration gradient. The balloon was then removed and its gas content analysed for NO.

The NO concentration in subjects with IBS was significantly higher than in the healthy control subjects (150 ppb, interquartile range [IQR] 53–200 vs 45 ppb, IQR 34–64; P <0.001). Concentrations of NO in patients with IBD and those with collagenous colitis (3475 ppb, IQR 575–8850 and 9950 ppb, IQR 4475–19 750, respectively) were much higher than those in patients with IBS (P <0.001). (Fig. 4.2). IBD with complete remission showed significant reduction in NO on repeat tests, compared to IBD patients with only partial remission and those with IBS, both of which showed no significant reduction in NO. However, there was a significant reduction in rectal NO concentration in patients with IBD who sustained complete remission after 4 weeks of therapy. The NO concentration correlated with disease activity in patients with IBD and collagenous colitis. The concentration of NO in the rectum can be assessed by minimally invasive means. The levels are high in inflammatory conditions affecting the gut, and can be used to distinguish between IBD and IBS. NO levels were higher in IBS patients than in healthy controls.

Comment

While the main message of this study is that rectal NO can be used to distinguish IBD from IBS, the other interesting point is the increased level of NO in IBS

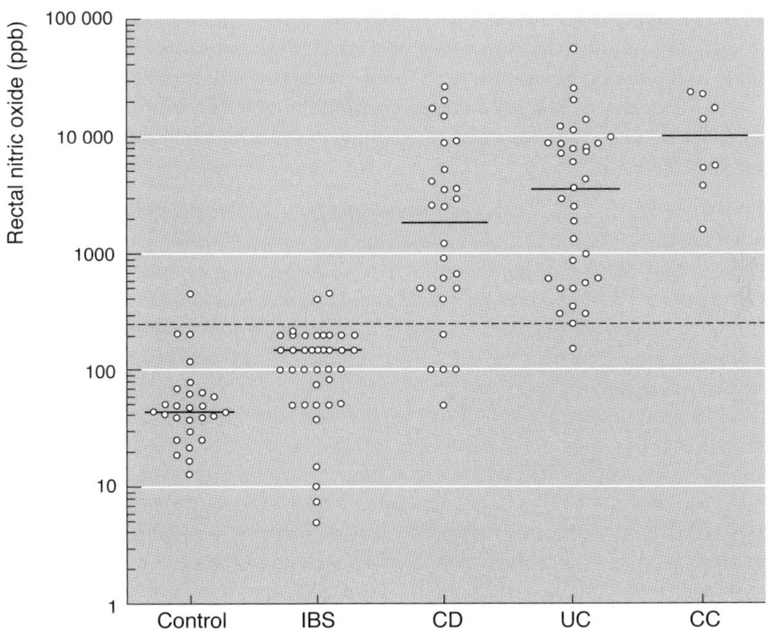

Fig. 4.2 Rectal NO levels in healthy subjects (controls) and in patients with irritable bowel syndrome (IBS), active Crohn's disease (CD), active ulcerative colitis (UC) or active collagenous colitis (CC). The horizontal lines show the median for each group. The dotted line represents a cut-off value for rectal NO at 250 ppb. Source: Reinders *et al.* (2005).

patients compared with healthy controls. Post-infectious IBS is an established clinical entity, and inflammatory changes were documented in rectal samples from IBS patients. It is possible that NO levels would have been even higher if patients with IBS had been screened, and selected, for the presence of rectal inflammation. The NO level thus has the potential to serve as a marker in those patients with IBS who have a clinical or histological background of gut inflammation.

Dyspepsia and irritable bowel syndrome after a Salmonella gastroenteritis outbreak: one-year follow-up cohort study

Mearin F, Pérez-Oliveras M, Perelló A, *et al. Gastroenterol* 2005; **129**: 98–104

BACKGROUND. In IBS, the focus has been on gut hypersensitivity and psychology. It is now recognized that in most cases neither stress nor psychology is the cause of or a contributor to the gastrointestinal complaints in IBS. This change is due in part to recent discoveries of an altered intestinal flora in IBS. One burgeoning area of research is the relationship between acute gastroenteritis and the precipitation of IBS. Essentially, acute gastroenteritis is the heralding event that results in the development of IBS. The initial reaction to these studies was that this was not IBS but rather a prolonged recovery from the infective event. However, recent evidence from long-term studies demonstrates that the symptoms persist for years—for the duration of the follow-up in most cases; hence the term 'post-infectious IBS' was adopted. There is thus a growing body of evidence demonstrating the link between acute infection and IBS but no such link has been reasonably defined for other functional gastrointestinal disorders.

INTERPRETATION. This was a case–control study of 1201 subjects with *Salmonella* enteritis after eating cream cakes during a celebration in a Spanish town, who were compared with 677 controls. The Rome II questionnaire, addressing symptoms of IBS and dyspepsia, was sent to these individuals at baseline and 3, 6 and 12 months after infection. On the initial questionnaire, 96.1% of the patients with gastroenteritis reported that they had eaten the cream cakes. The prevalence rates of dyspepsia before the gastroenteritis were 3.8% in the control group and 2.5% in the gastroenteritis group. The prevalence of IBS was 2.3 and 2.9% for the control and gastroenteritis groups respectively at baseline. Dyspepsia had increased 3-fold over the baseline. Twelve months after infection, the rate of dyspepsia in the gastroenteritis group was 13.4% vs 2.6% for controls. The prevalence of IBS at 12 months was 10.0% for the group with gastroenteritis and 0.7% for the controls (Fig. 4.3). Interestingly, vomiting and abdominal pain during the acute gastroenteritis were risk factors for the development of functional dyspepsia. *Salmonella* infection is a risk factor for precipitating both dyspepsia and IBS. Prolonged vomiting and abdominal pain during acute infection portend an increased risk of developing dyspepsia.

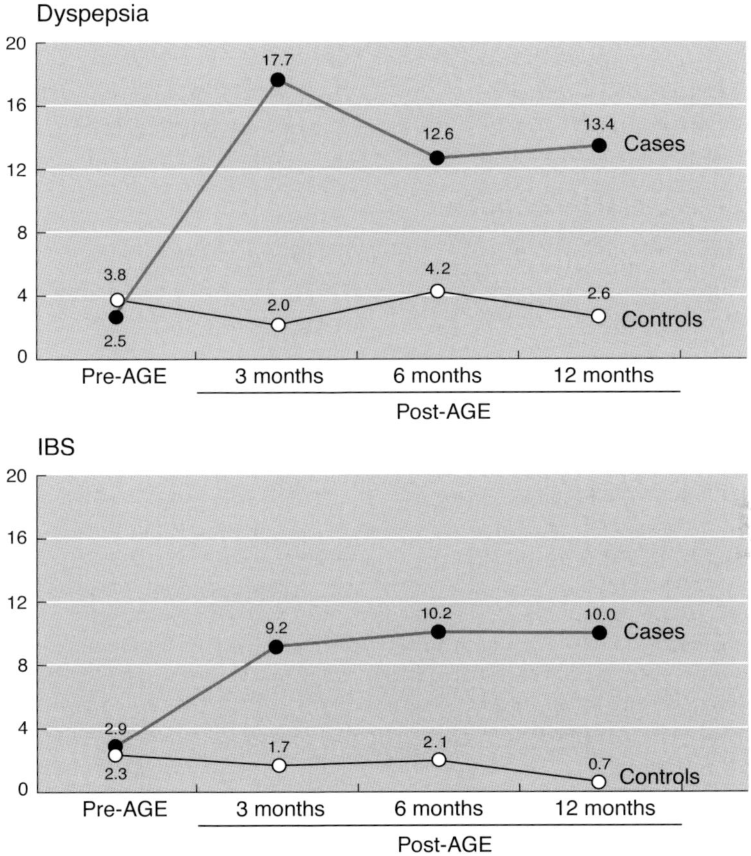

Fig. 4.3 Changes in the prevalence of dyspepsia and IBS during the 1-year follow-up. Source: Mearin *et al.* (2005).

Comment

There is a growing literature on the association between acute gastroenteritis and IBS. This is the first large cohort of subjects showing an association between acute gastroenteritis and functional dyspepsia. An important aspect of this study is the uniformity of infection. This was a unimicrobial infection, and thus allowed a comparison of manifestations. The most interesting aspect of this study is that vomiting portends an increased risk of dyspepsia. In other studies, diarrhoea was a risk factor for the development of IBS. Since the infection was with a single pathogen, it hints that the location in the gastrointestinal tract mostly affected by the bacteria can dictate the clinical outcome. This remains to be determined.

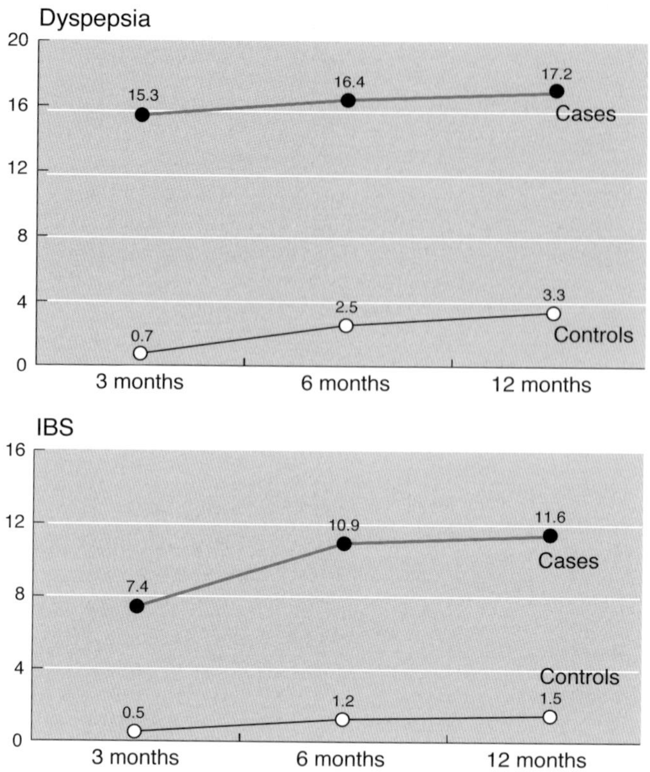

Fig. 4.4 Cumulative incidence (new cases) of dyspepsia and IBS at each point of the study during the 1-year follow-up. Source: Mearin *et al.* (2005).

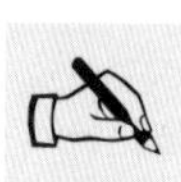

Food-specific IgG4 antibody-guided exclusion diet improves symptoms and rectal compliance in irritable bowel syndrome

Zar S, Mincher L, Benson MJ, Kumar D. *Scand J Gastroenterol* 2005; **40**: 800–7

BACKGROUND. Patients with IBS commonly tend to associate symptoms with certain food products that 'do not agree with them'; hence the attempt to treat IBS with exclusion diets. These were traditionally diets eliminating food products suspected by the patient to produce symptoms; alternatively, using a more aggressive approach, patients were started on a small number of food ingredients deemed less allergenic, with gradual introduction of other food items over time. Food exclusion based on the immunological response to specific food antigens is attractive as it appears to target specific food items suspected of being responsible for inducing

symptoms. The purpose of this study was to test this concept by putting patients with IBS on an exclusion diet based on titres of immunoglobulin G4 (IgG4) to specific food ingredients, and assessing its effect on symptoms and rectal motor and sensory responses to balloon distension.

INTERPRETATION. Twenty-five patients with IBS, of different subgroups based on Rome II criteria, were enrolled. Serum IgG4 titres against 16 different food antigens were assessed in each subject. A symptom severity questionnaire was administered and anxiety and depression scores were obtained at baseline and 3 and 6 months after the initiation of a diet that eliminated food ingredients associated with a serum IgG4 titre greater than 250 μg/l. Twelve patients also underwent assessment of rectal compliance and sensitivity to balloon distension by a barostat at baseline and 6 months.

Elevated titres against milk, cheddar cheese, eggs, beef, pork, lamb, wheat and tomatoes were observed in more than 50% of the patients. The number of foods excluded by each patient ranged from three to 13, with an average of eight. Data at 3 months were available from 21/25 patients with significant improvement in individual symptoms, such as pain and bloating, as well as total score (123, IQR ±215 vs 309, IQR ±104; P <0.001). Symptom score was separated from the anxiety and depression scores. Symptom severity score assessed: 1) pain severity; 2) pain frequency; 3) bloating severity; 4) bowel habits, and effect on life in general. These 5 scores composed the total score. Similar improvement was noted at 6 months; however, data from only 15 patients were available. A significant improvement in anxiety and depression scores was noted at 6 months. A significant increase in rectal compliance was observed at the end of 6 months (5.42 ± 2.33 vs 7.75 ± 4.22 ml/mmHg at baseline; P = 0.011). Diet had no effect on variables of perception of balloon distension. An exclusion diet, based on food-specific IgG4 antibody titres, improves symptoms in patients with IBS and results in an increase in rectal compliance.

Comment

The concept that changing what patients consume can modulate symptoms is intuitively attractive. Studies of dietary exclusion, however, have inherent problems, such as the impracticality of blinding and the difficulty in maintaining such diets over an extended period, as was obvious in this study from the significant dropout rate at 6 months. Nonetheless, an exclusion diet based on quantifiable criteria offers a more objective method of patient selection and may be easier to follow. Hopefully, future studies, perhaps with clearer definition of the antibody titres used for exclusion, will clarify the role of such diets in IBS.

Genetic influences in irritable bowel syndrome: a twin study

Mohammed I, Cherkas LF, Riley SA, *et al. Am J Gastroenterol* 2005; **100**: 1340–4

BACKGROUND. Genetics is among a variety of pathophysiological factors that may play a role in IBS. Clues about genetic aetiology are considered when studies show a prevalence of the disease in specific populations or geographic areas or among ethnic

or racial groups, or if familial aggregation is documented. For the most part, however, it is difficult to separate genetic from environmental factors in such studies. Twin studies offer a more precise approach. Monozygotic twins share the same genetic make-up while dizygotic twins share only 50% of their genes. If a higher proportion of co-twins of affected monozygotic twins have the disease compared with dizygotic twins (higher concordance) and if there is a higher probability that a monozygotic twin is affected when his or her co-twin has the disease compared with dizygotic twins (casewise concordance), there is a strong case for a genetic basis for the disease. In this study the authors determined these variables in a large group of monozygotic and dizygotic twins with IBS.

Interpretation. A total of 4480 pairs of twins from a large twin registry in the UK were asked to participate. They were asked to fill in questionnaires concerning demographic details and psychosomatic symptoms, and were selected according to the Rome II criteria for IBS. Concordance rates were then determined and genetic modelling was performed. Of 5032 subjects who returned the questionnaires, 1870 complete twin pairs fulfilled the criteria for evaluation, comprising 888 monozygotic pairs and 982 same-gender dizygotic pairs. There was no significant difference in casewise concordance between monozygotic and dizygotic twins (Table 4.1). Multivariate logistical regression analysis showed that younger age and higher psychosomatic score were independently associated with IBS. Genetic factors are of minor importance in the pathogenesis of IBS.

Table 4.1 Concordance rates for irritable bowel syndrome in the monozygotic and dizygotic twins

Twin type	Total pairs	Discordant pairs	Concordant affected pairs	Casewise concordance rate*
Monozygotic	888	220	42	28 (21–34)%
Dizygotic	982	224	42	27 (21–34)%

*95% confidence intervals in parentheses.
Source: Imityaz *et al.* (2005).

Comment

A few twin studies in IBS have been reported, with conflicting results. The strengths of this study are the large number of subjects evaluated and the use of validated questionnaires and Rome II criteria for the selection of patients. The results strongly favour environmental factors over genetics in the pathophysiology of IBS.

The placebo effect in irritable bowel syndrome trials: a meta-analysis

Patel SM, Stason WB, Legedza A, *et al.* *Neurogastroenterol Motil* 2005; **17**: 332–40

BACKGROUND. Therapeutic trials in functional gut disorders such as IBS invariably show a high placebo response, ranging between 40 and 70%. Such a placebo effect influences the design of drug studies and the interpretation of results, since the response in the active arm has to be sufficiently high in order to detect a therapeutic benefit over placebo. The purpose of this study was to systematically review therapeutic trials of IBS in order to assess the variability of the placebo response and to identify factors that predict such variability.

INTERPRETATION. The authors performed a meta-analysis of randomized control trials in patients with IBS published in the English literature that comprised 20 or more patients treated for at least 2 weeks and had an active medication and placebo. They searched a number of databases, spanning various periods, starting in 1960. Of 96 studies that met these initial criteria, 45 that had a well-defined global response outcome were included in the final analysis. The following variables were assessed as potential modifiers of the placebo response: study design, study duration, use of a run-in phase, Jadad score, entry criteria, number of office visits, and number of office visits/study duration, the use of diagnostic testing, gender, age and type of medication. A total of 7101 subjects were included, and 3352 of these received placebo. The population-weighted mean response to placebo was 40.2%, with a range of 16–71%. In the active treatment arm the mean response was 54.1%, with a range of 28–93.3%. The odds ratio of response to placebo versus response to active medication was 0.55. The placebo response declined significantly with increasing number of office visits and in studies that enrolled patients according to Rome II criteria. Therapeutic trials in IBS have a substantial placebo response rate that is affected by enrolment criteria and the frequency of office visits.

Comment

The study has some limitations, as pointed out by the authors, including significant heterogeneity among studies and the lack of epidemiological and clinical data in some of the studies. However, it is the first meta-analysis addressing the issue of the placebo response in therapeutic trials of IBS. The finding of a decreased placebo effect with the use of accepted criteria for IBS should encourage the use of stringent criteria when enrolling patients in IBS studies.

Abnormal breath tests to lactose, fructose and sorbitol in irritable bowel syndrome may be explained by small intestinal bacterial overgrowth

Nucera G, Gabrielli M, Lupascu A, *et al. Aliment Pharmacol Ther* 2005; **21**: 1391–5

BACKGROUND. Patients with IBS frequently complain of intolerance to carbohydrates such as lactose and sorbitol. The difficulty lies in finding an accurate method of non-invasive testing to identify patients with true intolerance. One way to do this is to use the hydrogen breath test. Within this context are recent studies pointing to an association between bacterial overgrowth and IBS, and an improvement in IBS after treatment with antibiotics that depends on the normalization of the lactulose breath test. In the case of bacterial overgrowth, a common substrate for breath testing is lactulose. If bacterial overgrowth is common in IBS and contributes to the symptoms, it may render the diagnosis of maldigestion of other carbohydrates inaccurate. Breath testing requires a substrate which, when fermented by gut bacteria, produces hydrogen that can then be quantified in the breath. Under ideal circumstances the carbohydrate in question, such as lactose or fructose, is not digested in the small bowel; it then passes intact to the colon and undergoes fermentation there with the production of hydrogen. However, in the presence of bacterial overgrowth, the same carbohydrate can be fermented by bacteria in the proximal small bowel before it is fully digested, resulting in excess hydrogen production that can be interpreted as evidence of carbohydrate maldigestion, even if maldigestion does not occur. This study was designed to evaluate whether, in IBS and bacterial overgrowth, the breath test for other substrates is confounded.

INTERPRETATION. Ninety IBS subjects positive for the Rome II criteria, recruited from internal medicine and general gastrointestinal clinics, underwent a lactulose breath test (10 g lactulose) to determine whether bacterial overgrowth was present. This was considered positive if there were two peaks, each producing a rise of at least 10 ppm (parts per million) above baseline, the first increase in hydrogen occurring less than 90 min into the test. About a week later, subjects underwent a breath test using sorbitol (20 g), lactose (20 g) and fructose (25 g). Any rise greater than 20 ppm was considered abnormal. Subjects with small intestinal bacterial overgrowth (SIBO) were then given an antibiotic (rifaximin, metronidazole or fluoroquinolone) for 1 week and the tests were repeated.

Of the 98 subjects with IBS, 65 had a positive lactulose breath test, suggesting the presence of bacterial overgrowth (SIBO). An abnormal breath test for sorbitol was seen in 70% of SIBO-positive subjects versus 36% of SIBO-negative subjects ($P < 0.01$). The lactose breath test was positive in 83% of subjects with SIBO compared with 64% for subjects without SIBO ($P < 0.05$). Similarly, the fructose breath test was positive in 70% of subjects with SIBO versus 36% of subjects without SIBO ($P < 0.01$). Importantly, when the lactulose breath test was normalized by antibiotics, there was a much lower prevalence of sorbitol, lactose and fructose intolerance. There was a greater elimination of IBS symptoms among IBS patients whose breath test became normal after antibiotics. The authors conclude that bacterial overgrowth is very common in IBS and can therefore confound the carbohydrate testing that is commonly used in assessing the maldigestion of carbohydrates. They recommend breath testing with lactulose and treating any bacterial overgrowth before attempting other carbohydrate breath tests.

Comment

This is an interesting study because it points to some of the inherent problems with breath testing. For example, in the use of breath testing to diagnose lactose intolerance we assume that the bacteria of the intestine are relegated to those of the colon since this is the only way this test will give an accurate result (i.e. lactose is ingested, the small bowel does not absorb it all, it gets to the colon, and the bacteria of the colon ferment it, producing symptoms and an abnormal breath test result). However, this does not account for the possibility of bacterial overgrowth. This article tries to eliminate the variable of bacterial overgrowth. The most relevant finding is that subjects with SIBO have a higher rate of positivity with other carbohydrates. The problem with the study is the interpretation of breath testing after the antibiotic treatment. When an antibiotic is given before any breath test, the results will be altered since there will be a reduction in both small bowel and colonic bacteria. Even if the carbohydrate were truly maldigested, there would be fewer enteric organisms to ferment them. Nevertheless, the study does highlight possible pitfalls in the diagnosis and then treatment of carbohydrate malabsorption if one does not account for the possibility of bacterial overgrowth.

Do interventions which reduce colonic bacterial fermentation improve symptoms of irritable bowel syndrome?

Dear KLE, Elia M, Hunter JO. *Dig Dis Sci* 2005; **50**: 758–66

BACKGROUND. The aetiology of IBS remains poorly understood but there is growing evidence that the enteric flora play a role. Studies have addressed various aspects, from excessive bacteria, such as in bacterial overgrowth, to the effect of alteration of the intrinsic flora by probiotics such as bifidobacteria. Ultimately, one of the by-products of bacterial alterations is an alteration in intestinal gas, the product of luminal fermentation. In some studies the type of gas (e.g. methane) may also be important. The purposes of this study were to quantify the effects of diet and antibiotics on gas production and to determine whether the effects on symptoms can vary according to the manipulation of the quantity of gas by each of these two factors.

INTERPRETATION. The study recruited subjects with IBS according to the Rome criteria after exclusion of other aetiology. Subjects were enrolled for a 6-week study. In the first 2 weeks, all subjects received a standard 1905 kcal balanced diet. During the second 2 weeks, subjects were randomized to receive either a fibre-free diet or the same diet as in the first 2 weeks but with the addition of metronidazole. During the final 2 weeks patients were asked to eat as usual. Subjects were asked to keep a symptom diary in the second week of each 2-week interval. Whole-gut transit was assessed using radio-opaque markers during both dietary periods. The diary was completed during the weeks of each of the 3 two-week periods. At the end of each 2-week period, subjects stayed in a calorimeter for 24 h to measure all fermented gases produced. In addition, a hydrogen breath test and methane assessments every 30 min after 10 g of lactulose were performed at the conclusion of the 24-h calorimetry period. Stool culture was performed at the end of each 2-week period.

Thirteen IBS patients underwent the study protocol; twelve completed all components of study. Using calorimetry, total hydrogen and methane production was reduced from 564 to 205 ml after the fibre-free diet ($P<0.05$). Likewise, metronidazole reduced the total volume of these gases from 671 to 422 ml ($P<0.05$). Both the fibre-free diet and metronidazole resulted in a reduction in IBS symptoms. The overall symptom score was reduced from 8.0 to 5.5 ($P<0.05$) while on metronidazole. Similarly, a fibre-free diet reduced the score from 9.6 to 6.6 ($P<0.05$). Furthermore, bloating and wind scores as well as pain scores were improved significantly with both interventions. Stool cultures demonstrated almost a 10-fold reduction in anaerobes with both metronidazole and the fibre-free diet. Transit was not affected by the interventions. The authors conclude that IBS symptoms may be in part due to gases accumulating in the digestive tract. The reduction of these gases using antibiotics or fibre-reduced diets may help reduce symptoms.

Comment

This is an interesting study since it demonstrates that a diet that restricts the amount of lumen carbohydrates is effective in reducing IBS symptoms. By reducing the access of bacteria to orally ingested carbohydrates, the food source is reduced, leading to a reduction in gas. This in turn leads to improvement of symptoms. Diet may be an alternative to antibiotics in reducing symptoms in IBS.

Lactobacillus and bifidobacterium in irritable bowel syndrome: symptom responses and relationship to cytokine profiles

O'Mahony L, McCarthy J, Kelly P, *et al.* *Gastroenterology* 2005; **128**: 541–51

BACKGROUND. The focus of IBS research has been on gut motility and visceral afferent function, but there is growing evidence for alterations in gut bacteriology as another possible pathophysiological mechanism for IBS. This research includes post-infectious IBS, the role of bacterial overgrowth and now the use of probiotics. The hypothesis that probiotics may be of benefit in IBS stems from stool culture studies in IBS demonstrating a relative lack of bifidobacteria and acidophilus compared with controls. In addition, these same organisms are known to have prokinetic effects on the gut as well as anti-inflammatory properties. The hypothesis of this study is that these probiotics may have a positive influence on gastrointestinal symptoms in IBS.

INTERPRETATION. This was a double-blind, randomized, placebo-controlled study comparing 8 weeks of therapy with *Lactobacillus salivarius* UCC4331, *Bifidobacterium* *infantis* 35624 and placebo, in three separate groups. The quantity of each probiotic was 10^{10} colony-forming units. Symptoms were tracked with a Likert scale over the 8-week treatment phase and a 4-week washout phase. These included three symptom clusters of bloating and distension, abdominal pain and difficulty with bowel movement. Stool was collected at baseline and at the end of treatment to evaluate colonization with the probiotic, and blood was taken at the same time-points to evaluate levels of cytokines (IL-10 and IL-12). The subjects were 18–75 years old, had Rome II-positive IBS, and had no previous gastrointestinal disorder and no abdominal surgery. All IBS subtypes were included in the study.

Eighty patients were enrolled in the study and data were obtained from 75 subjects. Most of the dropouts were due to protocol violation of antibiotic use. Using a visual analogue score (VAS) and a Likert composite score for the three symptom clusters, there was a significant improvement in IBS with *Bifidobacterium infantis* in 7 out of 8 weeks for the VAS and in 6 out of 8 weeks for the Likert composite score, compared with placebo. No difference was seen with *Lactobacillus salivarius* compared with placebo. While individual symptoms of bloating, abdominal pain and bowel difficulty improved over time with *B. infantis*, the difference compared with the control was significant only in a small fraction of the weeks. There was also no durable effect beyond treatment for any symptom or score. The ratio of IL-10 to IL-12 was lower in IBS subjects than in controls. This abnormal profile was normalized to control levels with *Bifidobacterium* but not *Lactobacillus*.

Treatment with a single probiotic, *B. infantis*, but not with *L. salivarius* appears to have efficacy in improving the symptoms of IBS and this improvement is associated with normalization of the cytokine profile.

Comment

There is a growing number of probiotic studies in IBS. Most of these studies involve the use of the *Lactobacillus* genus. While there is much hype about lactobacillus-based probiotics in IBS on the basis of these initial studies, the reality is that in none of these studies did the probiotic demonstrate a statistically significant benefit in the primary end-point. Although this fact does not justify the use of *Lactobacillus* in IBS, subanalysis in these studies showed modest benefit in component symptoms of IBS, such as bloating. The present study adds to the data in three ways. This is one of the first studies to demonstrate the effectiveness of a probiotic (*Bifidobacterium*) in improving the primary end-point in IBS. Secondly, it adds to the growing list of studies demonstrating that *Lactobacillus* does not improve this same end-point and therefore may not have a role in IBS. Thirdly, the study takes the data one step further by trying to suggest that one means by which bifidobacteria may improve IBS is through the normalization of the cytokine profile. The hope is that there will be larger studies that will demonstrate this effect more definitively.

Conclusion

This has been an exciting year in the IBS arena. Of the various topics being researched, those that address the dynamics of intestinal gas and the role of the gut flora in the pathophysiology of IBS are perhaps the most intriguing. The latter topic in particular may have an important impact on IBS, by providing new therapeutic modalities that eradicate abnormal bacterial growth, or that can change the bacterial milieu of the gut.

5

Epidemiological studies in inflammatory bowel disease

BRET LASHNER

Introduction

Articles published last year provided a better understanding of the clinical epidemiology of inflammatory bowel disease (IBD). Bone mineral density is often diminished in patients with IBD, mostly as a result of steroid use and active inflammation. Bone loss can be minimized by using a steroid with high rate of first-pass metabolism (budesonide) or by controlling inflammation with an anti-inflammatory medication such as infliximab. Another study stressed the importance of supplementing IBD patients with calcium and vitamin D, which can counter the effects of bone loss in IBD even without bisphosphonate therapy.

Patients with IBD are prone to the development of malignancy of the gastrointestinal tract. A meta-analysis quantified this risk in Crohn's disease patients. Another meta-analysis quantified the increased risk of lymphoma in IBD patients, which is likely after the use of medications such as immunosuppressive agents and infliximab. Yet another meta-analysis examined the chemopreventive beneficial effect of 5-aminosalicylic acid compounds on the risk of colorectal cancer in IBD. IBD patients with primary sclerosing cholangitis should take ursodeoxycholic acid for the magnitude of its cancer chemopreventive effect and its important beneficial effect on mortality. Our methods of cancer surveillance colonoscopy can be improved if physicians perform high-quality examinations.

Since both arterial and venous thromboses are important complications of IBD, some epidemiological studies were devoted to this topic. Apparently, inherited mutations are not predisposing factors, but increased homocysteine (from active inflammation and/or folic acid deficiency) and platelet-derived microparticles are. A safe and accurate diagnostic test has yet to be developed in IBD. Magnetic resonance imaging (MRI) has promise, but wireless capsule endoscopy and single photon emission computed tomography (SPECT) scanning are of limited usefulness.

Quality of life measures can be improved in children with IBD with a specially designed summer camp sponsored by the Crohn's and Colitis Foundation of America. Narcotic use and chronic steroid use are associated with diminished quality of life. Studies this year have shown that patients on chronic steroids often turn to complementary and alternative medicine. Narcotic users need to work with pain management consultants. Interestingly, antibiotics may be protective against flares of IBD.

Bone mineral density in IBD

Bone mineral density in relation to efficacy and side effects of budesonide and prednisolone in Crohn's disease

Schoon EJ, Bollani S, Mills PR, *et al.*; Matrix Study Group. *Clin Gastroenterol Hepatol* 2005; **3**: 113–21

BACKGROUND. Low bone mineral density in patients with IBD is an important problem that is often unrecognized. Factors responsible for bone loss include active disease with excess cytokine formation, malabsorption of calcium and vitamin D, cigarette smoking, and corticosteroid use. Steroids, while effective, are limited in usefulness because of toxicity. Budesonide, a steroid with high first-pass metabolism, has been shown to be effective in patients with Crohn's disease with an acceptable toxicity profile, especially with regard to bone loss. The effect of long-term budesonide use on bone mineral density is an important question.

INTERPRETATION. In this randomized clinical trial, 272 patients with Crohn's disease of the terminal ileum and/or right colon were treated with sufficient prednisolone or budesonide to control symptoms over a 2-year period. The dose of the medication was

Table 5.1 Number (%) of patients with treatment-emergent corticosteroid side effects

Side effect	Budesonide (n = 138*)	Prednisolone (n = 134)	*P*-value
Any corticosteroid side effect	71 (51)	95 (71)	0.001
Insomnia	25 (18)	42 (31)	0.011
Mood swings	24 (17)	34 (25)	ns
Acne	21 (15)	35 (26)	0.026
Moon face	12 (9)	44 (33)	<0.0001
Depression	25 (18)	30 (22)	ns
Bruising easily	16 (12)	31 (23)	0.012
Swollen ankles	11 (8)	18 (13)	ns
Hirsutism	10 (7)	18 (13)	ns
Hair loss	7 (5)	13 (10)	ns
Skin striae	2 (1)	4 (3)	ns
Buffalo hump	1 (1)	3 (2)	ns

*In one patient, only adverse event evaluation was performed. ns, not significant
Source: Schoon *et al.* (2005).

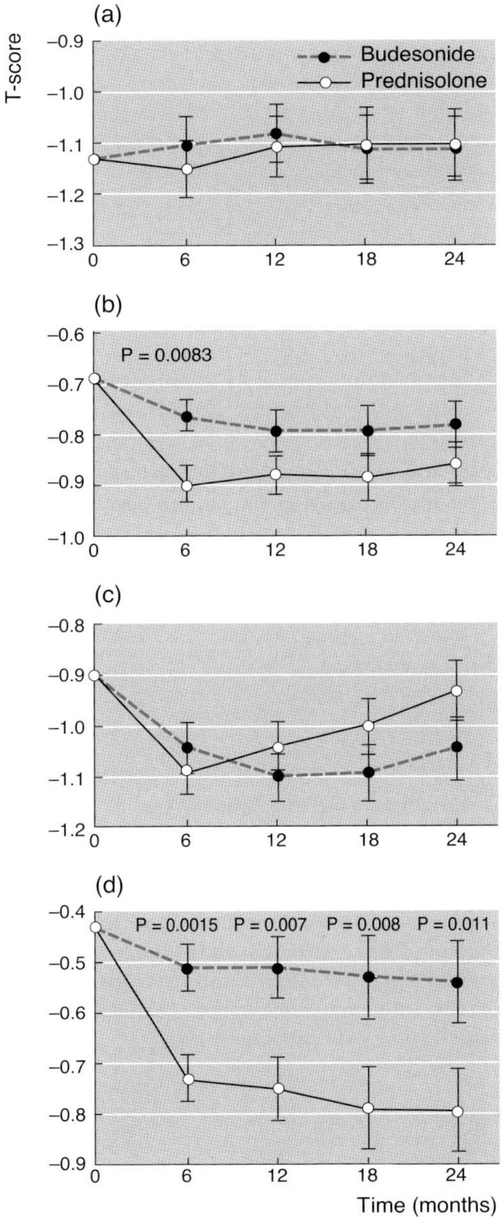

Fig 5.1 Mean BMD expressed as T-score (with SEM) during the 2-year study period in (a) corticosteroid-dependent ($n = 90$), (b) corticosteroid-free ($n = 181$), (c) corticosteroid-exposed ($n = 83$) and (d) corticosteroid-naive ($n = 98$) patients. Source: Schoon *et al.* (2005).

adjusted continuously to control symptoms. The mean dose of prednisolone was 14.9 mg daily and the mean dose of budesonide was 6.8 mg daily, and disease activity indices were similar during the course of the study. Among the 98 steroid-naive patients, the loss of bone mineral density over 2 years was 3.84% in the prednisolone group and 1.04% in the budesonide group (Fig. 5.1). In the other groups – steroid-dependent, currently on steroids, and previously exposed to steroids – bone mineral density was diminished at baseline and there was no significant difference in the change in bone mineral density over the 2 years of the study. Steroid-related side effects were seen about half as often in the budesonide-treated patients than in the prednisolone-treated patients (Table 5.1).

Comment

Budesonide is an important advance in the treatment of mildly to moderately active Crohn's disease. Indeed, it is the only drug approved by the US Food and Drugs Administration (FDA) for this indication. In recent years, budesonide has been used preferentially as first-line therapy for patients with mildly to moderately active disease because it is very effective. However, there has been reluctance to use the drug as maintenance therapy because of the well-known long-term side effects of conventional steroid use. Schoon *et al.* have shown that the long-term adverse effects of budesonide are relatively low and in the acceptable range—especially in patients who are steroid-naive. Largely from these data, in 2005 the FDA approved budesonide for maintenance therapy for Crohn's disease.

Maintenance infliximab treatment is associated with improved bone mineral density in Crohn's disease

Bernstein M, Irwin S, Greenberg GR. *Am J Gastroenterol* 2005; **100**: 2031–5

Background. Bone mineral density is decreased in Crohn's disease patients as a result of the effects of tumour necrosis factor (TNF). TNF is known to inhibit osteoblast formation and increase osteoclast activity through a p55-TNF receptor. It stands to reason that inhibition of TNF with infliximab, a monoclonal anti-TNF antibody, will improve bone mineral density if given over the long term.

Interpretation. Investigators from Mount Sinai Hospital in Toronto studied 43 patients with Crohn's disease who were given infliximab 5 mg/kg every 6–8 weeks for at least 1 year. Thirteen of these patients were receiving prednisone concurrently at a mean dose of 10 mg daily. Significant improvements in bone mineral density were found at 1 year in the lumbar spine (2.4%), the femoral trochanter (2.8%) and the femoral neck (2.8%) (Fig. 5.2). Baseline osteopenia and concurrent steroid use did not change the effect of infliximab on bone mineral density.

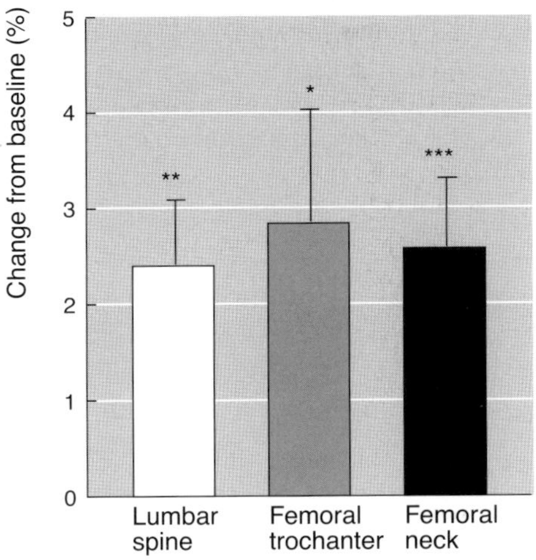

Fig. 5.2 Percentage change in bone mineral density from baseline to 1 year at the lumbar spine (L2–L4), left femoral trochanter and left femoral neck. Value are mean ± SEs. $*P = 0.03$; $**P = 0.002$; $***P = 0.001$ compared with baseline.
Source: Bernstein *et al.* (2005).

Comment

Infliximab has been approved by the FDA for induction therapy in moderately to severely active Crohn's disease (both inflammatory type and fistulizing type), maintenance therapy for Crohn's disease, and as induction and maintenance therapy for ulcerative colitis. The drug has been shown to be of great benefit in treating intestinal symptoms. Now, the effect of infliximab on bone metabolism has been shown. Patients with Crohn's disease need to pay attention to possible bone loss, but those on maintenance therapy with infliximab are less likely to run into serious problems with osteopenia and osteoporosis.

Randomized trial of etidronate plus calcium and vitamin D for treatment of low bone mineral density in Crohn's disease

Siffledeen JS, Fedorak RN, Kiminoski K, *et al. Clin Gastroenterol Hepatol* 2005; **3**: 122–32

BACKGROUND. IBD patients with low bone mineral density are often prescribed bisphosphonates as well as calcium and vitamin D supplements. The data supporting these recommendations are minimal, and it is generally felt that calcium and vitamin D supplements are not very effective.

Interpretation. One hundred and fifty-four patients with Crohn's disease and low bone mineral density were randomized to receive the bisphosphonate etidronate or placebo over a 2-year period. All patients were supplemented with 500 mg of calcium and 400 IU of vitamin D over the course of the study. After 2 years, bone mineral density of the lumbar spine, total hip, trochanter and ultradistal radius increased in all groups regardless of the use of bisphosphonates (Fig. 5.3).

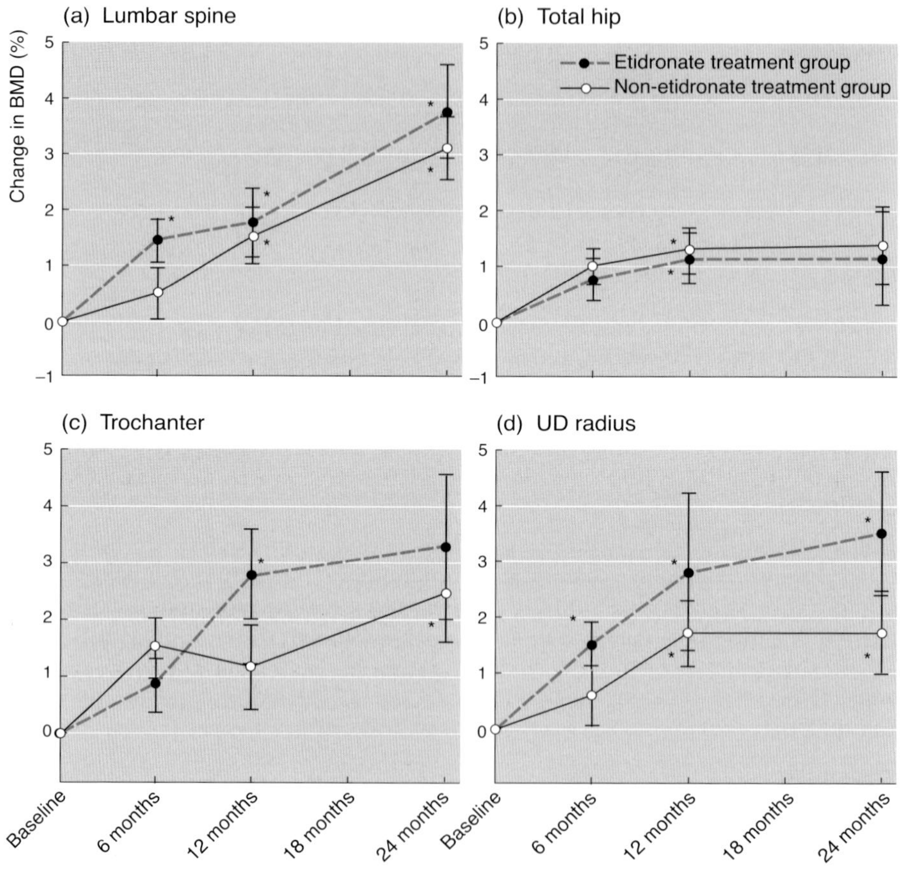

Fig. 5.3 Mean (± standard error of mean [SEM]) percentage change in the BMD from baseline to 24 months in 72 patients with Crohn's disease treated with etidronate plus daily calcium and vitamin D supplementation (*solid circles* and *dashed line*) (etidronate treatment group), and 71 Crohn's disease patients treated with daily calcium and vitamin D supplementation only (*open circles* and *solid line*) (non-etidronate treatment group). (a) Lumbar spine, (b) total hip, (c) trochanter, (d) ultradistal (UD) radius. *Significant change in BMD from baseline (P <0.05). Source: Siffledeen *et al.* (2005).

Comment

It is very reasonable to place all Crohn's disease patients on calcium and vitamin D supplements. Prior to this study, such supplementation was not believed to be effective. However, this study provides reasonable evidence that supplementation with calcium and vitamin D can improve bone mineral density over a 2-year period. It is also reasonable to conclude that, when started early in the course of Crohn's disease, supplements may prevent bone loss.

Malignancy in IBD

Increased risk of intestinal cancer in Crohn's disease: a meta-analysis of population-based cohort studies

Jess T, Gamborg M, Matzen P, Munkholm P, Sorensen TIA. *Am J Gastroenterol* 2005; **100**: 2724–9

BACKGROUND. It has been known for many years that patients with ulcerative colitis have an increased risk of colorectal cancer, with population-based relative risk estimates of at least 3. Controversy exists, though, about the risk of colorectal cancer in Crohn's disease. If the risk is markedly elevated, the cancer surveillance strategies recommended to Crohn's disease patients should be similar to those for ulcerative colitis patients.

INTERPRETATION. A meta-analysis was performed of six population-based studies to assess the risk of intestinal cancer among patients with Crohn's disease. Even though four of the six studies did not show a significant increase in the incidence rate of colorectal cancer, the pooled standardized incidence rate for colorectal cancer was 1.9 (95% confidence interval [CI] 1.7–3.5) (Fig. 5.4). The standardized incidence rate for small bowel cancer was 27.1 (95% CI 14.9–49.2).

Comment

It is generally believed that chronic inflammation leads to malignant transformation. Therefore, for patients with Crohn's disease to have an increase in the risk of colorectal cancer there should be a substantial portion of the colon with active disease. All of these studies, and consequently the meta-analysis, failed to adjust the risk for the extent of colonic disease. Therefore, in patients with extensive colonic disease (i.e. at least one-third of the colon involved), the standardized incidence rate of colorectal cancer is likely to be much higher than 1.9 and could approach that of ulcerative colitis patients. Cancer surveillance should be offered to such patients.

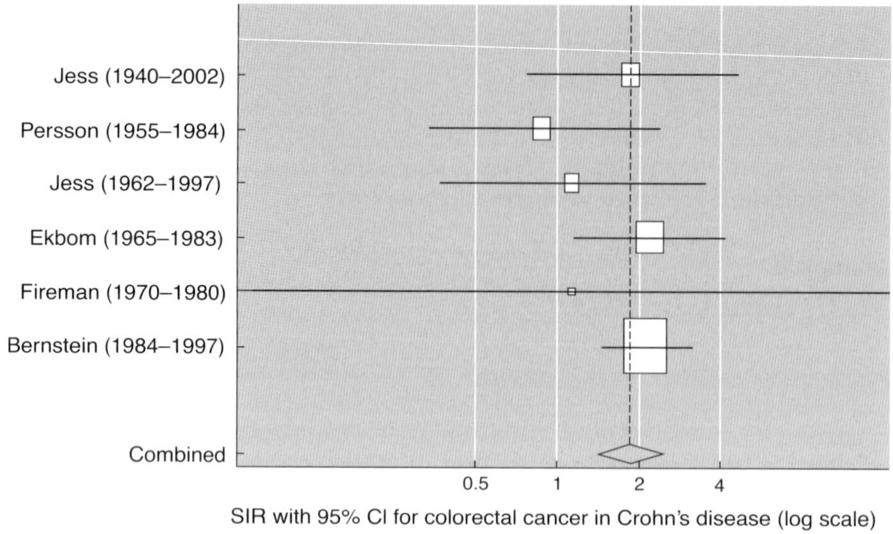

Fig. 5.4 Individual and combined standardized incidence ratios (with 95% confidence intervals) of colorectal cancer in Crohn's disease: a meta-analysis of six population-based cohort studies. The size of the boxes is proportional to the weight (1/SE) for each study. Source: Jess *et al.* (2005).

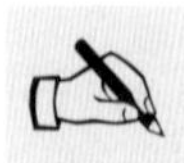

Increased risk of lymphoma among inflammatory bowel disease patients treated with azathioprine and 6-mercaptopurine

Kandiel A, Fraser AG, Korelitz BI, Bresinger C, Lewis JD. *Gut* 2005; **54**: 1121–5

BACKGROUND. Lymphomas have been reported in Crohn's disease patients treated with infliximab. Indeed, the risk of lymphoma is often a concern expressed by patients being considered for such therapy. However, other medications used to treat Crohn's disease (i.e. azathioprine and 6-mercaptopurine), which are often used in conjunction with infliximab, may account for the elevated risk of lymphoma.

INTERPRETATION. A meta-analysis was performed of six large cohort studies designed to evaluate the risk of lymphoma in patients with Crohn's disease treated with azathioprine or 6-mercaptopurine. Eleven cases of lymphoma were reported and 2.63 were expected (pooled relative risk 4.18; 95% CI 2.07–7.51). A sensitivity analysis showed little change in this estimate when it was adjusted for the size of the study or the magnitude of the risk.

Comment

The excess number of lymphomas seen in Crohn's disease patients treated with infliximab may not be due to infliximab but to the concomitant immunosuppression most of these patients are receiving. Studies need to be done to see if infliximab confers a synergistic risk of lymphoma.

Effect of 5-aminosalicylate use on colorectal cancer and dysplasia risk: a systemic review and meta-analysis of observational studies

Velayos FS, Terdiman JP, Walsh JM. *Am J Gastroenterol* 2005; **100**: 1345–53

BACKGROUND. Primary prevention of colorectal cancer in ulcerative colitis is an attractive option because treatment algorithms for colorectal cancer are less than ideal. 5-aminosalicylic acid (5-ASA) compounds offer a possible chemopreventive effect through a variety of mechanisms, which include the control of inflammation and the inactivation of reactive oxygen species. Epidemiological studies to date have not shown a consistent chemopreventive effect of 5-ASA agents.

INTERPRETATION. Nine studies (three cohort and six case–control) studies were included in the meta-analysis, which included a total of 1932 patients with ulcerative colitis, 334 of whom developed colorectal cancer. 5-ASA was chemoprotective for colorectal cancer (odds ratio [OR] 0.51; 95% CI 0.37–0.69) or the combined outcome of cancer or dysplasia (OR 0.51; 95% CI 0.38–0.69) (Fig. 5.5). The authors could not demonstrate a dose–response effect.

Comment

Long-term 5-ASA use is known to be effective maintenance therapy for patients with ulcerative colitis. Unfortunately, patients who are usually feeling well are not compliant with their maintenance therapy. The added benefit of cancer chemoprevention from 5-ASA may encourage patients to comply better with their therapy. Still, chemoprevention with 5-ASA is not sufficient to eliminate the risk of cancer. Patients will still need regular surveillance colonoscopy for cancer.

The impact of ursodeoxycholic acid on cancer, dysplasia, and mortality in ulcerative colitis patients with primary sclerosing cholangitis

Wolf JM, Rybicki LA, Lashner BA. *Aliment Pharmacol Ther* 2005; **22**: 783–8

BACKGROUND. Ulcerative colitis patients with primary sclerosing cholangitis (PSC) are at particularly high risk of colorectal cancer. The relative risk for such patients is at least 3 times the risk in ulcerative colitis patients without PSC. Ursodeoxycholic

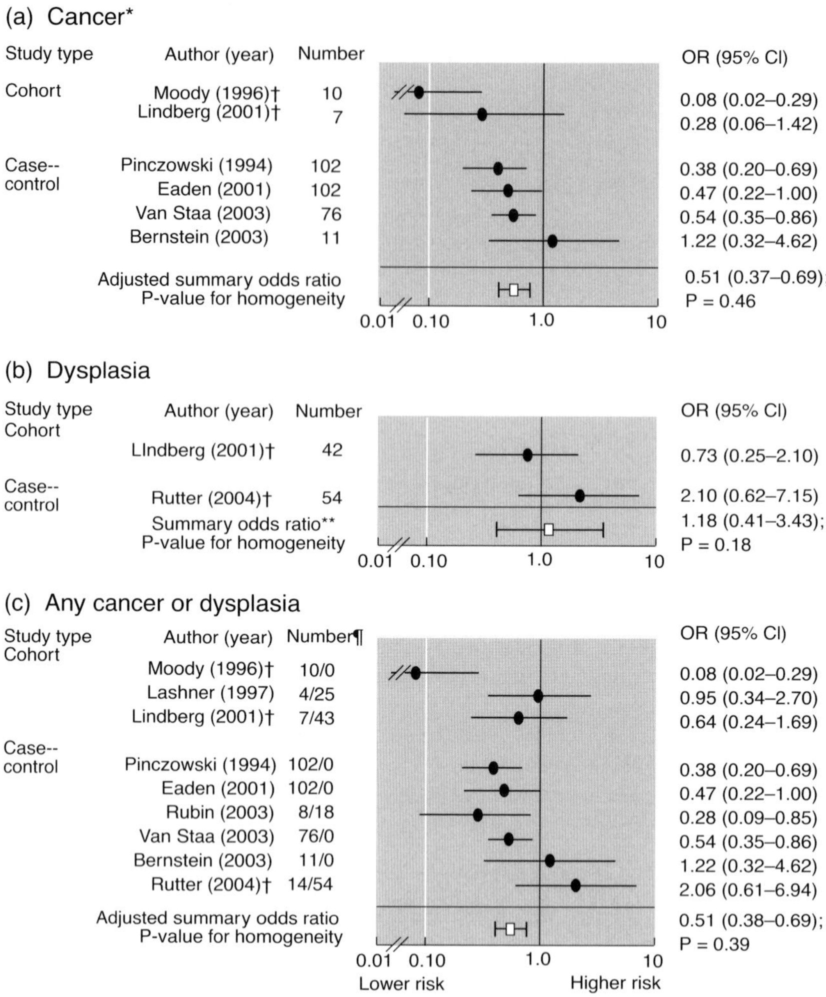

Fig. 5.5 Summary of studies assessing the risk of colitis-associated colorectal neoplasia with any 5-aminosalicylate use. All reported odds ratios (OR) are adjusted for confounding variables, unless otherwise noted. *All cancer patients in the study by Rutter *et al.* had taken 5-ASA for at least 3 months and therefore there was no reference group. †Only unadjusted odds ratio reported. **Pooled odds ratios unadjusted for confounding variables. ¶Number of cancer cases/number of dysplasia cases. Source: Velayos *et al.* (2005).

acid (UDCA) is a primary bile acid that, when given orally, displaces carcinogenic secondary bile acids from the bile and may decrease the risk of cancer. Two previous studies have demonstrated a significant beneficial chemopreventive effect of UDCA.

Interpretation. A historical cohort study was performed on 120 ulcerative colitis patients with PSC, 28 of whom were taking UDCA. Among the patients taking UDCA, the adjusted relative risk of developing cancer or dysplasia was 0.59 (95% CI 0.26–1.36). However, the relative risk of death among UDCA users was 0.44 (95% CI 0.22–0.90). Even though UDCA did not significantly reduce the risk of neoplasia in IBD, it is recommended because of the magnitude of the reduction of the risk of neoplasia and its beneficial effect on mortality, probably from its beneficial effects on the liver.

Comment

5-ASA agents as well as folic acid are recommended for the chemoprevention of cancer in IBD. UDCA can be added to this list for PSC patients since it appears to have some beneficial effect in cancer prevention and an important beneficial effect on liver disease.

Endoscopic factors in the diagnosis of colorectal dysplasia in chronic inflammatory bowel disease

Toruner M, Harewood GC, Loftus EV, *et al. Inflamm Bowel Dis* 2005; **11**: 428–34

Background. Cancer surveillance colonoscopy in patients with IBD is a time-consuming procedure. Careful examination of the colon and extensive biopsies are required. Biopsies are taken randomly and of raised lesions. A histological diagnosis of dysplasia often prompts a recommendation of colectomy since the risk of cancer being present or developing in the near future is inordinately high. Although dysplasia is rarely found, there may be factors related to the endoscopist that determine the detection rate for dysplasia.

Interpretation. Among 635 patients with IBD who were having surveillance colonoscopy, 24 (3.8%) had dysplasia in flat mucosa, twelve (1.9%) had a dysplasia-associated lesion or mass and 28 (4.4%) had a sporadic adenoma identified. The longer the colonoscopy time, the higher was the rate of detection of dysplasia in flat mucosa ($P < 0.02$). The number of biopsies was not associated with detection rate of dysplasia.

Comment

It is critically important to identify dysplasia if it exists. The rate of progression to higher grades of dysplasia or to cancer has been estimated to be as high as 50% at 5 years. To maximize the sensitivity of such testing, endoscopists must perform high-quality examinations by allotting added time to this procedure and must carefully biopsy all regions of the colon.

Thrombosis in IBD

Thrombosis in inflammatory bowel disease: role of inherited thrombophilia

Spina L, Saibeni S, Battaglioli T, *et al. Am J Gastroenterol* 2005; **100**: 2036–41

Homocysteine triggers mucosal microvascular activation in inflammatory bowel disease

Danese S, Sgambato A, Papa A, *et al. Am J Gastroenterol* 2005; **100**: 886–95

Elevated circulating platelet-derived microparticles in patients with active inflammatory bowel disease

Andoh A, Tsujikawa T, Hata K, *et al. Am J Gastroenterol* 2005; **100**: 2042–8

Background. The risk of arterial and venous thrombosis in IBD is greater than that in the general population. The consequences of thrombosis and thromboembolism can be severe and even fatal. The causes of thrombosis in IBD patients are unknown, but may be related to genetic mutations such as factor V Leiden mutations, elevated homocysteine from chronic inflammation or folic acid deficiency, or from platelet-derived microparticles.

Interpretation. Spina *et al.* tested for the most common factor V Leiden mutations among 47 IBD patients with a history of thrombosis and two controls per case. Mutations were found significantly less frequently in the IBD patients (12.8 vs 29.8%; $P < 0.04$), putting to rest this theory. Danese *et al.* showed that homocysteine from both plasma and mucosa was associated with active inflammation in IBD and that treatment with folic acid can decrease homocysteine levels, reduce inflammation and decrease the risk of thrombosis. Andoh *et al.* demonstrated that platelet-derived microparticles were significantly elevated in ulcerative colitis and Crohn's disease patients with active disease. These levels decreased following successful therapy.

Comment

Thrombosis in IBD is very much related to active inflammation. Both homocysteine and platelet-derived microparticles are likely to be involved in the pathogenesis of both inflammation and thrombosis. Fortunately, the level of homocysteine can be decreased by folic acid supplementation. It is unlikely that genetic mutations leading to an elevated risk of thrombosis are involved in the pathogenesis of thrombosis in patients with IBD.

Advances in diagnostic testing in IBD

Capsule endoscopy versus enteroclysis in the detection of small-bowel involvement of Crohn's disease

Marmo R, Rotondano G, Piscopo R, *et al. Clin Gastroenterol Hepatol* 2005; **3**: 772–6

A prospective comparison study of MRI versus small bowel follow-through in recurrent Crohn's disease

Bernstein CN, Greenberg J, Boult I, Chubey S, Leblanc C, Ryner L. *Am J Gastroenterol* 2005; **100**: 2493–502

Technetium-99m-HMPAO labeled leukocyte single photon emission computerized tomography (SPECT) for assessing Crohn's disease extent and intestinal infiltration

Biancone L, Schillaci O, Capoccetti F, *et al. Am J Gastroenterol* 2005; **100**: 344–54

BACKGROUND. There is no gold standard test to diagnose Crohn's disease or to measure the extent and severity of disease. Many new tests are being developed, some of which were studied this year. Compared with older tests, the newer tests will increase the sensitivity of testing at the expense of lower specificity. There will be more true-positive results, but also more false-positive results, with the use of newer diagnostic techniques.

INTERPRETATION. Marmo *et al.* compared wireless capsule endoscopy (WCE) with small bowel enteroclysis in 31 patients with Crohn's disease. Lesions suggestive of active Crohn's disease were found in 25.8% of patients by small bowel enteroclysis, compared with 71% by WCE ($P < 0.001$). Superiority of WCE was found for both ileal and jejunal lesions. Bernstein *et al.* compared MRI with small bowel follow-through in 30 patients with known Crohn's disease. Both tests gave normal results in ten patients; the two tests showed similar results in eight patients; small bowel follow-through showed additional results in four patients (stricture and ileosigmoid fistulas); and MRI showed additional results in eight patients (active inflammation in strictures and lymphadenopathy). The lack of radiation is another advantage for MRI. SPECT uses radiolabelled leucocytes to identify areas of inflammation. Biancone *et al.* studied SPECT for 22 patients with IBD. SPECT scanning was particularly sensitive for detecting inflammation in the ileocaecal region and in the perianum.

Comment

There are certain advantages to each of these diagnostic tests compared with more conventional diagnostic testing. WCE is highly sensitive, but its low specificity (for example, WCE detects aphthous ulcers in patients taking non-steroidal anti-inflammatory drugs) makes the test of limited usefulness. Furthermore, because of the risk of obstruction from the capsule in Crohn's disease patients with a stricture, a radiographic study is necessary prior to WCE. It is doubtful that WCE will be a commonly used diagnostic test in the coming years. MRI, on the other hand, has the advantages of added sensitivity in detecting inflammation, the possibility of finding extra-intestinal lesions, and no radiation exposure. Such testing, if available and affordable, could be very useful clinically. SPECT, at this point, offers only crude estimates of the site of inflammation and does not provide enough detailed information for clinical decisions to be made.

Factors related to improved quality of life in IBD

Antibiotic use and the risk of flare of inflammatory bowel disease

Aberra FN, Brensinger CM, Bilker WB, Lichtenstein GR, Lewis JD. *Clin Gastroenterol Hepatol* 2005; **3**: 459–65

BACKGROUND. Both Crohn's disease and ulcerative colitis are recurring–remitting diseases. The aetiology of a flare is rarely known, but factors suspected to induce a flare are systemic infection, stress, the season of the year, and the use of antibiotics. Antibiotic use can alter the delicate balance of commensal bacteria in the gut. Patients with IBD are often advised to avoid antibiotics if possible.

INTERPRETATION. Using a large database which includes about eight million people, Aberra *et al.* found that antibiotic use was protective against flares from Crohn's disease but had no effect in patients with ulcerative colitis. In the 1205 patients with Crohn's disease, a short course of antibiotics gave a 22% reduction in the risk of flare, defined by a new prescription of steroids or mesalamine (OR 0.78; 95% CI 0.64–0.98). The protective effect was strongest with recent antibiotic exposure. The effect among 2230 patients with ulcerative colitis was not significant (OR 0.96; 95% CI 0.82–1.12).

Comment

When needed, patients with IBD need not avoid antibiotics. However, because of the risk of antibiotic-associated colitis, patients should avoid antibiotics for non-serious infections.

Narcotic use in patients with Crohn's disease

Cross RK, Wilson KT, Binion DG. *Am J Gastroenterol* 2005; **100**: 2225–9

BACKGROUND. Chronic abdominal pain is a clinical feature of Crohn's disease. The pain is commonly treated with narcotics, but such treatment does nothing for the Crohn's disease activity. Chronic narcotic use is certain to decrease the quality of life both in the workplace and at home.

INTERPRETATION. Among 291 patients with Crohn's disease seen in two medical centres, 13.1% were chronic users of narcotic medications. Narcotic users were more likely to be female (72 vs 49% in non-narcotic users), have worse disease activity (Harvey-Bradshaw index 9.1 vs 5.0), have higher rates of disability (15.4 vs 3.6%), exhibit polypharmacy (6.97 vs 4.7 medications), use neuropsychiatric drugs more often (37 vs 19%), and be cigarette smokers. Furthermore, there was a decreased quality of life score in patients on chronic treatment with narcotics.

Comment

Relief of pain and suffering is the prime charge of physicians. However, it is not always in the patient's best interest to prescribe narcotics to treat the pain of Crohn's disease. Working with pain management and psychiatric services and maximizing medical and surgical therapy are all essential components of the therapy of patients with Crohn's disease.

Health-related quality of life improves in children and adolescents with inflammatory bowel disease after attending a camp sponsored by the Crohn's and Colitis Foundation of America

Shepanski MA, Hurd LB, Culton K, Markowitz JE, Mamula P, Baldassano RN. *Inflamm Bowel Dis* 2005; **11**: 164–70

BACKGROUND. Children with IBD are different from their peers. Medication use, frequent visits to doctors and hospitals, and inability to participate fully in activities are a few of the problems these children encounter. The Crohn's and Colitis Foundation of America (CCFA) sponsored a 1-week overnight summer camp for children with IBD to see if their quality of life could be improved.

INTERPRETATION. Completed questionnaires were received from 61 individuals, 47 with Crohn's disease and 14 with ulcerative colitis. Fifty were girls and eleven were boys. Compared with pre-camp scores, post-camp scores reflected an improvement in overall quality of life, including bowel symptom scores, social functioning scores and treatment intervention scores.

Comment

The CCFA is to be commended for this innovative effort. Children with IBD can improve their quality of life in these summer camps by improving their social functioning and by better accepting IBD symptoms and treatment. This programme needs to be supported by industry, physicians and philanthropists to ensure that children with IBD have the best opportunity to normalize their quality of life.

Amount of systemic steroid medication is a strong predictor for the use of complementary and alternative medicine in patients with inflammatory bowel disease: results from a German national survey

Langhorst J, Anthonisen IB, Steder-Neukamm U, *et al. Inflamm Bowel Dis* 2005; **11**: 287–95

BACKGROUND. Complementary and alternative medicines (CAMs) are often used by IBD patients, usually without the knowledge of their physicians. For the most part, CAMs are ineffective and are taken by patients who are desperate for relief of their symptoms.

INTERPRETATION. Questionnaires focusing on CAMs were returned by 671 of 1000 IBD patients given the opportunity of participating. CAMs were used more frequently in patients with ulcerative colitis than in patients with Crohn's disease (59.8 vs 48.3%). Homeopathy and herbal medicine were the most often used CAMs. CAMs were used by 63.8% of patients to enable them to stop using steroids, and steroid use was a strong predictor of CAM use (OR 2.40; 95% CI 1.26–4.56). Other predictors of CAM use were a history of psychotherapeutic support, the use of relaxation techniques and an academic education.

Comment

Quality of life is greatly diminished in patients given long-term treatment with steroids. Patients seeking relief often resort to CAMs, which are largely ineffective. Physicians need to treat patients vigorously with as much steroid-sparing medication as is required.

Conclusion

The complications of IBD, such as osteoporosis, cancer and thrombosis, are plentiful. Patients and physicians need to pay careful attention to treatment and any reversible risk factors that could minimize the risk. For example, calcium and vitamin D supplements should be given to all IBD patients at risk of osteopenia, and cigarette smoking needs to be strongly discouraged. Chemoprevention of colorectal cancer with 5-ASA products and UDCA should be strongly considered in patients who are at risk. Control of chronic inflammation may decrease the risk of osteopenia, colorectal cancer and thrombosis. Also, folic acid supplementation has several beneficial effects by decreasing homocysteine levels and by acting as a chemopreventive agent against cancer. Finally, the quality of life of IBD patients can be improved by reducing the use of narcotics and steroids. CCFA summer camps seem to be a good idea. In all, there is much that can and should be done for IBD patients.

Further reading

1. Tursi A, Giorgetti GM, Brandimarte G, Elisei W. High prevalence of celiac disease among patients affected by Crohn's disease. *Inflamm Bowel Dis* 2005; **11**: 662–6.
2. Reguiero M, Kip KE, Cheung O, Hegazi RA, Plevy S. Cigarette smoking and age at diagnosis of inflammatory bowel disease. *Inflamm Bowel Dis* 2005; **11**: 42–7.
3. Reddy SI, Friedman S, Telford JJ, Strate L, Ookubo R, Banks PA. Are patients with inflammatory bowel disease receiving optimal care? *Am J Gastroenterol* 2005; **100**: 1357–61.
4. Gupta G, Gelfand JM, Lewis JD. Increased risk for demyelinating diseases in patients with IBD. *Gastroenterology* 2005; **129**: 819–26.
5. Bernstein CN, Wajda A, Blanchard JF. The clustering of other chronic inflammatory diseases in inflammatory bowel disease: a population-based study. *Gastroenterology* 2005; **129**: 827–36.
6. Auslander JN, Lieberman DA, Sonnenberg A. Lack of seasonal variation in the endoscopic diagnoses of Crohn's disease and ulcerative colitis. *Am J Gastroenterol* 2005; **100**: 2233–8.
7. Basu D, Lopez I, Kulkarni A, Sellin JH. Impact of race and ethnicity on inflammatory bowel disease. *Am J Gastroenterol* 2005; **100**: 2254–61.
8. Schroder O, Mickisch O, Seidler U, de Weerth A, Dignass AU, Herfarth H, Reinshagen M, Schreiber S, Junge U, Schrott M, Stein J. Intravenous iron sucrose versus oral iron supplementation for the treatment of iron deficiency anemia in patients with inflammatory bowel disease—a randomized, controlled, open-label, multicenter study. *Am J Gastroenterol* 2005; **100**: 2503–9.
9. Harty S, Fleming P, Rowland M, Crushell E, McDermott M, Drumm B, Bourke B. A prospective study of the oral manifestations of Crohn's disease. *Clin Gastroenterol Hepatol* 2005; **3**: 886–91.

10. Moolsintong P, Loftus EV Jr, Chari ST, Egan LJ, Tremaine WJ, Sandborn WJ. Acute pancreatitis in patients with Crohn's disease: clinical features and outcomes. *Inflamm Bowel Dis* 2005; **11**: 1080–4.

11. Achkar JP, Al-Haddad M, Lashner B, Remzi FH, Brzezinski A, Shen B, Khandwala F, Fazio V. Differentiating risk factors for acute and chronic pouchitis. *Clin Gastroenterol Hepatol* 2005; **3**: 60–6.

12. Farhadi A, Keshavarzian A, Van de Kar LD, Jakate S, Domm A, Zhang L, Shaikh M, Banan A, Fields JZ. Heightened responses to stressors in patients with inflammatory bowel disease. *Am J Gastroenterol* 2005; **100**: 1796–804.

13. Sechi LA, Scanu AM, Molicotti P, Cannas S, Mura M, Dettori G, Fadda G, Zanetti S. Detection and isolation of *Mycobacterium avium* subspecies *paratuberculosis* from intestinal mucosal biopsies of patients with and without Crohn's disease in Sardinia. *Am J Gastroenterol* 2005; **100**: 1529–36.

14. Cosnes J, Nion-Larmurier I, Beaugerie L, Afchain P, Tiret E, Gendre JP. Impact of the increasing use of immunosuppressants in Crohn's disease on the need for intestinal surgery. *Gut* 2005; **54**: 237–41.

15. Calabrese E, La Seta F, Buccellato A, Virdone R, Pallotta N, Corazziari E, Cottone M. Crohn's disease: a comparative prospective study of transabdominal ultrasonography, small intestine contrast ultrasonography, and small bowel enema. *Inflamm Bowel Dis* 2005; **11**: 139–45.

16. Lawrence IC, Hall A, Leong R, Pearce C, Pearce C, Murray K. A comparative study of goblet cell and pancreatic exocrine autoantibodies combined with ASCA and pANCA in Chinese and Caucasian patients with IBD. *Inflamm Bowel Dis* 2005; **11**: 890–7.

17. Gupta A, Derbes C, Sellin J. Clinical indications of the use of antineutrophil cytoplasmic antibodies and anti-Saccharomyces cerevisiae antibodies in the evaluation of inflammatory bowel disease at an academic medical center. *Inflamm Bowel Dis* 2005; **11**: 898–902.

6

Update on medical therapy for inflammatory bowel disease

AARON BRZEZINSKI, JEAN-PAUL ACHKAR

Introduction

The aetiology of the inflammatory bowel diseases, Crohn's disease and ulcerative colitis, is multifactorial, and some hypotheses may appear to be contradictory. The most commonly accepted hypothesis is that there is a trigger or triggers causing an abnormal immune reaction primarily in the gastrointestinal tract of genetically predisposed individuals. Given the billions of bacteria present in the gastrointestinal tract, it is believed that the intrinsic immune system of the gastrointestinal tract is in a 'controlled state of inflammation', and reacts primarily to inactivate noxious antigens while tolerating non-pathogenic bacteria. There is also the possibility that the main abnormality in inflammatory bowel disease is alteration of the innate intestinal immune defence, allowing increased exposure to luminal antigens. The trigger or triggers for the development of chronic inflammation in inflammatory bowel disease have not been identified, but in recent years our understanding of some of the genetic mutations that are related to an increased risk of developing Crohn's disease [1] and the immune abnormalities that occur in inflammatory bowel disease have been better defined. With such advances, more effective and targeted treatments have been developed. Currently, most medical treatments for inflammatory bowel disease are geared towards ameliorating the immune response, either with topical anti-inflammatory medications such as 5-aminosalicylic acid (5-ASA) products and some halogenated corticosteroids, or with systemic treatments with corticosteroids, immunosuppressive agents or antibodies against pro-inflammatory cytokines. In this chapter we will review significant advances in the treatment of inflammatory bowel disease over the past year.

Sargramostatim for active Crohn's disease

Korzenik JR, Dieckgraefe BK, Valentine JF, Hausman DF, Gilbert MJ; Sargramostim in Crohn's Disease Study Group. *N Engl J Med* 2005; **352**: 2193–201

Background. The current treatment of Crohn's disease is with agents that cause immunosuppression. However, there is some evidence that suggests that patients with Crohn's disease may have an abnormality in the function of the intestinal immune defence leading to a breakdown in the epithelial defence barrier, leading to persistent exposure of lamina propria cells to bacterial antigens and bacterial products. In turn, persistent exposure to bacteria and bacterial antigens leads to an abnormal chronic inflammatory process mediated by T cells. If this is true, treatment with an agent that stimulates the mucosal immune response would lead to less exposure to luminal antigens and would decrease the antigenic stimulation. Sargramostim (Leukine, Berlex) is a yeast-derived recombinant human granulocyte–macrophage colony stimulating factor (GM-CSF) that is used to stimulate myeloid recovery after chemotherapy. There is evidence that GM-CSF may play an important role in helping maintain the integrity of the intestinal immune barrier, thus decreasing the exposure of the lamina propria to luminal antigens. A pilot study on the use of sargramostim in 15 patients reported in 2002 [2] showed beneficial effects.

Interpretation. Patients eligible for this clinical trial had moderately to severely active Crohn's disease defined by a Crohn's disease activity index (CDAI) of 220–475, had not received immunosuppressive medication within a predefined period, and had no contraindication, such as pregnancy, breast-feeding, infections, or other serious medical diseases. Patients were randomized in a 2:1 ratio to receive either sargramostim 6 μg/kg or placebo subcutaneously daily for 56 days. Efficacy and safety were evaluated every 2 weeks for the duration of the trial and for 30 days after the end of treatment. Patients who met the primary end-point of clinical response, defined by a decrease in the CDAI by at least 70 points, were followed up for 6 months. Secondary end-points included a decrease in the CDAI by at least 100 points, clinical remission defined by a CDAI below 150, and an improvement in quality of life, defined by an increase in the inflammatory bowel disease questionnaire (IBDQ) score. A total of 127 patients in 28 centres were randomized, and 124 started treatment (81 with sargramostim, 43 with placebo). Nineteen patients in the treatment group and ten in the placebo group underwent colonoscopy and were evaluated with the Crohn's Disease Endoscopic Index of Severity (CDEIS).

There was no significant difference in response, defined by the primary end-point of a decrease of at least 70 points in the CDAI by day 57. However, the treatment group did significantly better than the placebo group when evaluated by the secondary end-points; these included a decrease in the CDAI of at least 100 points, clinical remission, and an improvement in quality of life (Fig. 6.1). Furthermore, there was a significant improvement in mucosal healing in patients who underwent endoscopic evaluation compared with patients in the placebo group. Patients receiving sargramostim had more reactions at the injection site and more bone pain.

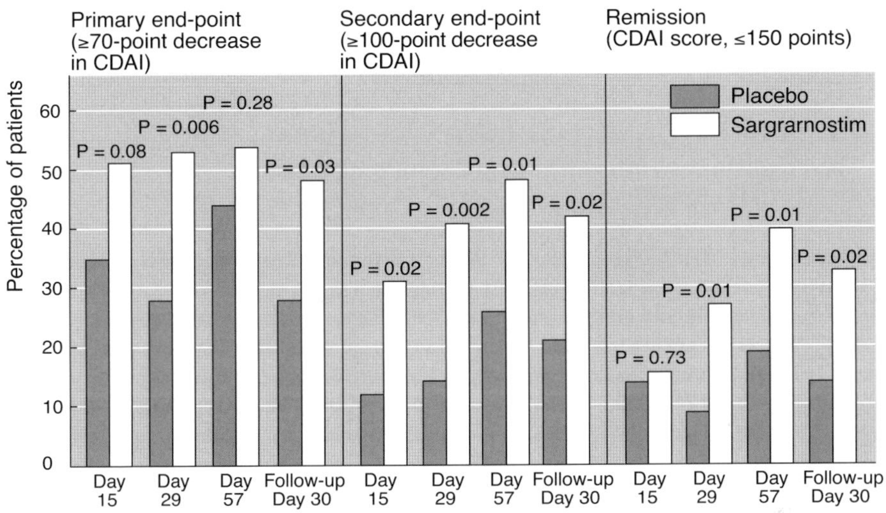

Fig. 6.1 Percentage of patients who had a clinical response, as defined by a decrease from baseline of at least 70 or at least 100 points in the CDAI score, or remission up to 30 days of follow-up. The analysis included all patients who received at least one dose of assigned treatment, with the last observation carried forward in the case of missing values. Patients who prematurely discontinued treatment for any reason were considered to have had no response from that point onward. There was no significant difference between groups in the percentage of patients who reached the primary end-point of a decrease from baseline of at least 70 points in the CDAI score on day 57 ($P = 0.28$). Source: Korzenik *et al.* (2005).

Comment

Crohn's disease is a heterogeneous disease. The hypothesis that it may be a result of a defect in the intrinsic innate immune defence in the intestinal epithelium and in the lamina propria is a concept that has evolved from better understanding of the pathophysiology of the disease. The current conventional treatments available for Crohn's disease are designed to cause immunosuppression, and if the problem is that of an immune defect the current treatments would not be the optimal treatments. With the current information it cannot be recommended that immune-stimulating drugs should be used as the primary treatment for Crohn's disease patients, though this approach may be an acceptable one for patients with refractory disease. However, it is important to recognize that such an approach is not free of potential side effects. The frequency and severity of side effects are difficult to quantify, given that the main use of sargramostim is in the treatment of patients with acute myelogenous leukaemia and after transplantation. Side effects such as injection site reactions, headache and bone pain can usually be treated with paracetamol (acetaminophen). One patient in the treatment group in this clinical trial had a central nervous system event, and it is unclear whether this was secondary to sargramostim treatment.

Autologous hematopoietic stem cell transplantation in patients with refractory Crohn's disease

Oyama Y, Craig RM, Traynor AE, *et al. Gastroenterology* 2005; **128**: 552–63

BACKGROUND. The natural history of Crohn's disease is variable. Some patients follow a benign course over their life, but others run a very aggressive course that is refractory to medical and surgical treatment—the so-called malignant Crohn's disease. There are factors that can improve prognosis, such as discontinuation of cigarette smoking and abstaining from using non-steroidal anti-inflammatory drugs. Once a patient fails to respond to a variety of medications, including corticosteroids, immunomodulators such as azathioprine/6 mercaptopurine or methotrexate, tumour necrosis factor-α (TNF-α) antibodies, home total parenteral nutrition and resections, the treatment options are limited to clinical trials. The rationale for this proposed treatment is that, in a genetically susceptible individual, exposure to an antigen or antigens triggers an abnormal immune cell response, primarily an excessive Th1-mediated inflammatory response of the gastrointestinal system. However, Crohn's disease is a multisystem disease with numerous extra-intestinal manifestations. By performing autologous stem cell transplantation, the immune system is 'reset' to its status at birth—the genetic susceptibility is still present but the abnormal immune response has not been triggered, so it is expected that the patient will achieve clinical remission.

INTERPRETATION. There are anecdotal reports of patients with Crohn's disease who undergo haematopoietic stem cell transplantation for malignancy, and whose symptoms of Crohn's disease improve after this treatment. Given this background, it seemed logical to test autologous stem cell transplantation in patients with severely active Crohn's disease in spite of maximal medical treatment. The rationale of performing autologous stem cell transplantation rather than donor stem cell transplantation was that the former prevents problems with graft-versus-host disease and improves the success rate of engraftment. This article reports the results of a pilot study in which twelve such patients were treated with autologous haematopoietic stem cell transplantation at the Northwestern University Medical Center. The patients' clinical characteristics are described in the article, and it is clear that these patients had aggressive disease that had failed to respond to conventional medical and surgical treatment. All patients had moderate to severely active Crohn's disease at the time of transplantation, defined by a CDAI of 250–400 (values ≤150 are considered to indicate remission). Patients were followed up for 7–37 months, with a median follow-up of 18.5 months. The outcome was very good. The patients had the complications expected of an autologous stem cell transplant and neutropenia; one patient had an episode of haematemesis secondary to a Mallory–Weiss tear, and no significant complications occurred. After transplantation there was a rapid and dramatic improvement in the clinical status of the patients, as evidenced by a rapid and sustained decrease in the CDAI (Fig. 6.2).

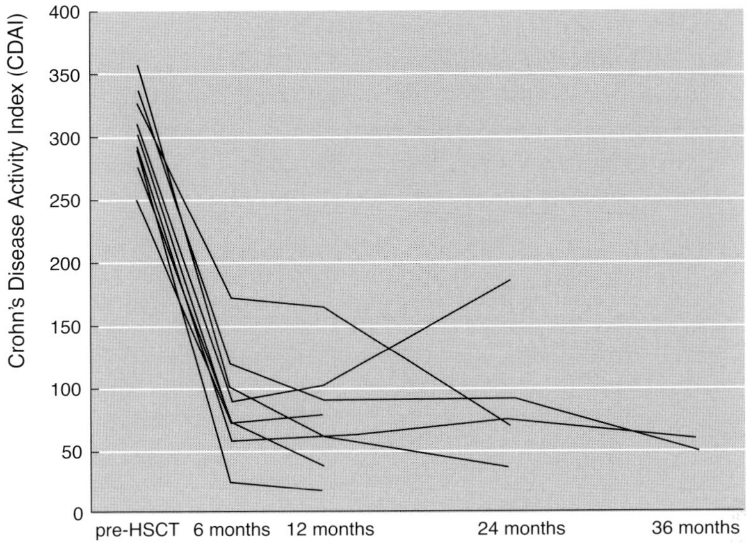

Fig. 6.2 Clinical and laboratory results before and after haematopoietic stem cell transplantation for CDAI. Source: Oyama *et al.* (2005).

Comment

The results of this pilot study are very encouraging, especially because the patients had prolonged remission and were off treatment for Crohn's disease after undergoing the procedure, and hence they had decreasing morbidity associated with the disease and the treatment of the disease. Interestingly, one patient developed recurrent symptoms 15 months after transplantation and had to resume treatment with prednisone and methotrexate 21 months after transplantation. This observation is in keeping with previous studies that have shown that smokers have a lesser response to the treatment of Crohn's disease, including infliximab; and it may be appropriate to demand that patients discontinue cigarette smoking for a defined period of time prior to undergoing autologous stem cell transplantation. Autologous stem cell transplantation is an interesting treatment alternative that for the time being should be reserved for patients with malignant Crohn's disease and be done in tertiary care centres. The short-term complications of transplantation, including death, and long-term complications, such as premature ovarian failure and infertility, should be discussed thoroughly with the patient and, if appropriate, the patient's parents.

Safety and efficacy of adalimumab (D2E7) in Crohn's disease patients with an attenuated response to infliximab

Papadakis KA, Shaye OA, Vasiliauskas EA, *et al. Am J Gastroenterol* 2005; **100**: 75–9

Background. Treatment of Crohn's disease with infliximab, a chimeric human–mouse monoclonal TNF-α antibody, has revolutionized the treatment of Crohn's disease patients. Infliximab is approved by the US Food and Drugs Administration (FDA) for the induction and maintenance of remission in patients with moderate to severely active inflammatory disease and for fistulizing Crohn's disease. It is effective, safe and well tolerated; the response rate in clinical practice has been very similar to that reported in clinical trials; the response rate has been ~70% and the remission rate ~50% in patients with inflammatory disease. However, patients may develop anti-infliximab antibodies; the patients who are at higher risk of developing these antibodies are those who receive episodic treatment, with rates reported between 30 and 61%. Patients on maintenance treatment have a lower frequency of anti-infliximab antibodies, with rates between 7 and 10%. Patients with anti-infliximab antibodies have a higher frequency of infusion reactions, particularly those who have high levels of anti-infliximab antibodies. In patients who have had an adequate response to infliximab previously, this infusion reaction may preclude the ongoing use of infliximab. Furthermore, patients may lose their response and require more frequent administration and/or a higher dose of infliximab [3–5]. It is believed that the anti-infliximab antibodies are directed against the murine region of the molecule. Adalimumab is a recombinant humanized monoclonal immunoglobulin G1 TNF-α antibody that has only human peptide sequences. Its mechanism of action is similar to that of infliximab; it binds TNF-α with high affinity and neutralizes its activity by blocking the interaction between this cytokine and the cell surface receptors. Both infliximab and adalimumab are FDA-approved for clinical use in the treatment of patients with rheumatoid arthritis.

Interpretation. The study is a retrospective analysis of 15 patients with Crohn's disease who had been responders to infliximab and had lost their response to infliximab in spite of increasing the dose to 10 mg/kg IV every 8 weeks. The patients received adalimumab 80 mg SC once followed by 40 mg SC every 2 weeks. In patients in whom the response was not durable for the 2-week interval, the dose was adjusted; in three patients the dose was increased to 80 mg every 2 weeks, in two patients to 80 mg/week and in one patient to 120 mg every 2 weeks. Patients were evaluated with the Harvey–Bradshaw index. Of the fifteen patients, two did not have adequate follow-up, seven (54%) had a complete response, four (31%) had a partial response and 2 (15%) were non-responders (Fig. 6.3). The mean time to response was 5.3 ± 3 weeks. There was no relation between smoking status and response. There was a steroid-sparing effect; eleven patients were receiving concomitant steroids at the time of initiation of treatment with adalimumab, five discontinued steroids by week 14, and three were able to decrease the dose. There were no significant adverse events; the most common side effect was pain at the injection site in two patients that lasted less than 24 h.

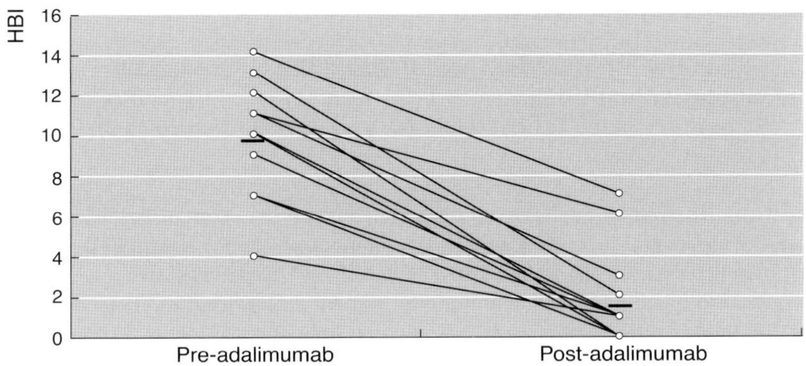

Fig. 6.3 Harvey–Bradshaw index (HBI) at baseline and following treatment with adalimumab in eleven complete and partial responders. Source: Papadakis *et al.* (2005).

Comment

Since the FDA approval of infliximab, there have been over 630 000 patients worldwide with either Crohn's disease or rheumatoid arthritis who have been treated with infliximab. There is a great deal of information from academic and non-academic practices, case series, case reports of adverse events to regulatory agencies, and from registries kept by the manufacturer. The effectiveness reported in controlled clinical trials has been confirmed; we understand better when to initiate treatment, how to evaluate the patient and tests to be done prior to starting treatment, what is the best mode of administration, the risks and management of infusion reactions, and the short- and long-term safety of infliximab. It has become clear that the optimal way to administer infliximab is on a scheduled and not on an episodic basis. Patients receiving infliximab on an episodic basis have a higher risk of developing anti-infliximab antibodies; this leads to infusion reactions and loss of response. On the basis of this report, two previous abstracts on the use of adalimumab in a similar group of patients and an abstract on a randomized clinical trial on the effectiveness of adalimumab in the induction and maintenance of remission in patients with moderately to severely active Crohn's disease ($n = 299$), it appears that adalimumab is a viable alternative for the treatment of patients who lose their response to infliximab |**6,7**|. There is a large multicentre clinical trial being done, and this will hopefully answer questions such as the optimal dose and regimen of administration and the long-term effectiveness of the drug.

Infliximab for induction and maintenance therapy for ulcerative colitis

Rutgeerts P, Sandborn WJ, Feagan BC, *et al. N Engl J Med* 2005; **353**: 2462–76

BACKGROUND. Ulcerative colitis is a mucosal disease of the colon; it begins in the rectum and spreads proximally. The pharmacological treatment is with anti-inflammatory medications such as 5-aminosalicylates, corticosteroids and immunosuppressive medications. The colectomy rate for patients with extensive disease at the time of presentation is 20% in the first year and as high as 35% in the first 5 years of the disease. Unfortunately, colectomy is not curative, there are risks associated with surgery, including mortality, impotence and sepsis, and in those who undergo total proctocolectomy with ileal–pouch–anal anastomosis there is a risk of pouchitis. Furthermore, for some patients who have surgery for ulcerative colitis it is found over time that the underlying disease was Crohn's disease rather than ulcerative colitis; therefore it is clear that more effective treatments with less long-term side effects are needed to decrease symptoms and improve quality of life in patients with ulcerative colitis. Infliximab is an accepted treatment for the induction and maintenance of remission in patients with moderately to severely active Crohn's disease and for patients with fistulizing Crohn's disease; however, its role in the treatment of patients with ulcerative colitis is unclear. Whereas it is well accepted that TNF-α is a key player in the inflammatory process in Crohn's disease, its role in ulcerative colitis is felt to be less significant. However, TNF-α has also been found to be elevated in the mucosa, blood and stool of ulcerative colitis patients, though to a lesser degree. Over the years there have been small case series and case reports that have provided conflicting information in regard to the effectiveness of infliximab in the treatment of ulcerative colitis patients, with response rates reported as low as 33% and as high as >90%. To answer the questions about effectiveness, dosing and safety, two large multicentre, randomized, double-blind, placebo-controlled trials were conducted.

INTERPRETATION. The clinical trials are known as Active Ulcerative Colitis 1 and 2 (ACT 1 and ACT 2). These studies were conducted between March 2002 and March 2005; there were 62 sites and a total of 364 patients in ACT 1 and 55 sites and 364 patients in ACT 2. The design of the two trials was very similar: eligible patients had a confirmed diagnosis of ulcerative colitis, with moderate to severe active disease on sigmoidoscopy, a Mayo score of 6–12 (Table 6.1) despite treatment with corticosteroids alone or in combination with azathioprine or 6-mercaptopurine, and no contraindications, such as ongoing sepsis. The design was very straightforward: patients were randomly assigned to placebo, infliximab 5 mg/kg or 10 mg/kg in a 1:1:1 ratio at weeks 0, 2 and 6 and then every 8 weeks until week 46 in ACT 1 and week 22 in ACT 2. Patients were evaluated at weeks 0, 2, 6, 8, 14, 22 and 30 in both studies, and in ACT 1 patients were also evaluated at weeks 38, 46 and 54. The Mayo score was determined at weeks 0, 8 and 30 for patients in both trials, and at week 54 in patients in ACT 1.

The primary end-point was clinical response at week 8. Secondary end-points were a clinical response or clinical remission off steroids at week 30 in both studies, and in

ACT 1 also at week 54; a clinical remission and mucosal healing at weeks 8 and 30 in both studies and at week 54 in ACT 1; and a clinical response at week 8 in those patients who were refractory to treatment with corticosteroids. Clinical response was defined as a decrease by at least 3 points and 30% in the Mayo score, with a decrease in the subscore of rectal bleeding of at least 1 point or in the absolute subscore for this parameter of 0 or 1. Clinical remission was defined by a total Mayo score of 2 or less and no subscore above 1. Mucosal healing was defined as subscore of 0 or 1. The results showed that significantly fewer patients receiving treatment withdrew from the trial (61.2% of those receiving placebo, 37.2% of those receiving 5 mg/kg and 40.2% of those receiving 10 mg/kg infliximab). In ACT 1, 84/121 (69.4%) of patients receiving infliximab 5 mg/kg and 75/122 (61.5%) of patients receiving 10 mg/kg had a clinical response compared with 45/121 (37.2%) in the placebo group; $P < 0.001$ (Fig. 6.4). In ACT 2, 78/121 (64.5%) of patients receiving infliximab 5 mg/kg, 83/120 (69.2%) of

Table 6.1 Mayo scoring system for assessment of ulcerative colitis activity*

Stool frequency†
0: Normal number of stools for this patient 1: 1 to 2 stools more than normal 2: 3 to 4 stools more than normal 3: 5 or more stools more than normal Subscore, 0 to 3
Rectal bleeding‡
0: No blood seen 1: Streaks of blood with stool less than half the time 2: Obvious blood with stool most of the time 3: Blood alone passes Subscore, 0 to 3
Findings on endoscopy
0: Normal or inactive disease 1: Mild disease (erythema, decreased vascular pattern, mild friability) 2: Moderate disease (marked erythema, lack of vascular pattern, friability, erosions) 3: Severe disease (spontaneous bleeding, ulceration) Subscore, 0 to 3
Physician's global assessment§
0: Normal 1: Mild disease 2: Moderate disease 3: Severe disease Subscore, 0 to 3

*The Mayo score ranges from 0 to 12, higher scores indicating more severe disease.
†Each patient serves as his or her own control to establish the degree of abnormality of the stool frequency.
‡The daily bleeding score represents the most severe bleeding of the day.
§The physician's global assessment covers the three other criteria, the patient's daily recollection of abdominal discomfort and general sense of well-being, and other observations, such as physical findings and the patient's performance status.
Source: Rutgeerts *et al.* (2005).

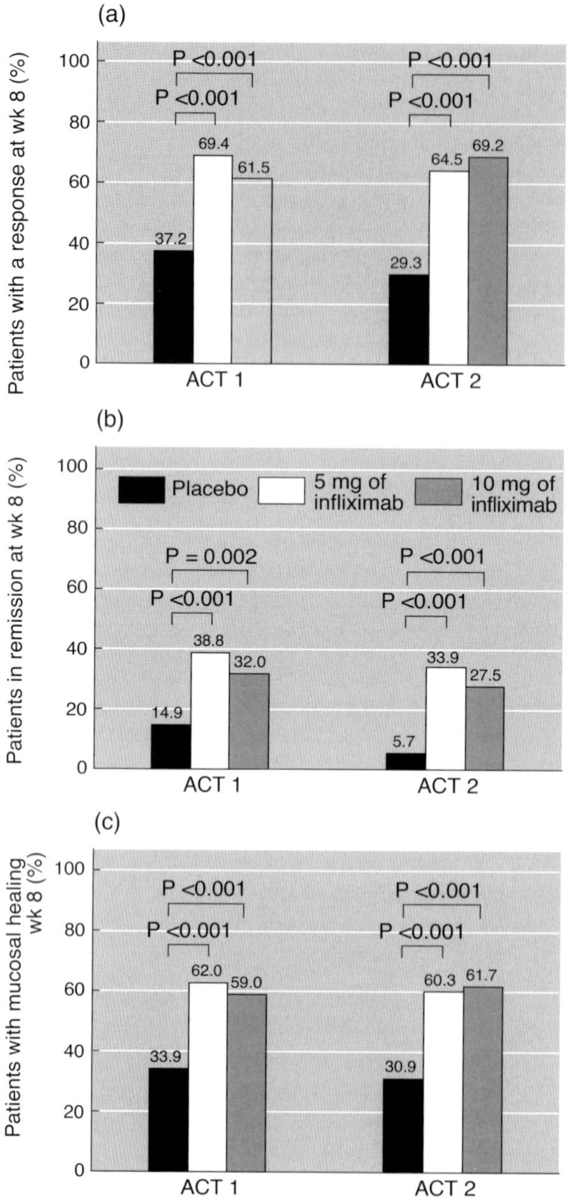

Fig. 6.4 Proportions of patients with a clinical response (a), in clinical remission (b) and with mucosal healing (c) at week 8 in ACT 1 and ACT 2. Source: Rutgeerts *et al.* (2005).

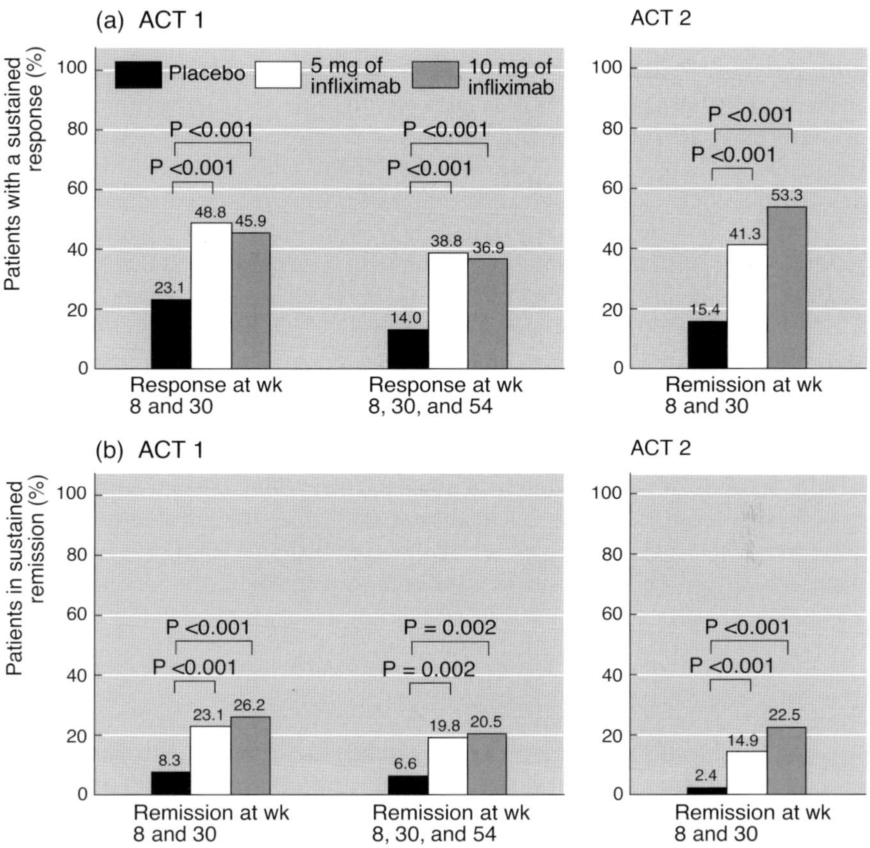

Fig. 6.5 Proportions of patients with a sustained clinical response (a) and in sustained clinical remission (b) in ACT 1 and ACT 2. Source: Rutgeerts *et al.* (2005).

patients receiving infliximab 10 mg/kg and 36/123 (29.3%) in the placebo group had a response (P <0.001). In both treatment groups, there were significantly more patients who achieved clinical remission, sustained response and mucosal healing and were able to discontinue steroids compared with placebo (Fig. 6.5). Side effects were uncommon; some were unlikely to have been associated with treatment, such as prostatic adenocarcinoma in a patient who had had an elevated prostate specific antigen (PSA) for 2 years, and a basal cell carcinoma. However, three neurological events occurred in patients on the treatment arm: one patient in ACT 1 receiving infliximab 5 mg/kg developed optic neuritis, one patient in ACT 2 receiving infliximab 5 mg/kg also developed optic neuritis, and after completion of ACT 2 one patient who had received infliximab 10 mg/kg developed multifocal motor neuropathy with conduction block syndrome. One patient receiving infliximab 10 mg/kg in ACT 1 developed tuberculosis and one patient in the extension treatment of ACT 2 who was receiving infliximab 5 mg/kg died from pulmonary complications of histoplasmosis.

Comment

Infliximab has had a significant impact in the treatment of patients with Crohn's disease, but until now its use in the treatment of ulcerative colitis patients has remained empirical, and frequently as 'a last resort' prior to deciding on colectomy. ACT 1 and ACT 2 have shown that infliximab is effective in the induction and maintenance of remission in ulcerative colitis patients with moderately to severely active disease. Whenever we use a medication, it is important to balance the pros and cons of each treatment; even though it was not statistically significant, it is difficult to ignore the fact that three patients had neurological events that have been associated with the use of TNF-α antibodies. These side effects are 'class-related' and not unique to infliximab, but it is important to remind patients that even though these side effects are rare, they are certainly a reality. The other note of caution is that even though there was no statistical difference in the number or septic events, a patient receiving infliximab died from pulmonary complications or histoplasmosis. We and others have reported that even though the number of infections is not increased in patients receiving infliximab compared with patients receiving other immunosuppressive medications, the infections appear to be more serious and a high index of suspicion is required to diagnose these infections early and treat them appropriately. Lastly, even though patients in this trial had severe disease, they were ambulatory patients and not patients who had failed treatment with oral steroids requiring hospitalization.

Infliximab as rescue therapy in severe to moderately severe ulcerative colitis: a randomized, placebo-controlled study

Järnerot G, Hertervig E, Friis-Liby I, *et al.* *Gastroenterology* 2005; **128**: 1805–11

BACKGROUND. Patients with severe ulcerative colitis require hospitalization and are treated with IV corticosteroids; in general, if there is no response after 4–5 days the options are to continue medical treatment with IV cyclosporine or with colectomy. The colectomy rate in patients with severe disease has been quoted as between 38 and 47%, patients with extensive disease have a higher colectomy rate, and patients with a moderately severe attack have a 20% colectomy rate [8]. Cyclosporine A has been used as rescue treatment in patients who have failed to respond to IV steroids, and a clinical trial comparing treatment with IV steroids and treatment with cyclosporine as the initial treatment in patients hospitalized with severe ulcerative colitis showed that it was effective and safe. However, there is significant morbidity with the use of cyclosporine A, and this treatment has not been universally accepted for patients with severe ulcerative colitis who fail on IV steroids [9,10].

INTERPRETATION. Patients with a severe or moderately severe attack of ulcerative colitis by the Seo index were admitted to hospital and treated with betamethasone 4 mg IV twice per day. Patients underwent the usual tests to exclude infectious aetiologies and also underwent a colonoscopy to determine the extent and severity of the disease

Table 6.2 Number of patients with colectomy during the first 90 days after infliximab/placebo treatment

Variable	Infliximab (colectomy/total)	Placebo (colectomy/total)	*P*-value (Fisher's exact test, 2-sided)
All patients	7/24 (29%)	14/21 (67%)	0.017
Inclusion based on fulminant colitis index	7/15 (47%)	9/13 (69%)	0.276
Seo index	0/9 (0%)	5/8 (62%)	0.009
Severe endoscopy	2/9 (22%)	4/6 (67%)	0.136
Moderately severe endoscopy	5/15 (33%)	10/15 (67%)	0.143

Source: Järnerot *et al.* (2005).

according to the Groupe d'Étude Thérapeutique des Affections Inflammatories Digestives (GETAID). On day 4 the fulminant colitis index was calculated, and if it was 8 or greater the patients were randomized to receive additional treatment with either infliximab 5 mg/kg or placebo. If the fulminant colitis index was below 8, patients continued with IV steroids alone and the Seo index was calculated daily for the previous day in the mornings of days 6, 7 and 8; if the index was above 150 on any of those days, patients were also randomized to receive additional treatment with either infliximab 5 mg/kg or placebo. Responders were discharged home on a regimen of prednisone 40 mg/day, tapering by 5 mg once per week, and a 5-ASA medication for maintenance; in some patients azathioprine was also started. These patients underwent repeat colonoscopy between days 10 and 14 and on days 30 and 90 after the infliximab or placebo infusion. During the first 90 days after randomization, a significantly greater number of patients in the placebo group underwent colectomy (14/21) compared with those who received infliximab (7/24; $P = 0.017$). The difference in colectomy rate in the patients who had a positive fulminant colitis index between those patients who received placebo and those who received infliximab did not reach statistical significance (69% in the placebo group and 47% in the infliximab group). When adjusting for treatment, the severity of inflammation on initial colonoscopy was not a predictor of outcome (Table 6.2).

Comment

This is a very valuable study. It shows that patients with moderately severe ulcerative colitis who fail to respond to IV steroids by day 4 have a good possibility of avoiding colectomy when infliximab is added to the regimen, but that infliximab should not be used as rescue treatment in patients with fulminant colitis. The timing of surgery in patients with severe colitis is very important—if a patient has a perforation before surgery the mortality rate is 50%.

Ornidazole for prophylaxis of post-operative Crohn's disease recurrence: a randomized, double-blind, placebo-controlled trial

Rutgeerts P, Van Assche GV, Vermeire S, *et al.* *Gastroenterology* 2005; **128**: 856–61

Background. Patients with Crohn's disease who undergo surgical resection have a significant risk of developing recurrent disease. Recurrence rates vary depending on whether endoscopic evidence of disease, clinical symptoms, or the need for further surgical resection is the measured end-point. Endoscopic recurrence rates as high as 93% within 1 year of surgery have been reported in some studies [11]. Reported rates of clinical recurrence after resection of all macroscopically diseased bowel with primary anastomosis are variable but range between 18 and 55% at 5 years and between 52 and 76% at 15 years [11]. When surgical recurrence rates are analysed, approximately 30% of patients will require subsequent resection within 10 years. Although the underlying pathophysiology of recurrent Crohn's disease is not well understood, there is some evidence that faecal stream and bowel continuity play an important aetiological role in this process. A previous study assessing the use of short-term metronidazole in the prevention of post-operative recurrence found a beneficial effect of metronidazole, but this was partially offset by a high rate of adverse effects [12]. In this study by the same investigators, ornidazole, another nitroimidazole antibiotic, which is thought to have fewer side effects than metronidazole, was studied in the post-operative setting as prophylaxis for Crohn's disease recurrence.

Interpretation. This was a randomized, double-blind, placebo-controlled trial to assess the efficacy of ornidazole in the prevention of post-operative recurrence of Crohn's disease. Eligible patients had just undergone surgical resection of all macroscopically involved bowel with anastomosis of the ileum to the colon and no diverting ileostomy. Eighty patients were randomized to receive either ornidazole 500 mg twice daily ($n = 40$, but two patients never started the drug) or an identical-appearing placebo ($n = 40$) for 54 weeks. Therapy was started within 1 week of surgery in 90% of subjects and within 2 weeks in all subjects. All other medications for Crohn's disease were discontinued. The primary end-point was clinical recurrence at 54 weeks and the secondary end-points were endoscopic recurrence at 3 and 12 months and radiographic recurrence at 12 months. Clinical recurrence at 2 and 3 years was also assessed. Results of the study are outlined in Table 6.3. Ornidazole therapy reduced the risk of clinical, endoscopic and radiographic recurrence 12 months after surgery. This benefit, however, lasted only while patients were on therapy, as demonstrated by the similar clinical recurrence rates in the two groups on longer-term follow-up. Side effects were significantly more common in the ornidazole-treated group than in the placebo group (68 vs 30%; $P = 0.0007$) and more patients discontinued therapy because of side effects in the ornidazole group than in the placebo group (32% vs 13%; $P = 0.041$).

Table 6.3 Recurrence rates for ornidazole and placebo groups

Recurrence	Ornidazole	Placebo	*P*-value	Odds ratio (95% CI)
Clinical				
12 months*	3/38 (8%)	15/40 (38%)	0.0046	0.14 (0.04–0.55)
24 months	11/37 (30%)	18/40 (45%)	0.17	–
36 months	17/37 (46%)	19/40 (48%)	0.53	–
Endoscopic				
3 months	11/32 (34%)	20/34 (59%)	0.047	0.37 (0.13–0.99)
12 months	12/28 (54%)	26/33 (79%)	0.037	0.31 (0.10–0.94)
Radiographic				
12 months	12/28 (43%)	21/28 (75%)	0.014	–

*Primary end-point.
CI, confidence interval.
Source: Rutgeerts *et al.* (2005).

Comment

On the basis of data regarding the impact of the faecal stream on post-operative recurrence, the use of post-operative antibiotics appears logical. The results of this study are similar to those of a previous shorter-term trial by the same group of investigators. In that study, 60 patients undergoing ileocolonic resection were randomized to treatment with metronidazole (20 mg/kg/day) or placebo within 1 week of surgery and treatment was continued for a total of 12 weeks **|12|**. Endoscopic recurrence rates at 3 months were 52% for metronidazole compared with 75% for placebo ($P = 0.09$), and clinical recurrence rates at 12 months were 4% for metronidazole versus 25% for placebo ($P = 0.046$). In both studies, the positive results were offset by prominent side effects related to the nitroimidazole antibiotics.

The results of this study are promising and lend support to the growing evidence for the potential role of enteric flora modulation in the treatment of inflammatory bowel disease. Potential limitations of prolonged antibiotic therapy include side effects and concerns about the development of bacterial resistance. Additional trials are needed to assess lower, more tolerable doses of nitroimidazole antibiotics as well as to evaluate alternative and perhaps better tolerated antibiotics.

A randomized, double-blind, controlled withdrawal trial in Crohn's disease patients on long-term remission on azathioprine

Lemann M, Mary JY, Colombel JF, *et al. Gastroenterology* 2005; **128**: 1812–18

BACKGROUND. Azathioprine and 6-mercaptopurine have been shown to be effective in the treatment of Crohn's disease. A meta-analysis of nine placebo-controlled trials of these agents in Crohn's disease revealed response rates for the induction of remission of 56% for the drug treatment versus 32% for placebo (odds ratio 3.09) and rates of maintenance of remission of 67% for drug treatment versus 53% for placebo (odds ratio 2.27) [13]. A question that comes up fairly frequently in clinical practice among patients who have had prolonged remission with azathioprine or 6-mercaptopurine is how long to continue therapy. Previous uncontrolled studies have suggested that the benefit of azathioprine may be sustained over many years and that relapse rates upon withdrawal of therapy may be as high as 40% within 1 year. The goal of this study was to perform a randomized controlled trial of azathioprine withdrawal among Crohn's disease patients who had had prolonged remission on this therapy.

INTERPRETATION. This study was a multicentre (France and Belgium), randomized, double-blind, non-inferiority withdrawal trial of patients with Crohn's disease who were in clinical remission induced by azathioprine for at least 42 months. The non-inferiority trial design tested the null hypothesis that ongoing treatment with azathioprine is superior to azathioprine withdrawal. Eighty-three patients were randomized to 18 months of double-blind therapy with either continued azathioprine (n = 43, but one patient never took the study medication) or placebo (n = 40). The primary end-point was the proportion of patients who experienced a clinical relapse, as assessed by the CDAI, over the 18-month period.

Baseline characteristics were similar in the two groups. Patients randomized to continued therapy had been on azathioprine for a mean of 64 months and had been in remission for a mean of 57 months compared with means of 67 months and 62 months respectively for the placebo group. Of note, the mean dose of azathioprine in both groups was 1.7 mg/kg, which is somewhat lower than the recommended dose of 2.0–2.5 mg/kg. At 18 months, relapse rates were 3/40 (mean relapse rate 7.9%) for the continued azathioprine group versus 9/43 (mean relapse rate 21.3%) for the placebo group, a difference of 13.4% between groups. Based on non-inferiority analysis, the upper limit of the one-sided 95% confidence interval for this difference does not lead to rejection of the null hypothesis, and thus the authors conclude that continued therapy with azathioprine is superior to withdrawal of therapy. Adverse events consisted of myelodysplastic syndrome developing and leading to death in one patient in the azathioprine group and a facial rash in one patient in the placebo group.

Comment

The results of this study demonstrate that continued azathioprine therapy among patients with prolonged remission leads to lower relapse rates over an 18-month follow-up period compared with withdrawal of azathioprine therapy. Interestingly, the relapse rate of 16.5% at 1 year after withdrawal (and 21.3% at 18 months) in this study was lower than the relapse rates of approximately 40% reported in previous uncontrolled or retrospective studies. This could be related partly to the fact that patients in this study were in a prolonged remission of at least 42 months prior to randomization. The difference between groups of 13.4% in relapse rates in this study has to be balanced against the unclear but probably small risk of long-term toxicity, including lymphoma, with azathioprine therapy.

Delayed-release oral mesalamine at 4.8 g/day (800 mg tablet) for the treatment of moderately active ulcerative colitis: the ASCEND II trial

Hanauer SB, Sandborn WJ, Kornbluth A, *et al. Am J Gastroenterol* 2005; **100**: 2478–85

BACKGROUND. Agents containing 5-ASA are first-line therapies for mildly to moderately active ulcerative colitis. Oral preparations consist of either mesalamine encapsulated in controlled release form, or as 5-ASA acid linked by an azo bond to sulphapyridine (sulphasalazine), an inert carrier (balsalazide) or to itself (olsalazine). All oral 5-ASA agents have been shown to be effective in the treatment of mild to moderate ulcerative colitis in dose-dependent fashion, with remission rates as high as 70–80%. The goal of this study was to determine whether initial treatment with a higher dose of mesalamine (4.8 g/day) would be more effective than the standard FDA-approved dose of 2.4 g/day in patients with moderately active ulcerative colitis. Patients in the higher-dose group received tablets containing 800 mg mesalamine, which are currently not available commercially, while those in the lower-dose group received the standard 400 mg tablets. The study was a multicentre trial from the USA and Canada, originally designed to study both mild and moderate ulcerative colitis. However, when the results of a parallel trial (ASCEND I) revealed no added benefit for higher-dose mesalamine in the mild ulcerative colitis subgroup, the inclusion criteria for this study, which had already begun, were modified to include only patients with moderately active ulcerative colitis.

INTERPRETATION. Three hundred and eighty-six patients were randomized, of whom 268 had moderate disease at baseline. Patients were randomly assigned to receive either 2.4 or 4.8 g/day of mesalamine for 6 weeks in double-blind fashion. The primary end-point was overall improvement (either complete remission or clinical response from baseline) at week 6, as assessed by stool frequency, rectal bleeding, the patient's functional assessment, endoscopy findings and the physician's global assessment. Secondary end-points were overall improvement at week 3, improvement from baseline in each of the clinical assessment subscores, overall improvement at week 6 in the subgroup with left-sided disease, time to normalization of stool frequency or to resolution of rectal bleeding, and change from baseline in the ulcerative colitis disease activity index (UCDAI). The primary analysis was based on intention to treat all patients with moderate disease who took at least one dose of medication and for whom treatment outcome could be determined (n = 254; 130 patients in the 2.4 g/day group and 124 patients in the 4.8 g/day group).

For the primary end-point at week 6, 59.2% of patients in the 2.4 g/day group compared with 71.8% of patients in the 4.8 g/day group were classified as having overall improvement (P = 0.036). Most of this difference related to the clinical response from baseline (41.5% in the 2.4 g/day group versus 51.6% in the 4.8 g/day group) and to a lesser extent to achievement of clinical remission (17.7 % in the 2.4 g/day group versus 20.2% in the 4.8 g/day group). Time to cessation of rectal bleeding was shorter in the 4.8 g/day group (9 days) than in the 2.4 g/day group (16 days; P = 0.035). For most of the other secondary end-points, there were numerical trends to better outcome in the 4.8 g/day group that did not achieve statistical significance. Analysis of the 110 patients with mild ulcerative colitis confirmed previous findings that the higher dose of 4.8 g/day did not provide added benefit over a dose of 2.4 g/day. The incidence of adverse events was similar for the two groups. There were two serious adverse events in the 2.4 g/day group (cholecystitis, pancreatitis) and one in the 4.8 g/day group (pericarditis).

Comment

The results of this study validate what many clinicians who treat a lot of patients with ulcerative colitis already do in practice: use higher than the label-recommended doses of mesalamine to induce remission in patients with moderately active ulcerative colitis. On the basis of the results of this study, the authors suggest that patients with mildly active ulcerative colitis (fewer than four bowel movements per day with or without blood) can be treated with an initial mesalamine dose of 2.4 g/day, while those with moderately active disease (more than four bowel movements per day and no evidence of systemic toxicity) should be treated with an initial dose of 4.8 g/day. These recommendations certainly make sense and can be easily applied to daily practice. In addition, dosing will be facilitated and adherence hopefully improved once the 800 mg tablets are approved and available for routine clinical use; patients will only need to take six pills per day instead of the current twelve to get a dose of 4.8 g/day.

Trichuris suis **therapy for active ulcerative colitis: a randomized controlled trial**

Summers RW, Elliott DE, Urban JF Jr, Thompson RA, Weinstock JV.
Gastroenterology 2005; **128**: 825–32

BACKGROUND. It has long been known that there are geographic differences in the prevalence of inflammatory bowel disease. The high rate of helminth colonization in developing countries has been suggested as a potential explanation for the relative infrequency of inflammatory bowel disease in these countries. Potential benefits from helminth colonization could include down-modulation of the host immune response and

reduction of inflammation, as demonstrated in experimental mouse models of colitis. This study is a follow-up to successful open-label studies in which *Trichuris suis*, the pig whipworm, was shown to be effective therapy for both ulcerative colitis and Crohn's disease |14,15|.

INTERPRETATION. The study was a double-blind, placebo-controlled trial of *T. suis* ovum therapy in 54 adult patients with active ulcerative colitis, as assessed by the UCDAI. The primary end-point was clinical improvement at 12 weeks, defined as a decrease in the UCDAI by at least 4 points. The secondary end-point was clinical remission, defined as an UCDAI of 2 or less. Baseline characteristics among the two groups were similar. Of note, 59% of patients randomized to placebo and 46% of those randomized to *T. suis* therapy were on corticosteroids and/or azathioprine/ 6-mercpatopurine at study entry. Based on an intention-to-treat analysis, 43.3% of *T. suis*-treated patients versus 16.7% of the placebo group achieved the primary end-point of clinical improvement at 12 weeks ($P = 0.04$). There was no statistically significant difference in the number of patients who achieved clinical remission (10% of *T. suis*-treated patients versus 4% of the placebo group). On *post hoc* analysis of the individual components of the UCDAI, patients in the *T. suis* group had significant improvements from baseline for all the components (stool frequency, blood in stool, endoscopic appearance, and physician's overall assessment), whereas patients in the placebo group had improvement only in the stool frequency component. Furthermore, overall decreases in the mean UCDAI from baseline to 12 weeks were from 8.77 ± 0.35 to 6.1 ± 0.61 ($P = 0.0004$) for the *T. suis* group and from 8.75 ± 0.46 to 7.5 ± 0.66 ($P = 0.12$) for the placebo group. No side effects attributable to the study agent were noted and no worms or ova were detected in stools 2 weeks after each dose of *T. suis*.

Comment

The results of this study demonstrate that *T. suis* therapy can lead to improvement in clinical symptoms and endoscopic appearance in patients with ulcerative colitis. Of note, however, the mean UCDAI score at the end of the study in the treatment group was still relatively high (6.1) and rates of remission were not different between groups. Importantly, 59% of patients randomized to placebo and 46% of those randomized to *T. suis* therapy were on corticosteroids and/or azathioprine/ 6-mercpatopurine at study entry, with ongoing active symptoms of disease.

Overall, these results are interesting and suggest some benefit for this therapy. Additional trials with larger numbers of patients and assessment of different dosing regimens are needed. Further studies will also help address the issue of safety, especially in terms of whether treatment with *T. suis* could lead to infection in humans. The authors do note that there has been no evidence for this among over 100 patients they have treated with this agent over the past several years.

Impact of the increasing use of immunosuppressants in Crohn's disease on the need for intestinal surgery

Cosnes J, Nion-Larmurier I, Beaugerie L, Afchain P, Tiret E, Gendre JP. *Gut* 2005; **54**: 237–41

BACKGROUND. Long-term medical therapy remains a mainstay for patients with ulcerative colitis or Crohn's disease, because of the chronic inflammatory nature of these diseases. As our understanding of the pathogenesis of inflammatory bowel disease has expanded, so have therapeutic options targeted to different components of the inflammatory cascade. Most recently, biological agents have been developed to target very specific parts of the inflammatory pathways. With better therapies available, one would expect to be able to influence the natural history of disease, especially by avoiding surgery. In this study, the authors reviewed the experience of a referral group in France with the aim of evaluating the effect of the increasing use of immunosuppressants on the need for surgical resection in patients with Crohn's disease.

INTERPRETATION. Patients seen over a 25-year period were divided into two groups: those seen at the unit within the first 3 months after diagnosis (group 1; $n = 565$) and those seen more than 3 months after diagnosis (group 2; $n = 2008$). Within each group, patients were also divided into five consecutive 5-year cohorts according to their date of diagnosis: 1978–1982; 1983–1987; 1988–1992; 1993–1997; and 1998–2002. The main outcome evaluated was the time to first intestinal resection (surgery for stricturoplasty, bypass and elective treatment of abscess were not considered). The typical use of immunosuppressants consisted of: (i) azathioprine at 2 mg/kg for maintenance therapy for patients with steroid-dependent or poorly steroid-responsive disease, the dose being escalated to 2.5–3.0 mg/kg in case of repeated flare-ups; (ii) methotrexate 20–25 mg IM weekly for patients unresponsive or intolerant to azathioprine, the dose being tapered to 10–15 mg if the clinical course allowed; and (iii) infliximab after June 1999 at 5 mg/kg IV for steroid-refractory disease.

In group 1, immunosuppressants were used earlier and more frequently, with a 5-year cumulative probability for use of 0 in the 1978–1982 cohort versus 0.56 in the 1998–2002 cohort (Fig. 6.6). Despite this change in medical therapy, the cumulative rate of surgery was not different across the different time cohorts (Fig. 6.7). The indications for surgery also did not change significantly, except for the fact that a 'failure of medical treatment' indication was less common in the 1998–2002 cohort compared with the other four cohorts (13 vs 22–38%). It is important to note that when the authors analysed the time relation between the prescription of immunosuppressant and first surgery, they found that most patients in all cohorts were operated on without having first received immunosuppressants because surgery was done within 3 months of diagnosis (43% of cases) or had been on immunosuppressants for less than 3 months prior to surgery (49% of cases). Only 16 patients from group 1 (9%) had to be operated on after having received immunosuppressants for more than 3 months. Findings for group 2 were similar to those described above.

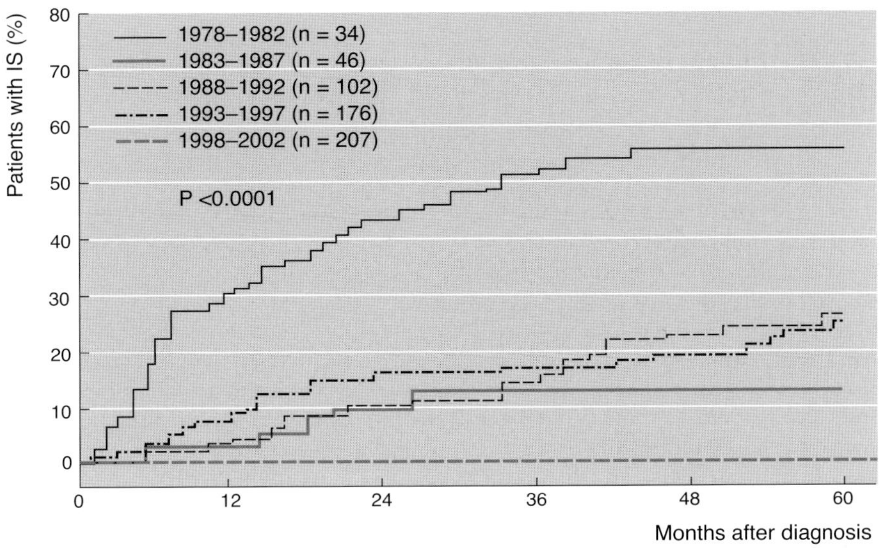

Fig. 6.6 Kaplan–Meier estimates of the cumulative risk of receiving immunosuppressants in five chronological cohorts of patients with Crohn's disease. Source: Cosnes *et al.* (2005).

Comment

In this study, the authors find that, although the use of immunosuppressants increased over the 25-year cohort period, the rate of surgery did not change. This finding is of interest as it suggests that our therapies may not affect the need for first surgery. However, these results need to be interpreted with some caution as most of the patients (92%) who went to first surgery were either not on immunosuppressants or were on them for less than 3 months prior to surgery. This could suggest that the medications were started too late to prevent first surgery. In addition, only 25 patients in group 1 required a second surgery over the 25-year follow-up period compared with 165 patients who needed an initial surgery. Putting together the findings of increased use of immunosuppressants over time and the fact that most people were started on these medications after first resection surgery, one could ask whether these medications are indeed having an impact on the prevention of second surgery.

Conclusion

In this chapter we have summarized the results of recent important therapeutic studies in inflammatory bowel disease. To summarize our review, we will categorize the studies based on therapy of Crohn's disease or ulcerative colitis.

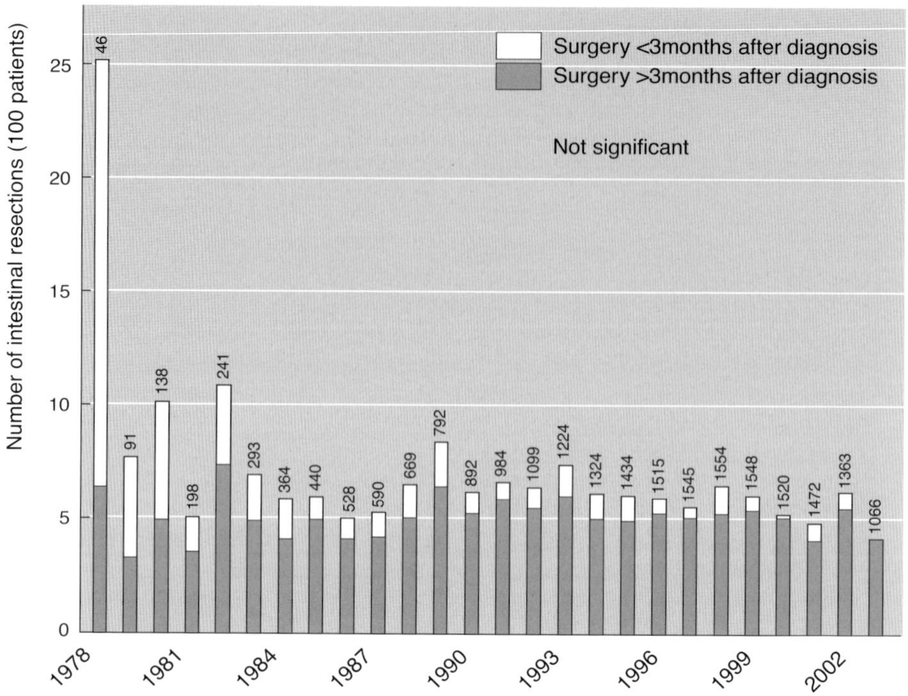

Fig. 6.7 Evolution of the annual rate of intestinal resections from 1978 to 2003 in 2573 patients with Crohn's disease. The numbers above the columns indicate the number of patients at risk of intestinal resection at the beginning of the year. Source: Cosnes *et al.* (2005).

Crohn's disease

1. In a placebo-controlled trial, treatment with granulocyte–macrophage colony stimulating factor did significantly better than treatment with placebo when evaluated by the secondary end-points of a decrease in the CDAI of at least 100 points, clinical remission, improvement in quality of life, and improvement in mucosal healing.
2. In a pilot study evaluating 12 patients with severely active Crohn's disease, autologous stem cell transplantation led to significant improvement. Until further studies are available, such therapy should be reserved for patients with malignant Crohn's disease and should be done in tertiary care centres.
3. In a retrospective analysis of 15 patients with Crohn's disease who had lost their response to infliximab in spite of increasing the dose to 10 mg/kg IV every 8 weeks, adalimumab was shown to lead to complete response in 54% and partial response in 31%, with a mean time to response of 5.3 ± 3 weeks.

4. In a placebo-controlled trial, ornidazole therapy reduced the risk of clinical, endoscopic and radiographic recurrence of Crohn's disease following surgical resection. This benefit, however, lasted only while patients were on therapy and was partially offset by frequent side effects.
5. In a placebo-controlled withdrawal study in Crohn's disease patients with prolonged remission, continued therapy with azathioprine led to lower relapse rates over an 18-month follow-up period compared with withdrawal of azathioprine therapy.

Ulcerative colitis

1. ACT 1 and ACT 2 have shown that infliximab is effective in the induction and maintenance of remission in ulcerative colitis outpatients with moderately to severely active disease.
2. Inpatients with moderately severe ulcerative colitis and who fail to respond to 4 days of IV steroids have a good chance of avoiding colectomy if treated with infliximab. However, infliximab should not be used as rescue treatment in patients with fulminant colitis.
3. Patients with mildly active ulcerative colitis (fewer than four bowel movements per day with or without blood) can be treated with an initial mesalamine dose of 2.4 g/day while those with moderately active disease (greater than four bowel movements per day and no evidence of systemic toxicity) should be treated with an initial dose of 4.8 g/day.
4. Treatment with *Trichuris suis*, the pig whipworm, led to improvement in clinical symptoms and endoscopic appearance in patients with ulcerative colitis but did not affect the achievement of remission.

References

1. Ogura Y, Bonen DK, Inohara N, Nicolae DL, Chen FF, Ramos R, Britton H, Moran T, Karaliuskas R, Duerr RH, Achkar JP, Brant SR, Bayless TM, Kirschner BS, Hanauer SB, Nunez G, Cho JH. A frameshift mutation in NOD2 associated with susceptibility to Crohn's disease. *Nature* 2001; **411**: 603–6.
2. Dieckgraefe BK, Korzenik JR. Treatment of active Crohn's disease with recombinant human granulocyte–macrophage colony-stimulating factor. *Lancet* 2002; **360**: 1478–80.
3. Rutgeerts P, D'Haens G, Targan S, Vasiliauskas E, Hanauer SB, Present DH, Mayer L, Van Hogezand RA, Braakman T, DeWoody KL, Schaible TF, Van Deventer SJ. Efficacy and safety of retreatment with anti-tumor necrosis factor antibody (infliximab) to maintain remission in Crohn's disease. *Gastroenterology* 1999; **117**: 761–9.

4. Hanauer SB, Feagan BG, Lichtenstein GR, Mayer LF, Schreiber S, Colombel JF, Rachmilewitz D, Wolf DC, Olson A, Bao W, Rutgeerts P; ACCENT I Study Group. Maintenance infliximab for Crohn's disease: the ACCENT I randomized trial. *Lancet* 2002; **359**: 1541–9.

5. Hanauer SB, Wagner CL, Bala M, Mayer L, Travers S, Diamond RH, Olson A, Bao W, Rutgeerts P. Incidence and importance of antibody responses to infliximab after maintenance or episodic treatment in Crohn's disease. *Clin Gastroenterol Hepatol* 2004; **2**: 542–53.

6. Sandborn WJ, Hanauer S, Loftus EV Jr, Tremaine WJ, Kane S, Cohen R, Hanson K, Johnson T, Schmitt D, Jeche R. An open l-label study of the human anti-TNF monoclonal antibody adalimumab in subjects with prior loss of response or intolerance to infliximab for Crohn's disease. *Am J Gastroenterol* 2004; **99**: 1984–9.

7. Sandborn W, Hanauer S, Lucas M, Wolf DC, Isaacs KL, MacIntosh DG, Panaccione R, Rutgeerts P, Pollack PF. Induction and maintenance of clinical remission and response in subjects with Crohn's disease treated during a 6-month open-label period with fully human anti-TNF-alpha monoclonal antibody adalimumab (Humira). *Gastroenterology* 2005; **128**: A111–12.

8. Järnerot G, Rolny P, Sandberg-Gertzén H. Intensive intravenous treatment of ulcerative colitis. *Gastroenterology* 1985; **89**: 1005–13.

9. Lichtiger S, Present DH, Kornbluth A, Gelernt I, Bauer J, Galler G, Michelassi F, Hanauer S. Cyclosporine in severe ulcerative colitis refractory to steroid therapy. *N Engl J Med* 1994; **330**: 1841–5.

10. Sandborn WJ. A critical review of cyclosporine therapy in inflammatory bowel disease. *Inflamm Bowel Dis* 1995; **1**: 48–63.

11. Achkar JP, Hanauer SB. Medical therapy to reduce post-operative Crohn's disease recurrence. *Am J Gastroenterol* 2000; **95**: 1139–46.

12. Rutgeerts P, Hiele M, Geboes K, Peeters M, Penninckx F, Aerts R, Kerremans R. Controlled trial of metronidazole treatment for prevention of Crohn's recurrence after ileal resection. *Gastroenterology* 1995; **108**: 1617–21.

13. Pearson DC, May GR, Fick GH, Sutherland LR. Azathioprine and 6-mercaptopurine in Crohn's disease. A meta-analysis. *Ann Intern Med* 1995; **122**: 132–4.

14. Summers RW, Elliott DE, Qadir K, Urban JF Jr, Thompson R, Weinstock JV. *Trichuris suis* appears safe and effective in the treatment of inflammatory bowel disease: a possible example of Th2 conditioning of the mucosal immune response. *Am J Gastroenterol* 2003; **98**: 2034–41.

15. Summers RW, Elliott DE, Urban JF Jr, Thompson R, Weinstock JV. *Trichuris suis* therapy in Crohn's disease. *Gut* 2005; **54**: 87–90.

7

Inflammatory bowel disease in children

ROBERT WYLLIE, MARSHA KAY

Introduction

There have been significant advances in our knowledge of the genetics of inflammatory bowel disease (IBD) in the last 5 years. A number of known mutations and a growing list of putative mutations have been reported since the initial association of the *NOD2* gene on chromosome 16, now designated *CARD15*, with Crohn's disease in 2001 [**1,2**]. The most common Crohn's disease-associated polymorphisms in the *CARD15* gene are two missense mutations (R702W, G908R) and one frame-shifting cytosine insertion, 3020insC (also known as Leu1007- fsinsC), encoding truncated *CARD15* [**2,3**]. It is believed that the *CARD15* gene product confers susceptibility to Crohn's disease by altering the intracellular recognition of microbial pathogens or by altering activation of nuclear factor κB (NF-κB) in monocytes [**1,2**]. These mutations may result in increased susceptibility of the intestinal epithelium to bacterial invasion [**4**]. *CARD15* may also be important in the regulation of defensin expression [**3**]. The presence of a single *CARD15* variant increases susceptibility to Crohn's disease by 2–3 times, and two mutant genes (in the homozygous or compound heterozygous state) increase susceptibility 28–40 times [**4**]. Other, rarer *CARD15* mutations also may be associated with Crohn's disease, especially in European patients [**4**].

Studies confirm that paediatric patients with IBD have both a high frequency (12–38%) and a higher likelihood of having a family member with IBD than adults [**5–7**]. The most recent data suggest that there are at least nine IBD susceptibility loci (*IBD1–9*) and that *CARD15/NOD2* is the Crohn's disease susceptibility gene at the *IBD1* locus [**3,8**]. The most common *CARD15* mutations appear to be phenotypically relevant as they are associated with earlier onset of disease, increased frequency of ileal involvement, and possibly with more aggressive stricturing disease, although the data are conflicting [**3,5,8–10**]. A recent paediatric study in primarily Jewish patients found that the specific G908R mutation was the mutation most likely to be associated with ileal disease [**10**]. Another study suggests that paediatric patients with Crohn's disease and mutations of *CARD15* may have a trend towards a more severe course (higher Pediatric Crohn's Disease Activity Index

[PCDAI], long-term and intermittent steroid use, the need for supplementary feeding and the use of tumour necrosis factor α [TNF-α] antagonist), although a number of these outcome variables did not reach statistical significance [8].

The frequency of *CARD* mutations in paediatric patients also differs among different ethnic groups. *CARD15* mutations may be found in 26–52% of Caucasian paediatric patients with Crohn's disease, the highest rates being found in patients of Ashkenazi Jewish descent, but in only 1.6% of African-American and 2.2% of Hispanic children with Crohn's disease respectively [5,9–11]. *CARD15* mutations were found in the USA in 9.1, 2.1 and 4.4% of newborn Caucasian, African-American and Hispanic controls respectively [11].

CARD15 mutations have also been found at a higher but not statistically significant rate in paediatric patients with ulcerative colitis compared with paediatric controls (12 vs 5%) [9]. Therefore, although these *CARD15* mutations may be important in Caucasian children with IBD, especially Crohn's disease, their contribution in non-Caucasian children remains to be determined and other genetic factors may play a role.

Polymorphisms of the TNF-α promoter gene located on chromosome 6 have been found to be associated with IBD, and may alter disease phenotype or activity. In paediatric patients, one polymorphism of the TNF-α promoter gene, 863A, appears to be positively associated with isolated colonic Crohn's disease and negatively associated with ileal disease. The effect of TNF-α promoter 863A on disease location in one series was comparable to the joint effect of the three primary *CARD15* mutations [10]. The presence of TNF-α promoter gene 863A also appears to be significantly associated with having a first-degree relative with Crohn's disease [10]. The TNF-α 863A polymorphism is associated with decreased TNF transcription, which may impair the local response to colonic bacteria [10].

Environmental exposures in early life have been implicated in the development of IBD in susceptible individuals. In an evaluation of 140 variables in 222 children with Crohn's disease and 60 with ulcerative colitis, Baron *et al.* [12] demonstrated that an increased risk of Crohn's disease was associated with a family history of IBD, breast-feeding, vaccination with bacillus Calmette-Guerin or a history of eczema. Increased risk factors for the development of ulcerative colitis included a family history of IBD, disease during pregnancy and the sharing of a bedroom. Identified protective factors for ulcerative colitis were appendectomy, and regular drinking of tap water for Crohn's disease [12]. A family history with early-onset ulcerative colitis may be especially common [6]. In family clusters of Crohn's disease, risk factors for the development of the disease included exposure to cigarette smoke, diets with less oats, rye and bran or more unpasteurized cheese and well water [13].

Limited data are available regarding the epidemiology of IBD in paediatric patients. Ulcerative colitis and Crohn's disease presenting before the age of 20 years account for 25–30% of all patients with IBD [14]. In paediatric patients, Crohn's disease is more common than ulcerative colitis, especially in older paediatric patients. This represents a change from the past, when the two diseases were thought to be more similar in distribution [6,7,15,16]. Incidence rates of paediatric

Crohn's disease range from 1.2 to 4.9 per 100 000 and those of paediatric ulcerative colitis range from 0.57 to 2.2 per 100 000 [7]. However, some series document similar incidence rates and it appears that incidence and prevalence rates vary significantly with geographic location, ethnic background and age at diagnosis [6,17]. The incidence rates and prevalence rates of IBD are both increasing in paediatric patients [7]. Indeterminate colitis accounts for a significant fraction of paediatric IBD, the rates in some series approaching 12–24% [6]. Most cases of indeterminate colitis in paediatric patients can ultimately be classified as Crohn's disease or ulcerative colitis. Children less than 8 years old at the time of diagnosis are significantly more likely to be diagnosed as having ulcerative colitis or indeterminate colitis compared with those older than 8 years [6].

The diagnosis of IBD in children depends on a constellation of compatible symptoms and laboratory, endoscopic and radiological findings. Improved diagnostic methods include routine ileal intubation and biopsy at the time of colonoscopy, the introduction of wireless capsule endoscopy, small-bowel enterography and abdominal magnetic resonance imaging (MRI). In a study in which gadolinium-enhanced MRI with oral opacification using 5% mannitol solution was compared with endoscopy and ultrasound, MRI demonstrated a sensitivity of 83% and specificity of 100%. This non-invasive technique may be useful as a first-line diagnostic modality, particularly in young patients with suspected IBD [18].

Ileocolonic disease continues to be the most frequent presentation of Crohn's disease in paediatric patients (43–71%); the next most common presentations are isolated colonic disease and isolated ileal disease [7,10,11]. A higher prevalence of isolated colonic Crohn's disease has been found in young children [6]. The expression of disease in the ileum in Crohn's disease may be an age-related phenomenon. In a retrospective review of French and Swedish children presenting with Crohn's disease, the likelihood of finding ileal disease was age-related, the incidence rates per 100 000 population ranging from 0.19 at 8 years up to 0.61 at 16 years of age. This may reflect the development of Peyer's patches, which grow in size and number until puberty, when they undergo involution [19]. Inflammatory disease rather than stricturing or fistulizing disease appears to be the most common presentation of Crohn's disease in the paediatric age group, but this finding is not consistent in all studies [5,11]. Crohn's disease appears to be phenotypically similar in Caucasian, African-American and Hispanic children in the USA [11]. Most paediatric patients with ulcerative colitis are found to have left-sided or pan-colitis if a full colonoscopy is performed at the time of diagnosis. Isolated proctitis appears to be relatively uncommon in young children with ulcerative colitis but accounts for approximately 12% of ulcerative colitis cases in older children [6,7].

The treatment of IBD in infants and children presents special challenges. The goals of therapy are to achieve and maintain remission while promoting growth and normal social development. A number of medical therapies have been used to help induce remission, including 5-aminosalicylates and corticosteroids. More recently, immune modulators, including azathioprine, 6-mercaptopurine and methotrexate, have been used to maintain remission. Traditionally, methotrexate has been given by subcutaneous injection, which is a particularly challenging mode of administration in children. Recently, however, the bioavailability of oral methotrexate has been found to be similar to that of subcutaneous methotrexate in children with Crohn's disease [20]. Side effects of immune modulators are related to underlying drug metabolism. The side effects, but not the efficacy, of methotrexate have been associated with a single mutation in the *MTHFR* gene [21].

Biological agents, particularly inhibitors of TNF, such as infliximab, have had a significant impact on the quality of life of children with IBD. Infusion reactions and possible long-term complications remain a concern for most families. The use of infliximab during pregnancy has not been evaluated rigorously but its use following conception has not been associated with fetal abnormalities and it seems to enhance the mother's ability to maintain remission during gestation [22]. Premedication (typically antipyretics, antihistamines or corticosteroids) does not seem to prevent the development of infusion reactions but may be useful in preventing subsequent infusion reactions in children. Infliximab is typically used for children with Crohn's disease but may also be useful in young people with moderate to severe ulcerative colitis [23].

Families are usually anxious to avoid 'drugs', and probiotic therapies are widely used by families of children with IBD. In a recent randomized double-blind trial of Lactobacillus GG versus placebo, in addition to standard therapies, in children in remission with Crohn's disease, the use of Lactobacillus GG did not prolong time to relapse [24].

Growth failure is a common complication in children with Crohn's disease. Fifteen to forty per cent of children have growth retardation at the time of diagnosis and abnormal growth velocity may occur in up to 90% of teenagers. The aetiology of growth failure is multifactorial, and includes inadequate calorie intake, loss via malabsorption and the increased energy burden associated with chronic inflammation. Anorexia may be out of proportion to the severity of disease symptoms, including abdominal pain and diarrhoea. Basal and stimulated growth hormone levels are typically normal but insulin-like growth factor may be reduced. Intestinal inflammation associated growth failure may be mediated by the level of interleukin 6 (IL-6), which is determined by the IL-6-174 polymorphism [25]. Growth failure may be complicated by the prolonged use of corticosteroids, and treatment protocols in children centre around diminishing the use of growth suppressive drugs. Burnham *et al.* studied body composition and demonstrated lower height and body mass index for age in children with Crohn's disease compared with age-matched controls, and deficits in lean body mass [26].

There are few prospective studies examining the effects of different interventions for growth failure. Three randomized controlled trials [27] have been performed looking at interventions that would promote growth or assist in the reversal of growth failure. The use of 6-mercaptopurine as a steroid-sparing agent in a placebo-controlled trial was evaluated over an 18-month interval in children receiving steroids for the control of Crohn's disease. Although the total dose of steroids was reduced in the group receiving 6-mercaptopurine, there was no difference in linear growth. Two other trials evaluated the use of enteral nutrition versus steroids using the height velocity standard deviation at 6 months as an outcome measure. Both trials demonstrated improved height velocity in the enteral feeding group compared with the control group receiving corticosteroid treatment. A comparison of exclusive polymeric enteral nutrition therapy in 65 children with Crohn's disease demonstrated improvement after treatment only in children with evidence of ileal or ileocolonic disease. Those with isolated colonic disease did not improve [28]. The mechanism of action leading to improvement in children with IBD on polymeric enteral nutrition may be a change in the gut microflora [29] or reductions in the levels of inflammatory cytokines [30]. Evaluation of the actual energy requirement may be helpful before enteral therapy is begun [31] and there may be some synergy between immunosuppressive therapy and enteral nutrition in the management of children with Crohn's disease. Data concerning the use of growth hormone are limited, but at this time it does not appear to be of benefit [32]. The effect of newer biological therapies on growth has not been fully evaluated.

Bone health is a significant concern in children with IBD. Osteopenia may arise from inadequate calcium and vitamin D intake, excessive proinflammatory cytokine production, prolonged use of corticosteroids and physical inactivity. Recent studies have documented bone density abnormalities in newly diagnosed steroid-naive children [33]. Initial steps towards prevention and therapy involve increasing dietary calcium intake. Behavioural intervention programmes may enhance compliance with dietary supplementation [34].

Surgical intervention, particularly restorative proctocolectomy with ileal pouch–anal anastomosis, has become the surgical procedure of choice for children with ulcerative colitis. In a long-term evaluation of 140 children with ulcerative colitis, most of the children (61%) had one or more episodes of pouchitis. The median number of bowel movements per day was six and 95% of children were satisfied with the result of the operation [35]. Similar but shorter-term results were reported from Denmark [36].

Children with IBD face a variety of psychosocial challenges resulting from the symptoms and diagnosis of a chronic illness. One of the problems identified in adolescent males with IBD is with self-esteem [37], but children with mild IBD symptoms diagnosed for at least 1 year typically report normal psychosocial functioning [38]. Attending a camp may help children adjust to their chronic illness and increase social functioning [39]. Parents may also benefit from a holistic family approach to the disease process [40]. The treatment of IBD remains challenging in children but recent advances in medical and nutritional management have enhanced the quality of life and prognosis of our youngest patients. Hope for the future lies in further understanding of the genetics of IBD and how different mutations may affect the severity of the disease and the response to therapy.

References

1. Hugot JP, Chamaillard M, Zouali H, Lesage S, Cezard JP, Belaiche J, Almer S, Tysk C, O'Morain CA, Gassull M, Binder V, Finkel Y, Cortot A, Modigliani R, Laurent-Puig P, Gower-Rousseau C, Macry J, Colombel JF, Sahbatou M, Thomas G. Association of NOD2 leucine-rich repeat variants with susceptibility to Crohn's disease. *Nature* 2001; **411**: 599–603.
2. Ogura Y, Bonen DK, Inohara N, Nicolae DL, Chen FF, Ramos R, Britton H, Moran T, Karaliuskas R, Duerr RH, Achkar JP, Brant SR, Bayless TM, Kirschner BS, Hanauer SB, Nunez G, Cho JH. A frameshift mutation in NOD2 associated with susceptibility to Crohn's disease. *Nature* 2001; **411**: 603–6.
3. Newman B, Siminovitch KA. Recent advances in the genetics of inflammatory bowel disease. *Curr Opin Gastroenterol* 2005; **21**: 401–7.
4. Russell RK, Nimmo ER, Satsangi J. Molecular genetics of Crohn's disease. *Curr Opin Genet Dev* 2004; **14**: 264–70.
5. Weiss B, Shamir R, Bujanover Y, Waterman M, Hartman C, Fradkin A, Berkowitz D, Weintraub I, Eliakim R, Karban A. NOD2/CARD15 mutation analysis and genotype–phenotype correlation in Jewish pediatric patients compared with adults with Crohn's disease. *J Pediatr* 2004; **145**: 208–12.
6. Heyman MB, Kirschner BS, Gold BD, Ferry G, Baldassano R, Cohen SA, Winter HS, Fain P, King C, Smith T, El-Serag HB. Children with early-onset inflammatory bowel disease (IBD): analysis of a pediatric IBD consortium registry. *J Pediatr* 2005; **146**: 35–40.
7. Auvin S, Molinie F, Gower-Rousseau C, Brazier F, Merle V, Grandbastien B, Marti R, Lerebours E, Dupas JL, Colombel JF, Salomez JL, Cortot A, Turck D. Incidence, clinical presentation and location at diagnosis of pediatric inflammatory bowel disease: a prospective population-based study in northern France (1988–1999). *J Pediatr Gastroenterol Nutr* 2005; **41**: 49–55.
8. Roesler J, Thurigen A, Sun L, Koch R, Winkler U, Laass MW, Gahr M, Rosen-Wolff A, Henker J. Influence of CARD15 mutations on disease activity and response to therapy in 65 pediatric Crohn patients from Saxony, Germany. *J Pediatr Gastroenterol Nutr* 2005; **41**: 27–32.
9. Ferraris A, Knafelz D, Torres B, Fortina P, Castro M, Dallapiccola B. Analysis of CARD15 gene variants in Italian pediatric patients with inflammatory bowel diseases. *J Pediatr* 2005; **147**: 272–3.
10. Levine A, Karban A, Eliakim R, Shaoul R, Reif S, Pacht A, Wardi J, Yakir B, Silver EL. A polymorphism in the TNF-alpha promoter gene is associated with pediatric onset and colonic location of Crohn's disease. *Am J Gastroenterol* 2005; **100**: 407–13.
11. Kugathasan S, Loizides A, Babusukumar U, McGuire E, Wang T, Hooper P, Nebel J, Kofman G, Noel R, Broeckel U, Tolia V. Comparative phenotypic and CARD15

mutational analysis among African American, Hispanic, and White children with Crohn's disease. *Inflamm Bowel Dis* 2005; **11**: 631–8.

12. Baron S, Turck D, Leplat C, Merle V, Gower-Rousseau C, Marti R, Yzet T, Lerebours E, Dupas JL, Debeugny S, Salomez JL, Cortot A, Colombel JF. Environmental risk factors in paediatric inflammatory bowel diseases: a population based case control study. *Gut* 2005; **54**: 357–63.
13. Van Kruiningen HJ, Joossens M, Vermeire S, Joossens S, Debeugny S, Gower-Rousseau C, Cortot A, Colombel JF, Rutgeerts P, Vlietinck R. Environmental factors in familial Crohn's disease in Belgium. *Inflamm Bowel Dis* 2005; **11**: 360–5.
14. IBD Working Group of the European Society for Paediatric Gastroenterology, Hepatology and Nutrition. Inflammatory bowel disease in children and adolescents: recommendations for diagnosis—the Porto criteria. *J Pediatr Gastroenterol Nutr* 2005; **41**: 1–7.
15. Farmer RG, Michener WM, Mortimer EA. Studies of family history among patients with inflammatory bowel disease. *Clin Gastroenterol* 1980; **9**: 271–7.
16. Moyer MS. A collaborative effort to define the epidemiology of pediatric inflammatory bowel disease: what can we learn from children with early-onset disease? *J Pediatr* 2005; **146**: 7–8.
17. Oliva-Hemker M, Fiocchi C. Etiopathogenesis of inflammatory bowel disease: the importance of the pediatric perspective. *Inflamm Bowel Dis* 2002; **8**: 112–28.
18. Pilleul F, Godefroy C, Yzebe-Beziat D, Dugougeat-Pilleul F, Lachaux A, Valette PJ. Magnetic resonance imaging in Crohn's disease. *Gastroenterol Clin Biol* 2005; **29**: 803–8.
19. Meinzer U, Idestrom M, Alberti C, Peuchmaur M, Belarbi N, Bellaiche M, Mougenot JF, Cezard JP, Finkel Y, Hugot JP. Ileal involvement is age dependent in pediatric Crohn's disease. *Inflamm Bowel Dis* 2005; **11**: 639–44.
20. Griffiths DM. The physiology of continence: idiopathic fecal constipation and soiling. *Semin Pediatr Surg* 2002; **11**: 67–74.
21. Herrlinger KR, Cummings JR, Barnardo MC, Schwab M, Ahmad T, Jewell DP. The pharmacogenetics of methotrexate in inflammatory bowel disease. *Pharmacogenet Genomics* 2005; **15**: 705–11.
22. Mahadevan U, Kane S, Sandborn WJ, Cohen RD, Hanson K, Terdiman JP, Binion DG. Intentional infliximab use during pregnancy for induction or maintenance of remission in Crohn's disease. *Aliment Pharmacol Ther* 2005; **21**: 733–8.
23. Eidelwein AP, Cuffari C, Abadom V, Oliva-Hemker M. Infliximab efficacy in pediatric ulcerative colitis. *Inflamm Bowel Dis* 2005; **11**: 213–18.
24. Bousvaros A, Guandalini S, Baldassano RN, Botelho C, Evans J, Ferry GD, Goldin B, Hartigan L, Kugathasan S, Levy J, Murray KF, Oliva-Hemker M, Rosh JR, Tolia V, Zholudev A, Vanderhoof JA, Hibberd PL. A randomized, double-blind trial of Lactobacillus GG versus placebo in addition to standard maintenance therapy for children with Crohn's disease. *Inflamm Bowel Dis* 2005; **11**: 833–9.
25. Sawczenko A, Azooz O, Paraszczuk J, Idestrom M, Croft NM, Savage MO, Ballinger AB, Sanderson IR. Intestinal inflammation-induced growth retardation acts through IL-6 in rats and depends on the -174 IL-6 G/C polymorphism in children. *Proc Natl Acad Sci USA* 2005; **102**: 13260–5.

26. Burnham JM, Shults J, Semeao E, Foster BJ, Zemel BS, Stallings VA, Leonard MB. Body-composition alterations consistent with cachexia in children and young adults with Crohn disease. *Am J Clin Nutr* 2005; **82**: 413–20.

27. Newby EA, Sawczenko A, Thomas AG, Wilson D. Interventions for growth failure in childhood Crohn's disease. *Cochrane Database Syst Rev* 2005; (**3**): CD003873.

28. Afzal NA, Davies S, Paintin M, Arnaud-Battandier F, Walker-Smith JA, Murch S, Heuschkel R, Fell J. Colonic Crohn's disease in children does not respond well to treatment with enteral nutrition if the ileum is not involved. *Dig Dis Sci* 2005; **50**: 1471–5.

29. Lionetti P, Callegari ML, Ferrari S, Cavicchi MC, Pozzi E, de Martino M, Morelli L. Enteral nutrition and microflora in pediatric Crohn's disease. *JPEN J Parenter Enteral Nutr* 2005; **29**(4 Suppl): S173–5; discussion S175–8, S184–8.

30. Sanderson IR, Croft NM. The anti-inflammatory effects of enteral nutrition. *JPEN J Parenter Enteral Nutr* 2005; **29**(4 Suppl): S134–8; discussion S138–40, S184–8.

31. Gavin J, Anderson CE, Bremner AR, Beattie RM. Energy intakes of children with Crohn's disease treated with enteral nutrition as primary therapy. *J Hum Nutr Diet* 2005; **18**: 337–42.

32. Calenda KA, Schornagel IL, Sadeghi-Nejad A, Grand RJ. Effect of recombinant growth hormone treatment on children with Crohn's disease and short stature: a pilot study. *Inflamm Bowel Dis* 2005; **11**: 435–41.

33. Harpavat M, Greenspan SL, O'Brien C, Chang CC, Bowen A, Keljo DJ. Altered bone mass in children at diagnosis of Crohn disease: a pilot study. *J Pediatr Gastroenterol Nutr* 2005; **40**: 295–300.

34. Stark LJ, Hommel KA, Mackner LM, Janicke DM, Davis AM, Pfefferkorn M, Crandall W, Heubi J. Randomized trial comparing two methods of increasing dietary calcium intake in children with inflammatory bowel disease. *J Pediatr Gastroenterol Nutr* 2005; **40**: 501–7.

35. Krausz MM, Duek SD. Restorative proctocolectomy with ileal pouch–anal anastomosis for ulcerative colitis and familial adenomatous polyposis: twenty years follow-up in 174 patients. *Isr Med Assoc J* 2005; **7**: 23–7.

36. Wewer V, Hesselfeldt P, Qvist N, Husby S, Paerregaard A. J-pouch ileoanal anastomosis in children and adolescents with ulcerative colitis: functional outcome, satisfaction and impact on social life. *J Pediatr Gastroenterol Nutr* 2005; **40**: 189–93.

37. De Boer M, Grootenhuis M, Derkx B, Last B. Health-related quality of life and psychosocial functioning of adolescents with inflammatory bowel disease. *Inflamm Bowel Dis* 2005; **11**: 400–6.

38. Mackner LM, Crandall WV. Long-term psychosocial outcomes reported by children and adolescents with inflammatory bowel disease. *Am J Gastroenterol* 2005; **100**: 1386–92.

39. Shepanski MA, Hurd LB, Culton K, Markowitz JE, Mamula P, Baldassano RN. Health-related quality of life improves in children and adolescents with inflammatory bowel disease after attending a camp sponsored by the Crohn's and Colitis Foundation of America. *Inflamm Bowel Dis* 2005; **11**: 164–70.

40. Day AS, Whitten KE, Bohane TD. Childhood inflammatory bowel disease: parental concerns and expectations. *World J Gastroenterol* 2005; **11**: 1028–31.

8

Pathogenesis and management of pouchitis

IOANNIS OIKONOMOU, BO SHEN

Introduction

Restorative proctocolectomy with ileal pouch–anal anastomosis (IPAA) has become the surgical treatment of choice in patients with medically refractory ulcerative colitis, those with ulcerative colitis with dysplasia and those with familial adenomatous polyposis (FAP). Although IPAA significantly improves patients' health-related quality of life, complications can occur. The most common complication is pouchitis, which occurs almost exclusively in patients with underlying ulcerative colitis and is rarely seen in patients with FAP. The aetiology and pathogenesis are not entirely clear. The prevailing hypothesis is that alteration in the microflora of the pouch in genetically susceptible patients leads to abnormal mucosal immune responses, resulting in acute or chronic inflammation in the pouch reservoir.

Association between fecal hydrogen sulfide production and pouchitis

Ohge H, Furne KS, Springfield J, Rothenberger DA, Madoff RD, Levitt MD. *Dis Colon Rectum* 2005; **48**: 469–75

BACKGROUND. The microflora play an important role in the initiation and development of pouchitis. However, there is no consistent evidence suggesting that a specific bacterial pathogen is solely responsible for the pathogenesis of the disease. The authors hypothesized that bacteria-associated toxins might contribute to the disease process. The intestinal bacteria release large quantities of hydrogen sulphide (H_2S) through the reduction of inorganic sulphate to sulphide and the metabolism of organic sulphur-containing compounds. H_2S is a highly volatile compound that rapidly penetrates the mucosa. H_2S could be detrimental to the mucosa of the ileal pouch. Experimental animal models have shown tissue injury induced by H_2S. In tissues H_2S is a highly volatile compound that rapidly penetrates the mucosa and binds to the haem moiety of cytochrome a3, blocking the terminal step in electron transport.

INTERPRETATION. This case–control study involved 45 patients with ulcerative colitis and five patients with FAP. The release of H_2S, methylmercaptan, carbon dioxide and hydrogen from fresh faecal specimens was measured. Production of H_2S was significantly higher in patients with active pouchitis and in patients with previous episodes of pouchitis than in those without current pouchitis or no history of pouchitis. The release of H_2S was significantly lower in patients on antibiotic therapy and in patients with a history of FAP compared with patients not treated with antibiotics. The sulphate-reducing bacterial counts were significantly higher in patients with active pouchitis than in those who had never experienced pouchitis, and the count fell dramatically with antibiotic treatment. The production of hydrogen and carbon dioxide did not differ significantly among the non-antibiotic groups. Methylmercaptan production was lower and more variable than H_2S production and did not differ statistically significantly between the groups.

Comment

The authors of this study explored the potential role of H_2S in the development of pouchitis. They reported increased H_2S production after incubation of fresh faecal specimens from patients with active pouchitis. This finding pointed to bacterial by-products being associated with pouchitis. However, it is difficult to prove that H_2S is the cause or the result of pouchitis; it might just be an innocent bystander. In this study, the diagnosis of pouchitis was based on clinical symptoms with or without endoscopic documentation. In patients with repeat attacks of pouchitis, the diagnosis was made mainly on the basis of clinical symptoms, which weakens the power of the study. Previous studies have shown that endoscopic evaluation is a key component in the diagnosis of pouchitis, since patients with other pouch diseases, such as Crohn's disease of the pouch, cuffitis and irritable pouch syndrome, could have symptoms similar to those of patients with pouchitis. Further studies using *in vitro* or animal models would be helpful to further delineate the association between H_2S and pouchitis.

Persistence of high CD40 and CD40L expression after restorative proctocolectomy for ulcerative colitis

Polese L, Angriman I, De Franchis G, *et al. World J Gastroenterol* 2005; **11**: 5303–8

BACKGROUND. CD40 and CD40L belong to the tumour necrosis factor (TNF) receptor family and are expressed by antigen-presenting cells and T cells respectively. They are necessary for the activation of the immune response during antigen presentation. The protein expression of CD40 and CD40L by gut leucocytes is elevated in patients with active or quiescent Crohn's disease or ulcerative colitis. Several lines of evidence suggest that CD40L-positive T cells play a role in inducing the production of cell adhesion molecules and the expression of soluble mediators by CD40-positive human intestinal fibroblasts and microvascular endothelial cells. As a result, more T cells are recruited from the peripheral blood to the tissue, leading to the

amplification of intestinal inflammation. The roles of CD40 and CD40L in patients with pouchitis immunologically resembling Crohn's disease or ulcerative colitis warrant investigation.

INTERPRETATION. In this case–control study the authors analysed CD40 and CD40L protein expression in the pouch of 28 ulcerative colitis patients with IPAA (14 with pouchitis and 14 with healthy pouches), in the terminal ileum of six patients with ulcerative colitis but without ileitis, and in the terminal ileum of healthy controls, using immunohistochemistry. The flow cytometric quantification of CD40+ B lymphocytes and monocytes in the peripheral blood of 20 patients with ulcerative colitis and pouch (seven with pouchitis), 15 ulcerative colitis patients without colectomy and eleven healthy subjects was also performed. The authors found that CD40 and CD40L expression in mucosal leucocytes in the pouch correlated with pouchitis. However, CD40 and CD40L expression was also present in the normal terminal ileum in ulcerative colitis patients and in healthy pouches. CD40 and CD40L expression was significantly higher in the pouch mucosa compared with the ileal mucosa from healthy subjects. Peripheral blood B lymphocytes of ulcerative colitis and pouch patients expressed significantly more CD40 than controls. CD40 in peripheral blood B cells in pouch patients correlated with spondyloarthropathy. Expression of CD40 in blood monocytes was not associated with extraintestinal manifestations. Patients with pouchitis did not present a higher incidence of extraintestinal manifestations.

Comment

In contrast to previous studies, in this study pouchitis was not associated with extraintestinal manifestations. CD40 expression in the pouch mucosa was greater in patients with pouchitis than in patients with healthy pouches and ulcerative colitis patients with normal terminal ileum before colectomy. Extraintestinal manifestations (spondyloarthropathy, or pyoderma gangrenosum) seem to be related to CD40 levels on peripheral B cells. Upregulation of CD40 and CD40L expression in pouchitis appears to be non-specific, since it occurs in many other chronic inflammatory conditions. It would be interesting to know what factors may trigger the upregulation of CD40 and CD40L expression; for example, alteration in the bacterial composition of the pouch.

Implications of pouchitis on the functional results following stapled restorative proctocolectomy

Abdelrazeq AS, Lund JN, Leveson SH. *Dis Colon Rectum* 2005; **48**: 1700–7

BACKGROUND. Few studies in the past have evaluated the long-term functional outcomes in patients after restorative proctocolectomy with IPAA. Pouchitis is the most common long-term complication that adversely affects patients' health perception and satisfaction.

INTERPRETATION. In this study, 100 consecutive patients who underwent restorative proctocolectomy between 1988 and 2004 by a single surgeon were divided into three groups: patients with no pouchitis, acute pouchitis or chronic pouchitis. The mean duration of follow-up was 71 months (range 6–196 months). Sixty-seven patients never experienced pouchitis, and four of those experienced cuffitis. Seventeen patients had acute pouchitis and 16 patients had chronic pouchitis. Three patients with chronic pouchitis had pouch failure. Functional results, general health perception and satisfaction were compared between the three groups at the time when patients were in symptomatic remission. A 4-point scale was used to rate patients' satisfaction and perception of their general health. A combination of clinical, endoscopic and histological criteria was used at least once for the diagnosis of pouchitis for each patient. There were no significant differences in clinical characteristics between the three groups. The frequencies of pancolitis and backwash ileitis were higher in patients with pouchitis. The duration and severity of ulcerative colitis before surgery were similar among the three groups. Long-term functional results were similar between patients with acute pouchitis and patients with no pouchitis. Patients with chronic pouchitis had a significant increase in the frequency of bowel movements, looseness of stools, urgency, nocturnal seepage, perianal excoriation, and dietary restrictions ($P < 0.05$) compared with patients with healthy pouches or acute pouchitis. They also had worse perception of general health ($P < 0.05$). A history of chronic pouchitis did not affect continence, daytime soiling or gas–faeces discrimination. Most patients were satisfied with IPAA and would recommend the operation to someone else with ulcerative colitis.

Comment

The findings of this study involving 100 consecutive patients confirm the results of previous studies reporting that IPAA surgery provides significantly improved quality of life and that most patients are satisfied with the operation. Acute pouchitis can be treated with antibiotics and does not affect pouch function, according to the findings of this study and other studies. On the other hand, chronic pouchitis leads to poor general health perception and functional results. Nonetheless, most of the patients (>90%) with chronic pouchitis would still recommend the operation to someone else with ulcerative colitis.

One of the limitations of the study was the small number of patients, only 33 patients having pouchitis. The results of the study are based on data for a single hospital and a single surgeon. The learning curve of surgeons might have affected the outcome in the earlier patients of the study. Patient satisfaction and health perception could have been affected by other factors in addition to the disease status of the pouch, such as the individual's coping skills.

Serologic responses in indeterminate colitis patients before ileal pouch–anal anastomosis may determine those at risk for continuous pouch inflammation

Hui T, Landers C, Vasiliauskas E, *et al. Dis Colon Rectum* 2005; **48**: 1254–62

BACKGROUND. Distinguishing between ulcerative colitis and Crohn's colitis can be difficult, especially in the setting of fulminant colitis. Under these circumstances the term 'indeterminate colitis' is used. Patients with indeterminate colitis have a higher risk of the post-operative development of Crohn's disease of the pouch. The establishment of independent pre-operative clinical and laboratory factors in order to predict the post-operative course in patients with indeterminate colitis is a clinically relevant issue.

INTERPRETATION. A cohort of 28 consecutive patients with a pre- or post-colectomy diagnosis of indeterminate colitis and undergoing IPAA was assessed prospectively for the development of pouchitis or Crohn's disease. Fifteen patients (54%) had transmural inflammation on colectomy specimens, five had discontinuous inflammation, five had involvement of the small bowel and three had anal disease. Six of 25 patients (24%) with pancolitis had backwash ileitis. Median follow-up was 38 months (range 3–75 months). Patients were seen every 3 months for the first year after ileostomy closure and yearly afterwards. Sera of study patients were drawn immediately before colectomy and analysed for serum perinuclear antineutrophil cytoplasmic antibodies (pANCA) expression and characterization of ANCA subtypes. The pANCA-positive patients were stratified into three groups based on antibody level. Anti-*Saccharomyces cervesiae* antibodies (ASCA), human immunoglobulin A antibodies to I-2 (outer membrane porin C [OmpC] of *Escherichia coli*) and OmpC (against a CD-related antigen from *Pseudomonas flourescens*) were also measured. Sixteen patients (61%) developed pouchitis; among these four (25%) had acute pouchitis and twelve (75%) had persistent pouch inflammation. Among the last patient group, nine (32% of the cohort of 28) had chronic pouchitis and three (11% of the 28) had Crohn's disease. Median time to diagnosis of the first episode of pouchitis was 13 months (range 2–64). Sixteen patients (57%) had a positive antibody reactivity profile. Persistent pouch inflammation developed in 10 of 16 patients (63%) who had a positive antibody reactivity profile compared with only 2 of 12 patients (17%) who had a negative antibody reactivity profile ($P = 0.015$).

Comment

The authors used an antibody panel consisting of ANCA, ASCA, I-2 and OmpC to predict the post-operative outcome of patients with indeterminate colitis undergoing restorative proctocolectomy with IPAA. The positive antibody profile in combination with persistent pouch inflammation suggests that this antibody panel might be helpful in identifying patients who would be good candidates for IPAA with few post-operative complications. The inclusion of patients with transmural inflammation in the indeterminate colitis group might have contributed to an increased frequency of positive antibody reactivity, because these patients might have had Crohn's disease at the time of surgery. Unfortunately, there were no established diagnostic criteria for indeterminate colitis. Therefore, predictive models from different studies may give different results.

Probiotic therapy in the prevention of pouchitis onset: decreased interleukin-1β, interleukin-8, and interferon-γ gene expression

Lammers KM, Vergopoulos A, Babel N, *et al.* *Inflamm Bowel Dis* 2005; **11**: 447–54

BACKGROUND. Pouchitis is a common complication after restorative proctocolectomy. The microflora play a significant role in the inflammatory response of the pouch mucosa. In previous studies, probiotics appeared to be effective for the primary and secondary prophylaxis of flare-ups of pouchitis. However, the exact mechanisms of the effect of probiotics are not clear.

INTERPRETATION. In this case–control study, pouch biopsy specimens from 16 patients with IPAA, enrolled in a double-blind, placebo-controlled study, were evaluated for the effect of VSL#3, a probiotic agent containing lyophilized bacteria of eight probiotic strains: *Bifidobacterium longum, B. breve, B. infantis, Lactobacillus acidophilus, L. casei, L. bulgaricus, L. plantarum* and *Streptococcus salivarius* ssp. *thermophilus*. Eight patients received VSL#3 and eight received placebo. No patient had evidence of pouchitis at entry into the study. Biopsy specimens were obtained at study entry and after 6 months in the study. Expression of mRNAs for interleukin (IL)-1β, IL-8 and interferon γ in mucosal biopsy specimens from patients treated with the probiotic preparation decreased 4-, 8- and 2-fold respectively. IL-6 and IL-12p40 were hardly expressed and did not differ significantly. TNF-α mRNA expression did not differ between the groups. The immunoregulatory cytokines IL-10 and transforming growth factor β did not differ between the two groups. The genes for CD3 (a marker for T-cell infiltration) and CTLA-4 (a marker for regulatory T cells) were expressed equally in the two groups. There were significantly fewer polymorphic nuclear cells in tissue from patients receiving probiotic treatment than in tissue from patients in the placebo group.

Comment

The data from this study suggest that probiotic treatment could lead to reductions in IL-8 and polymorphic nuclear cell infiltration of the pouch mucosa. The decreased expression of IL-8 in the probiotic-treated group, associated with a decreased number of polymorphic nuclear cells, is consistent with the role of IL-8 as a chemokine with strong chemoattractant properties. Decreased IL-8 production may limit the influx of polymorphic neutrophils. Probiotics may have an immunoregulatory effect by regulating tissue IL-8. The pathogenesis of pouchitis is still not clear and the pharmacological effects of probiotics in pouchitis remain to be investigated. It would be interesting to find interacting mechanisms among

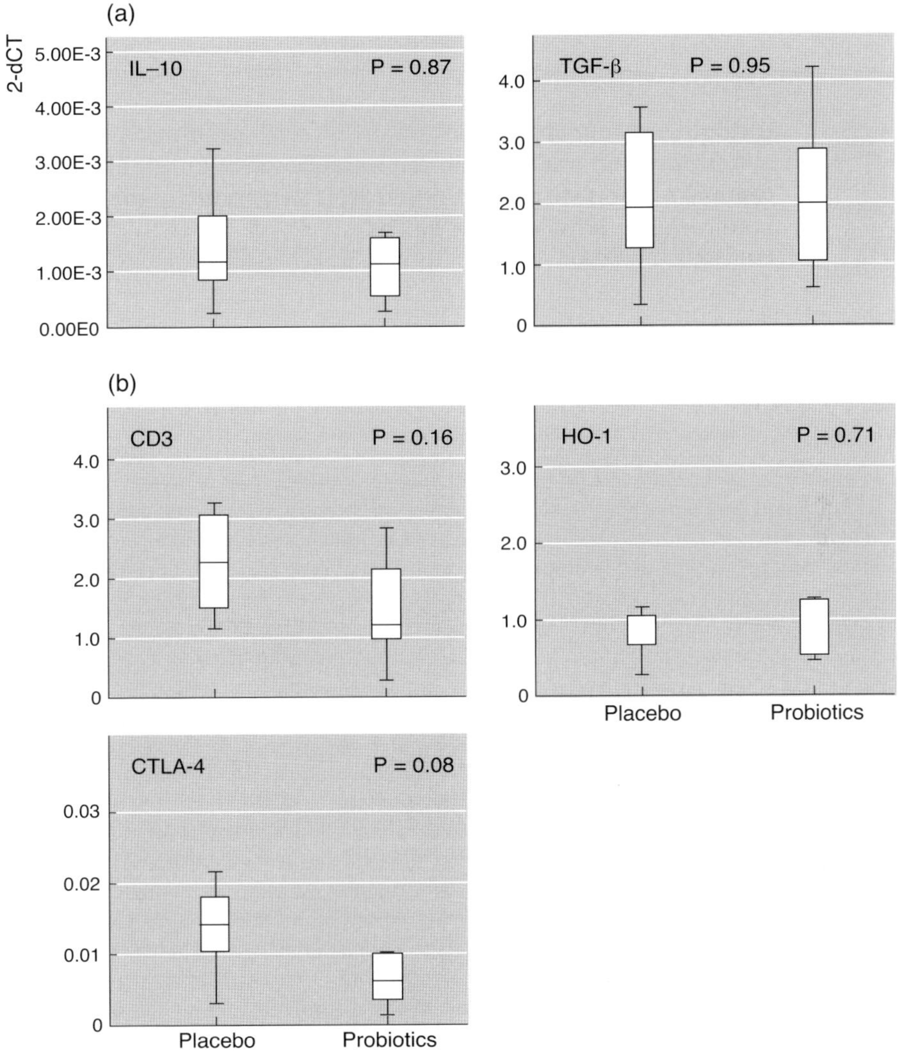

Fig. 8.1 Probiotic- and placebo-treated patients did not differ in expression in mucosa of genes for (a) regulatory cytokines IL-10 and TGF-β or (b) T-cell markers CD3 and CTLA-4 and macrophage stress protein HO-1. Source: Lammers *et al.* (2005).

probiotics, the commensal luminal bacteria of the pouch, mucosa-associated bacteria, and the local immune response.

Outcome of four weeks' intervention with probiotics on symptoms and endoscopic appearance after surgical reconstruction with a J-configurated ileal–pouch–anal anastomosis in ulcerative colitis

Laake KO, Bjorneklett A, Aamodt G, *et al. Scand J Gastroenterol* 2005; **40**: 43–51

BACKGROUND. The pathogenesis of pouchitis is still obscure. In pouchitis, lactobacilli and bifidobacteria species are decreased compared with patients with healthy pouches. An alternative to antibiotic treatment is the use of live bacteria in the form of probiotics that alter the microbial flora of the pouch.

INTERPRETATION. This was an open-label study that enrolled 69 patients with colectomy and IPAA surgery at least 1 year before study entry; 67 patients completed the study. Fifty-one patients had underlying ulcerative colitis, ten had underlying FAP, and six had ulcerative colitis and ileorectal anastomosis. Patients with or without symptoms and with or without pouchitis were included in the study. Five hundred millilitres of a fermented milk product (Cultura®) containing live lactobacilli (La-5) and bifidobacteria (Bb-12) was given daily for 4 weeks. Clinical characteristics were documented at the beginning of the intervention and at the end. Symptoms were documented using diary cards and in an interview at the beginning and the end of the study. Endoscopic inflammation was evaluated before and after the probiotic therapy. There was a significant reduction in symptoms on the diary cards in patients with ulcerative colitis/IPAA in regard to involuntary defaecation, leakage, abdominal cramps, number and consistency of stools, mucus and urge to defaecate. In FAP/IPAA patients symptoms decreased in regard to involuntary defaecation, leakage and abdominal cramps. In patients with ileorectal anastomosis there was no significant symptom improvement. The interviews indicated no significant symptom improvement. Stool samples were collected at the beginning and the end of the intervention and 1 week after the end. Faecal pH and counts of fungi remained unchanged. There were significant increases in faecal lactobacilli and bifidobacteria in the first week after intervention only in the ulcerative colitis/IPAA group, with non-significant change thereafter. The mean endoscopic score decreased significantly from 4.5 to 3.0 ($P = 0.0001$) in the ulcerative colitis/IPAA group. In the FAP and ulcerative colitis/ileorectal anastomosis groups the decrease did not reach statistical significance. In each group, clinical chemistry, antinuclear antibodies (ANA) and ANCA were similar before and after therapy. There were differences in fibre supplement and loperamide intake between the groups. Treatment with the probiotic led to symptom improvement and major joint improvement. Multivariable analysis showed that patients with a family history of irritable bowel disease (IBD) were significantly improved regarding stool frequency and consistency compared with patients without IBD in the family ($P = 0.01$). Mucus and the urge to evacuate, blood in the stool and morning fever were significantly improved in patients with ongoing pouchitis at the time of inclusion.

Comment

This open-label study provides valuable information on the effect of the probiotics. Improvement of the symptoms of patients with IPAA suggests that prolonged exposure to these probiotics might be beneficial. It is still not clear whether the probiotics stabilize the pouch microflora or have an immunomodulatory effect. The improvement in eye and major joint symptoms and the symptom improvement among patients with IBD in the family suggest a systemic action. The increase in the numbers of probiotic bacteria (bifidobacteria and lactobacilli) in the first week after the initiation of treatment indicates transient colonization and the improvement in the endoscopic score in patients with ulcerative colitis/IPAA indicates promise for treatment with this specific probiotic. However, this was an open-label study with a small number of patients.

Expression of keratinocyte growth factor and its receptor in adaptive changes of ileorectal pouch mucosa

Otte JM, Boser S, Brunke G, *et al. Scand J Gastroenterol* 2005; **40**: 1066–75

BACKGROUND. Growth factors can promote the migration and proliferation of intestinal epithelial cells to aid wound healing and tissue regeneration. Keratinocyte growth factor (KGF), an epithelial-specific growth factor of the fibroblast growth factor (FGF) family, has been shown to promote intestinal wound healing and re-epithelialization and to have immunomodulatory properties. KGF is a recognized mitogen for epithelial cells *in vitro*, and administration of exogenous KGF induces intestinal epithelial cell proliferation *in vitro* and *in vivo*. KGF elicits its effect by binding and activating its receptor (KGFR). Overexpression of KGF has been detected in intestinal mesenchymal cells in patients with Crohn's disease or ulcerative colitis.

INTERPRETATION. In this study, pouch biopsies were obtained from 45 age-matched and sex-matched individuals (30 patients with ulcerative colitis and 15 patients with FAP) and from the ileal and rectal mucosa of 16 healthy controls; the biopsies were stained with haematoxylin and eosin and scored for inflammation and morphological changes. KGF and KGFR mRNA, protein expression and phosphorylation were measured. Immunohistochemistry was used to localize KGF and KGFR in the tissue samples. KGF mRNA expression was not significantly different between non-inflamed pouch mucosa and the ileal mucosa of healthy controls. A similar result was obtained for KGFR mRNA in pouch mucosa and ileal mucosa of healthy controls. Inflamed and adapting mucosa demonstrated significant increases in the mRNA expression of KGF and KGFR compared with healthy ileal controls. The level of mRNA expression correlated positively with the extent of inflammation. Pouch mucosa of ulcerative colitis and FAP patients did not show significant differences in patterns of mRNA expression. KGF was detected on subepithelial cells, mainly on fibroblasts throughout the lamina propria, whereas KGFR was restricted to epithelial cells.

Comment

Animal experiments have shown that administration of recombinant KGF promotes the growth and differentiation of epithelial cells located in various organs, in particular gastrointestinal epithelial cells. Both mRNA and protein KGF and KGFR are over-expressed in intestinal tissue of patients with IBD, supporting their role in tissue repair. In addition, IL-1 and TNF-α appear to induce KGF gene expression. Further *in vivo* studies are needed to assess the role of KGF in the pathogenesis of pouchitis and whether the use of recombinant KGF might be an alternative approach to the treatment of pouchitis.

Combined carriership of TLR9–1237C and CD14–260T alleles enhances the risk of developing chronic relapsing pouchitis

Lammers KM, Ouburg S, Morré SA, *et al. World J Gastroenterol* 2005; **11**: 7323–9

BACKGROUND. The fact that pouchitis develops almost exclusively in patients with underlying ulcerative colitis and rarely in patients with FAP points to genetic or immunological factors. It is unclear whether single-nucleotide polymorphisms (SNPs) in innate immunity genes are associated with susceptibility to pouchitis.

INTERPRETATION. In this study, 157 ulcerative colitis patients with IPAA were analysed with regard to the SNPs *CD14* –260C→T, *CARD15/NOD2* 3020insC, Toll-like receptor 4 (*TLR4*) +896A→G, *TLR9* –1237T→C, *TLR9* +2848G→A and *IRAKM* + 22148G→A. The study enrolled 35 patients with chronic relapsing pouchitis (three or more episodes), 43 with infrequent pouchitis (up to two episodes) and 79 patients with a normal pouch (no episodes). The control group consisted of 224 Italian Caucasian healthy blood donors. There was no significant difference in SNP frequencies between controls and IPAA patients. There was a significantly higher carrier frequency of the *TLR9* –1237C allele in the chronic relapsing pouchitis group compared with the infrequent pouchitis group ($P = 0.028$; odds ratio 3.2; 95% confidence interval [CI] 1.2–8.6). There was no significant difference between the combined pouchitis groups and the patients with no pouchitis. This allele uniquely represented a four-locus *TLR9* haplotype comprising both of the *TLR9* SNPs studied in Caucasians. There was increased combined carriership of the alleles *TLR9* –1237C and *CD14* –260T in the chronic relapsing pouchitis and infrequent pouchitis groups ($P = 0.018$; odds ratio 4.1; 95% CI 1.4–12.3).

Comment

This is a useful study highlighting possible genetic susceptibility in the pathogenesis of pouchitis. A combination of SNPs such as *TLR9* –1237C and *CD14* –260T might be used as a genetic marker for development of chronic pouchitis. *TLR9* –1237C has been associated with Crohn's disease. This finding suggests that carriers of this allele are predisposed to an impaired immune response in ileal tissue. This could lead to pouchitis after restorative proctocolectomy. However, appropriate classification of clinical phenotypes is important in any genetic–phenotypic study. Unfortunately, there were no unified criteria for the classification of pouchitis. The classification of pouchitis in the present study appeared arbitrary. A larger number of patients and stricter patient selection based on the clinical, endoscopic and histological criteria for pouchitis would have been helpful in stratifying the different patient groups. The lifetime frequency of pouchitis episodes might give an indication but cannot define chronic pouchitis, given the different durations after IPAA. The possible inclusion of patients with irritable pouch syndrome (IPS) might also lead to invalid results. In future we hope to be able to assess the risk of pouchitis in patients considered for restorative proctocolectomy with IPAA on the basis of genetic analysis.

Table 8.1 Genotypes for *CD14*, *CARD15*, *TLR4*, *TLR9* and *IRAKM* polymorphisms in subgroups of patients with IPAA and controls

Polymorphism	Genotype	Controls	No pouchitis	Infrequent pouchitis	Chronic relapsing pouchitis
		n = 224 (%)	*n* = 79 (%)	*n* = 43 (%)	*n* = 35 (%)
CD14 –260 C→T	CC	55 (24.6)	24 (30.4)	11 (25.6)	7 (20)
	CT	102 (45.5)	34 (43)	21 (48.8)	22 (62.9)
	TT	67 (29.9)	21 (26.6)	11 (25.6)	6 (17.1)
CARD15 3020InsC	WT/WT	218 (97.3)	77 (97.5)	43 (100)	34 (97.1)
	WT/InsC	6 (2.7)	2 (2.5)	0 (0)	1 (2.9)
	InsC/InsC	0 (0)	0 (0)	0 (0)	0 (0)
TLR4 +896 A→G	AA	208 (92.9)	73 (92.4)	38 (88.4)	33 (94.3)
	AG	16 (7.1)	5 (6.3)	5 (11.6)	2 (5.7)
	GG	0 (0)	1 (1.3)	0 (0)	0 (0)
TLR9 –1237 T→C	TT	158 (70.5)	52 (65.8)	34 (79.1)	19 (54.3)
	TC	60 (26.8)	24 (30.4)	9 (20.9)	14 (40)
	CC	6 (2.7)	3 (3.8)	0 (0)	2 (5.7)
TLR9 +2848 G→A	GG	40 (17.9)	20 (25.3)	9 (20.9)	6 (17.1)
	GA	104 (46.4)	38 (48.1)	22 (51.2)	16 (45.7)
	AA	80 (35.7)	21 (26.6)	12 (27.9)	13 (37.2)
IRAKM +22148 G→A	GG	181 (80.8)	64 (81)	33 (76.7)	28 (80)
	GA	42 (18.8)	14 (17.7)	7 (16.3)	7 (20)
	AA	1 (0.4)	1 (1.3)	3 (7)	0 (0)

Source: Lammers *et al.* (2005).

Innate immune receptor genetic polymorphisms in pouchitis: is CARD15 a susceptibility factor?

Meier CB, Hegazi RA, Aisenberg J, *et al. Inflamm Bowel Dis* 2005; **11**: 965–71

BACKGROUND. It is not clear whether genetic polymorphism is associated with pouchitis. The occurrence of pouchitis in patients with ulcerative colitis but not in patients with FAP suggests an aberrant immunological response with increased inflammatory cytokine production. Immunogenetic determinants of host–microbe interactions probably influence the incidence and course of pouchitis after IPAA. The toll-like receptor (TLR) and nucleotide oligomerization domain 2 (NOD2)/caspase activation and recruitment domain (CARD) proteins are central immune sensors that detect microbes and initiate inflammatory responses. NOD2/CARD15 is an intracellular protein that recognizes bacterial muramyl dipeptide and activates inflammatory pathways through the transcription factor nuclear factor-kappa B (NF-κB). TLR4, a transmembrane protein that activates inflammatory pathways in the presence of extracellular bacterial lipopolysaccharide, has been associated with IBD.

INTERPRETATION. This cohort study comprised three groups of patients with ulcerative colitis, 5–12 years after restorative proctocolectomy. The first group had no pouchitis ($n = 52$), the second group ($n = 11$) had one or two episodes per year, and the third group ($n = 38$) had more than two episodes per year. Two SNPs in the *TLR4* gene were examined by a reverse transcription–polymerase chain reaction method with fluorogenic probes. Three Crohn's disease-associated SNPs in the *NOD2/CARD15* gene were determined with pyrosequencing assays. There was no correlation between *TLR4* polymorphisms and pouchitis. *NOD2/CARD15* mutations were more common in patients with pouchitis than in those without pouchitis (18 vs 8%; $P < 0.05$). The prevalence of *NOD2/CARD15* mutations was even greater among patients with more than two episodes of pouchitis per year (24%; $P < 0.01$ compared with the healthy group). The *NOD2/CARD15* insertion mutation L1007fsinsC was present in 14% of patients with pouchitis and in no patients without pouchitis ($P < 0.05$). All patients with this mutation were in the group with more than two episodes per year.

Comment

This study provides evidence that *NOD2/CARD15* genetic polymorphisms are more frequent in patients with pouchitis. Especially the L1007fsinsC insertion mutation may predispose to pouchitis after restorative proctocolectomy.

This study has limitations. Significant information about pouchitis was obtained by telephone interview, which limits the validity of the study. Not every patient had endoscopic and histological evaluation. Even in the group with more than two episodes per year, only 40% of patients had endoscopic and histological confirmation. Other inflammatory and non-inflammatory disease conditions of the pouch, such as Crohn's disease, cuffitis and irritable pouch syndrome, would have a presentation similar to that of pouchitis.

Since *NOD2/CARD15* genetic polymorphisms are frequently observed in patients with Crohn's disease, confounding factors such as the possible presence of Crohn's disease should have been considered.

A characterization of anaerobic colonization and associated mucosal adaptations in the undiseased ileal pouch

Smith FM, Coffey JC, Kell MR, O'Sullivan M, Redmond HP, Kirwan WO.
Colorectal Dis 2005; **7**: 563–70

BACKGROUND. The small bowel mucosa undergoes considerable changes as the pouch adapts to its new function as a faecal reservoir; this involves faecal stasis and alterations in bacterial colonization. During the adaptation period, incomplete colonic metaplasia develops and and the total anaerobic count increases. Sulphate-reducing bacteria of strictly anaerobic species colonize the pouch of ulcerative colitis patients and might play a role in the development of pouchitis. The clinically favourable response of patients with pouchitis to metronidazole therapy points to a possible aetiological and pathogenetic role of anaerobes.

INTERPRETATION. In this study, mucosal biopsies and faecal specimens from nine pouch patients with ulcerative colitis and five pouch patients with FAP were evaluated. For comparison, faecal samples and mucosal biopsies from ileostomies of seven of the nine patients with ulcerative colitis who underwent restorative proctocolectomy were collected. None of the study patients had pouchitis. Colonization by four types of strict anaerobe (sulphate-reducing bacteria, *Clostridium perfringens*, bifidobacteria and *Bacteroides*) as well as three types of facultative anaerobe (enterococci, coliforms and lactobacilli) was assessed. Strict anaerobes predominated over facultative anaerobes in the pouch patients with ulcerative colitis ($P = 0.041$). Sulphate-reducing bacteria were present in ulcerative colitis pouches exclusively and not in FAP pouches. Strict anaerobes still predominated after exclusion of sulphate-reducing bacteria. In the stoma specimens of ulcerative colitis patients, facultative anaerobes predominated ($P = 0.059$), sulphate-reducing bacteria were absent, and *C. perfringens* was present at significantly lower levels ($P = 0.005$) than the remaining species evaluated. In patients with FAP, strict and facultative anaerobes were present at similar levels ($P > 0.05$). Enterococci were present at significantly reduced levels in the pouch of ulcerative colitis patients when compared with the stoma of ulcerative colitis patients. There was no association between sulphate-reducing bacteria, other individual anaerobic species, and mucosal inflammation and morphology.

Comment

The authors of this study set out to assess the relationship between the bacterial flora, mucosa inflammation and mucosa morphology in patients without pouchitis and different underlying diseases. The remarkable finding was that sulphate-reducing bacteria were found to colonize only the pouches of patients with ulcerative colitis and not those of FAP patients. This finding suggests that genetic or immunological factors may contribute to the difference in sulphate-reducing bacteria in the setting of ulcerative colitis and FAP. However, this study included only 14 patients.

Maintenance therapy with a probiotic in antibiotic-dependent pouchitis: experience in clinical practice

Shen B, Brzezinski A, Fazio VW, *et al. Aliment Pharmacol Ther* 2005; **22**: 721–8

BACKGROUND. Most patients with pouchitis respond to antibiotics. Patients with antibiotic-dependent pouchitis often require long-term antibiotic treatment, raising concern about the development of bacterial resistance. Probiotics have frequently been used as antibiotic-sparing agents. VSL#3, a newly marketed probiotic agent, contains strains of *Lactobacillus*, three species of *Bifidobacterium* and *Streptococcus salivarius* ssp. *thermophilus*. In European randomized clinical trials, it has been shown to be effective in maintaining remission in patients with relapsing pouchitis and in preventing initial episodes of pouchitis after IPAA.

INTERPRETATION. This open-label study enrolled 31 patients from the USA with antibiotic-dependent pouchitis. All patients received 2 weeks of treatment with ciprofloxacin 500 mg twice daily followed by 8 months of VSL#3 at 6 g per day. The clinical symptoms of the patients were assessed at baseline, week 3 and at the end of the 8-month trial. Baseline Pouchitis Disease Activity Index (PDAI) scores were calculated. Some patients underwent repeat pouch endoscopy at the end of the trial. All patients responded to the ciprofloxacin treatment, as indicated by clinical symptoms. The mean duration of follow-up was 14.5 ± 5.3 months (range 8–26 months). At the 8-month follow-up, only six (19.4%) patients were still on VSL#3 therapy, and the remaining 25 patients had discontinued the therapy because of either recurrence of symptoms ($n = 23$) while on treatment or the development of adverse effects ($n = 2$). The mean duration of treatment in the discontinuation group was 1.2 ± 1.2 months (range 0.5–6.5 months). A subgroup of nine patients who discontinued VSL#3 by week 7 had a mean PDAI symptom score and a mean PDAI endoscopy score that were not statistically different from the baseline scores before initiation of treatment. At the time of repeat endoscopy all patients were back on antibiotics. The six patients who completed the 8-month course of treatment had repeat clinical and endoscopic evaluations at the end of the treatment course. Their symptom and endoscopic PDAI was not statistically different from their baseline PDAI.

Comment

The authors of this open-label treatment trial demonstrate less than optimal efficacy of VSL#3 in maintaining remission. The results contradict previous European studies in regard to the effectiveness of VSL#3. As in every open-label trial, there are some constitutional weaknesses. There is no control group, no blinding and no randomization. The results of the study are based mainly on clinical symptoms since the patients were instructed to start the VSL#3 if they had clinical resolution after treatment with ciprofloxacin. There was no endoscopic evaluation at the time of initiation of VSL#3 and immediately after discontinuation of the probiotic. In contrast to previous studies, in which patients received VSL#3 free of charge, in this study patients had to purchase the probiotic over the internet; this raises the question of adherence. Two patients experienced intolerable adverse effects, one having bloody bowel movements and one experiencing severe constipation, bloating, and gas. The difference in results between this study and previous studies favouring the use of VSL#3 might be due to the use of different diagnostic and classification criteria (e.g. for chronic refractory pouchitis). Previous trials have used 4 weeks of combination antibiotics. The question arises of the possibility of differences in the microbial flora and the immune response in the US population compared with the European population. Differences in diet on either side of the Atlantic could also play a role. Nonetheless, the post-market design of the trial probably reflected the practice patterns of the majority of the clinicians in the USA who manage pouchitis.

Rifaximin–ciprofloxacin combination therapy is effective in chronic active refractory pouchitis

Abdelrazeq AS, Kelly SM, Lund JN, Leveson SH. *Colorectal Dis* 2005; **7**: 182–6

BACKGROUND. Chronic refractory pouchitis can occur in patients with IPAA. Multiple treatment modalities have been used with poor results and often the occurrence of adverse reactions. Chronic refractory pouchitis can be treated with combination antibiotics. Ciprofloxacin has been widely used either alone or in combination with other antibiotics in the past. Rifaximin, a non-absorbable semisynthetic derivative of rifamycin, has bactericidal action by inhibiting bacterial RNA and protein synthesis. It covers gram-positive and gram-negative aerobic and anaerobic bacteria associated with gastrointestinal infections and it is often used in traveller's diarrhoea and IBD.

INTERPRETATION. This is an open-label study that enrolled eight patients with chronic active refractory pouchitis. All patients had chronic pouchitis (>4 weeks of symptoms or >2 weeks of treatment every month) with active symptoms, showed no response to at least 4 weeks of standard antibiotic treatment or relapsed immediately when antibiotic treatment was stopped or reduced. All patients had inflammation of the pouch diagnosed endoscopically and histologically without cuffitis, stricture, *Clostridium difficile*, cytomegalovirus, coeliac disease or Crohn's disease. They were treated with a combination of rifaximin 1 g twice daily and ciprofloxacin 500 mg twice daily for 2 weeks. The PDAI score, which includes clinical, endoscopic and histological assessments, was measured before and after treatment. Five patients went into remission (PDAI = 0) for at least 6 months, two patients responded to treatment (decrease in PDAI of at least 3 points) and one patient did not respond. Pouchitis recurred in two patients, 6 and 8 months after treatment respectively, but resolved after the use of the same combination treatment. The median PDAI score was 12 (range 9–18) before treatment and 0 (range 0–15) after treatment. The medication was well tolerated, with no side effects and no withdrawals. After 30 months the seven responding patients still had satisfactory pouch function.

Comment

This study was designed to assess the tolerability and effectiveness of rifaximin in combination with ciprofloxacin in patients with chronic pouchitis. It appears that rifaximin is well tolerated even at a large dose. The results confirm the previously reported efficacy of combination therapy with ciprofloxacin and rifaximin in treating chronic refractory pouchitis. The small number of patients limits the power of the study but it gives us useful data for clinical practice and the design of future trials. Another issue is the financial aspect. Ten 200-mg tablets of rifaximin in addition to ciprofloxacin could be a financial burden for some patients. Furthermore, maintenance of remission induced by ciprofloxacin and rifaximin therapy could be challenging.

Comprehensive evaluation of inflammatory and non-inflammatory sequelae of ileal pouch–anal anastomoses

Shen B, Fazio VW, Remzi FH, *et al. Am J Gastroenterol* 2005; **100**: 93–101

Background. IPAA leads to improvement of the health-related quality of life scores in ulcerative colitis patients. Complications such as pouchitis, cuffitis, Crohn's disease of the pouch and IPS can develop after surgery, adversely affecting the patient's quality of life.

Interpretation. This study enrolled 124 ulcerative colitis patients with IPAA, including 23 with Crohn's disease of the pouch, 22 with antibiotic-dependent or antibiotic-refractory pouchitis, 21 with cuffitis, 32 with IPS and 26 with normal pouches. Demographic and clinical data were compared between the disease groups and the group with a normal pouch. The use of non-steroidal anti-inflammatory drugs (NSAIDs) was more common in patients with pouchitis. Extraintestinal manifestations were more common in patients with cuffitis or IPS. Antidepressants were used more often in patients with IPS before the diagnosis of IPS. Endoscopic and histological inflammation of the afferent limb was the predominant feature of Crohn's disease of the pouch. Endoscopic and histological inflammation of the cuff was characteristic of cuffitis, but was also seen in some patients with Crohn's disease of the pouch or pouchitis. Bleeding occurred commonly in patients with cuffitis (20/21, 95.2%). Use of the PDAI instrument showed no significant difference in the symptom scores among the disease groups. Most of the symptoms overlapped in the disease groups. Obstructive symptoms occurred mainly in patients with Crohn's disease of the pouch. Endoscopy was useful in discriminating Crohn's disease of the pouch, pouchitis, cuffitis and normal pouches, and IPS. The Irritable Bowel Syndrome Quality of Life (IBS-QOL) scores were lower in the disease groups, and the IPS group had a significantly lower score than the pouchitis group. Patients with a diseased pouch had significantly worse Cleveland Global Quality of Life (CGQL) and IBS-QOL scores than patients with a normal pouch. The CGQL and IBS-QOL scores in all five groups were correlated (correlation coefficient from −0.38 to −0.64; P <0.03). The body image and social reaction domains were significantly poorer in patients with IPS than in patients with pouchitis.

Comment

This is the first study to compare different features and quality of life scores in patients with inflammatory and non-inflammatory sequelae of IPAA. Endoscopy is a useful means of discriminating between the different disease groups. The only difference in symptom scores between the groups was in rectal bleeding, which occurred almost exclusively in the cuffitis group. There are possible associations between NSAID use and pouchitis, extraintestinal manifestations and cuffitis, and antidepressant use and IPS. A longitudinal study is warranted to further delineate the natural history and clinical features of the pouch diseases.

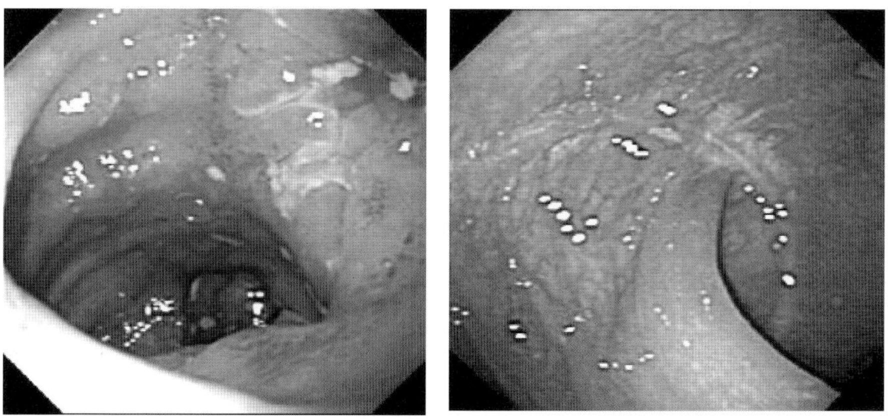

(a) (b)

Fig. 8.2 Endoscopic features of NSAID-induced pouchitis (a) and resolution of inflammation after the discontinuation of NSAID treatment (b). A 29-year-old female presented with antibiotic-refractory pouchitis, while taking ibuprofen daily. Pouch endoscopy showed inflammation of the afferent limb and pouch with oedema, superficial ulcers and aphthous ulcers. A repeat pouch endoscopy 4 weeks after she stopped ibuprofen revealed complete healing of ulcers and resolution of inflammation of the pouch and afferent limb. Her symptoms of abdominal pain and diarrhoea also resolved. Source: Shen *et al.* (2005).

Crohn's disease and indeterminate colitis and the ileal pouch–anal anastomosis: outcomes and patterns of failure

Brown CJ, MacLean AR, Cohen Z, MacRae HM, O'Connor BI, McLeod RS.
Dis Colon Rectum 2005; **48**: 1542–9

Background. Restorative proctocolectomy is indicated for patients with ulcerative colitis. Even though its role in patients with indeterminate colitis and Crohn's disease is controversial, it is often performed in patients with indeterminate colitis and is rare in patients with Crohn's disease. Previous studies have shown poor outcome and high frequency of pouch failure in patients with Crohn's disease. More studies are needed to further assess the long-term effects in patients with Crohn's colitis and indeterminate colitis in comparison with ulcerative colitis patients.

Interpretation. This study enrolled 1270 patients who underwent restorative proctocolectomy between 1982 and 2001 in a single institution. Among these patients, 1135 (89%) had ulcerative colitis, 36 (3%) had Crohn's disease, 21 (2%) had indeterminate colitis, and 78 (6%) had other diagnoses. The diagnosis of indeterminate colitis was based on pathological evaluation of the resected colon. The diagnosis of ulcerative colitis or Crohn's disease was based on clinical, pathological and endoscopic criteria. In all except one of the patients with Crohn's disease, the diagnosis was made after construction of the IPAA. Perioperative data were collected prospectively and functional outcomes were assessed with a 35-question survey (21 on pouch function and 14 on quality of life) mailed to all patients who had a functioning pouch of at least 6 months' duration. The mailed survey was responded to by 89% of the patients with ulcerative colitis, 75% of those with Crohn's disease and 53% of those with indeterminate colitis. Pouch-related complications were significantly more common in patients with Crohn's disease (64%) and indeterminate colitis (43%) compared with patients with ulcerative colitis (22%) ($P < 0.05$). Most of the patients with Crohn's disease (56%) had their pouch excised or defunctioned, compared with 10% of patients with indeterminate colitis and 6% of those with ulcerative colitis ($P < 0.01$). The main causes of pouch failure in Crohn's disease patients were pouch fistula, pelvic abscess/sepsis, small bowel inflammation and poor pouch function. Univariate analysis revealed a statistically significant association of pouch failure in patients with hand-sewn ileoanal anastomosis, females, younger patients, and those who had had their disease for a shorter time before restorative proctocolectomy. The functional results in patients with Crohn's disease with a successful pouch were not significantly different from those in patients with indeterminate colitis or ulcerative colitis. Multivariate analysis revealed that an initial pathology of ulcerative colitis and an increasing number of clinical, endoscopic and pathological features of Crohn's disease were significantly associated with pouch failure.

Comment

This study confirms the findings of previous studies showing that the overall pouch failure rate is similar in patients with indeterminate colitis and ulcerative colitis. In contrast, most patients with Crohn's disease required pouch excision or diversion.

This study supports the notion that restorative proctocolectomy with IPAA can be performed in patients with indeterminate colitis after rigorous evaluation to exclude Crohn's disease. Even though the complication rate in patients with indeterminate colitis was increased, the success rate was similar to that in patients with ulcerative colitis. Crohn's disease appears to be associated with significant complications and a high risk of pouch failure after restorative proctocolectomy. It is hard to explain why patients with a pre-operative pathological diagnosis of ulcerative colitis had an increased risk of developing pouch failure compared with patients with pre-operative pathological features of Crohn's disease.

Conclusion

Diseases of the ileal pouch, particularly, are common after restorative proctocolectomy and have a detrimental effect on the patient's quality of life. New genetic, immunological and bacterial factors associated with pouch inflammation, as well as treatment interventions such as probiotics and combination antibiotics, are presented in this review. Advances in genetic and serological studies may offer valuable information in regard to the identification of high-risk patients.

Further reading

1. Fazio VW, Ziv Y, Church JM, Oakley JR, Lavery IC, Milsom JW, Schroeder TK. Ileal pouch–anal anastomosis complications and function in 1005 patients. *Ann Surg* 1995; **222**: 120–7.
2. Carter MJ, Di Giovine FS, Cox A, Goodfellow P, Jones S, Shorthouse AJ, Duff GW, Lobo AJ. The interleukin 1 receptor antagonist gene allele 2 as a predictor of pouchitis following colectomy and IPAA in ulcerative colitis. *Gastroenterology* 2001; **121**: 805–11.
3. Duffy M, O'Mahony L, Coffey JC, O'Mahony L, Coffey JC, Collins JK, Shanahan F, Redmond HP, Kirwan WO. Sulfate-reducing bacteria colonize pouches formed for ulcerative colitis but not for familial adenomatous polyposis. *Dis Colon Rectum* 2002; **45**: 384–8.
4. Schmidt C, Giese T, Ludwig B, Menges M, Schilling M, Meuer SC, Zeuzem S, Stallmach A. Increased cytokine transcripts in pouchitis reflect the degree of inflammation but not the underlying entity. *Int J Colorectal Dis* 2005; **21**: 1–8.
5. Ulisse S, Gionchetti P, Alo S, Russo P, Pesce I, Ricci G, Rizzello F, Helwig U, Cifone MG, Campieri M, De Simone C. Expression of cytokine, inducible nitric oxide synthase, matrix metalloproteinases in pouchitis: effects of probiotic therapy. *Am J Gastroenterol* 2001; **96**: 2691–6.

6. Bulois P, Tremaine WJ, Maunoury V, Gambiez L, Hafraoui S, Leteurtre E, Cortot A, Sandborn WJ, Colombel JF, Desreumaux P. Pouchitis is associated with mucosal imbalance between interleukin-8 and interleukin-10. *Inflamm Bowel Dis* 2000; **6**: 157–64.

Part III

Gastrointestinal endoscopy

9

Endoscopic ultrasonography

JOHN VARGO

Introduction

Expanding the bounds of clinical applications and a critical assessment of established indications mark the progress of endoscopic ultrasonography (EUS) in recent times. The first article, by Rajan *et al.*, explores the EUS appearance of the ageing pancreas by asking whether specific findings are age-dependent and considering the implications of such observations in the diagnosis of chronic pancreatitis. The use of three-dimensional EUS in the evaluation of vessel invasion in the setting of pancreatic cancer is addressed in the article by Fritscher-Ravens and colleagues. In patients with equivocal findings on other imaging studies and the suspicion of a pancreatic malignancy, Klapman *et al.* determine the negative predictive value of EUS. Continuing the theme of comparison between endoscopic retrograde cholangiopancreatography (ERCP) and EUS, the diagnostic accuracies of EUS–fine-needle aspiration (FNA) and cytological brushings during ERCP are compared in subjects with biliary strictures. The emerging use of endobronchial ultrasound-guided transbronchial needle aspiration (EBUS-TBNA) will be compared with transoesophageal EUS-FNA in the evaluation of mediastinal lesions.

The diagnostic utility of oncogene and DNA analysis in the diagnosis of pancreatic cystic lesions will be reviewed. EUS-directed therapy of pancreatic cystic lesions with ethanol lavage will be reviewed through the work of Gan *et al.*

Zuccaro *et al.* tackle the vexing issue of staging errors during EUS for oesophageal cancer and identify clinical risk factors that are associated with an increased risk of errors. Larghi *et al.* attempt to improve the accuracy of staging with the combination of EUS and cap endoscopic mucosal resection. Finally, the issue of publication bias in the EUS staging of rectal cancer will be reviewed via the provocative article of Harewood.

Age-related changes in the pancreas identified by EUS: a prospective evaluation

Rajan E, Clain JE, Levy MJ, Norton ID, Wang KK. *Gastrointest Endosc* 2005; **62**: 401–6

BACKGROUND. Currently, certain parenchymal and ductal findings are used during EUS to diagnose chronic pancreatitis. Typically, the presence of five or more of these EUS findings has been felt to reliably predict the presence of chronic pancreatitis. This diagnostic threshold has never been addressed in an age- or gender-dependent fashion. Does the pancreas age? Can some of these age-related findings affect the sensitivity and specificity of EUS in the detection of chronic pancreatitis? Patients undergoing EUS for non-pancreaticobiliary indications were enrolled. Stratification by age (<40, 40–60, >60) was performed. Logistic regression analysis was used to identify factors associated with EUS abnormalities. Hyperechoic stranding was the most common EUS finding (22% of subjects). Though there was a trend to a higher number of abnormalities with advancing age, this did not reach statistical significance ($P = 0.12$). Male gender was found to be the only significant factor in predicting the presence of an EUS abnormality (odds ratio 2.9; 95% confidence interval 1.2–6.8). Other factors, such as smoking, low alcohol intake, endoscopic abnormalities and body mass index, were not found to be predictors of EUS abnormalities.

INTERPRETATION. The frequency of EUS abnormalities in subjects without clinical evidence may increase with age and is significantly higher in males than in females. Hyperechoic stranding is quite common and its value as a component of the EUS-based chronic pancreatitis score may be called into question.

Comment

If these findings are validated by other studies, gender- and age-specific thresholds for the EUS diagnosis of chronic pancreatitis will be needed. Of course, there may be concomitant, age-related exocrine pancreatic functional abnormalities, and future inquiries should consider this possibility.

Three-dimensional linear endoscopic ultrasound-feasibility of a novel technique applied for the detection of vessel involvement of pancreatic masses

Fritscher-Ravens A, Knoefel WT, Krause C, Swain CP, Brandt L, Patel K. *Am J Gastroenterol* 2005; **100**: 1296–302

BACKGROUND. A particular shortcoming of EUS lies in its use in the determination of malignant vascular involvement. Whereas in some cases it is relatively easy to demonstrate vascular invasion, when there is vascular compression or abutment the ability of EUS to detect invasion can be more problematic. The use of vascular

Table 9.1 Vascular involvement in patients with mass lesions of the pancreas

Staging modality	No vascular involvement	Vascular compression	Vascular invasion
Linear EUS	6	6	10
3D EUS	6	10	6
Surgery	6	9	7

Source: Fritscher-Ravens *et al.* (2005).

contrast agents for EUS has been explored but has met with little success. Fritscher-Ravens and colleagues used linear echoendoscopy coupled with a magnetically tracked 3D sensor. Patients were stratified after linear EUS as having no vascular involvement, vascular invasion or vascular compression. 3D image acquisition was performed with an electromagnetic positioning/tracking system that is commercially available for transabdominal ultrasonography. This also required post-procedure computer-generated image processing.

Interpretation. A series of 22 patients with mass lesions of the pancreas were included in the study. The endosonographer was blinded to the results of the previous imaging studies, but was informed about the presence of a pancreatic mass and its location in the pancreas. Surgical histology was the gold standard. Seventeen of the 22 patients were found to have adenocarcinoma and the remainder were diagnosed with chronic pancreatitis. The vascular invasion status is shown in Table 9.1. In two patients with pancreatic cancer, linear EUS suggested vascular invasion whereas 3D EUS found vascular compression. Surgery found vascular invasion in one patient and vascular compression in the other. In patients found to have no vascular involvement by linear EUS, one out of six was found to have vascular invasion at surgery. In the chronic pancreatitis group, vascular invasion was found in three out of five patients by linear EUS, whereas 3D EUS suggested vascular compression only. Surgery found one patient each with no vascular involvement, vascular compression and no vascular involvement. The authors conclude that 3D EUS is feasible for vascular assessment in patients with mass lesions after showing that one out of 22 patients exhibited a false-negative result when compared with linear EUS, which showed a false-negative result in four out of 22 patients and a false-positive result in an additional patient.

Comment

3D EUS may eventually have a role in determining vascular involvement, but it will require further refinements to improve its test characteristics. There is a learning curve and the endosonographer must perform a slow and deliberate examination in order to minimize blurring of images. 3D EUS allowed the identification of endoluminal tumour nodules and the detection of turbulent blood flow, which was also felt to be characteristic of vessel invasion. A more important basic question still needs to be answered: how can we improve the accuracy of EUS in the detection of non-malignant pancreatic masses such as chronic pancreatitis?

Negative predictive value of endoscopic ultrasound in a large series of patients with a clinical suspicion of pancreatic cancer

Klapman JB, Chang KJ, Nguyen P. *Am J Gastroenterol* 2005; **100**: 2658–61

BACKGROUND. Not infrequently, EUS is used to help clarify vague ERCP and CT scan findings in the setting of abdominal pain and/or weight loss. Klapman *et al.* attempted to determine the negative predictive value of EUS in patients with a suspicion of pancreatic malignancy.

INTERPRETATION. This is a retrospective database review of patients with any combination of the following constellation: *clinical findings*: abdominal pain/weight loss; *CT scan findings*: pancreatic enlargement/fullness; *ERCP findings*: narrowing of the bile/pancreatic duct; *laboratory findings*: elevated CA19-9. A total of 155 patients were identified and follow-up was available on 135 (87%). The mean follow-up was 25 months (range 8–48 months). By far the most common indication was abnormal imaging stemming from computed tomography, ultrasonography or ERCP (91 patients). The negative predictive value of EUS in excluding pancreatic cancer in this group of patients was 100%. The authors conclude that EUS is highly specific in the diagnosis of pancreatic cancer and should be considered as the initial modality.

Comment

In the expert hands of the authors, EUS was found to have a 100% negative predictive value in the setting of a suspicion of a pancreatic malignancy. This is the largest series of its kind in the literature. It is important to emphasize the experience of the authors and the possibility that operator dependency (i.e. lesser degrees of experience and/or EUS volume) may affect the test characteristics.

Comparative study of diagnostic value of cytologic sampling by endoscopic ultrasonography-guided fine-needle aspiration and that by endoscopic retrograde pancreatography for the management of pancreatic mass without biliary stricture

Wakatsuki T, Irisawa A, Bhutani MS, *et al. J Gastroenterol Hepatol* 2005; **20**: 1707–11

BACKGROUND. Pancreatic duct brushing can be quite problematic during ERCP. This technique requires a solid set of core skills, including the ability to perform a pancreatic sphincterotomy, traverse a ductal stricture with a guidewire, and (hopefully) minimize the risk of pancreatitis. This problem becomes even more challenging when dealing with masses of the proximal pancreas and a normal pancreatic duct.

INTERPRETATION. Wakatsuki *et al.* present a case–control study of patients in whom cytology brushing during endoscopic retrograde pancreatography or EUS-FNA were performed. All patients presented with solid pancreatic masses without biliary structuring. Thirty patients received cytological brushings during ERCP and 50 patients underwent EUS-FNA. Amazingly, there was a 100% rate of adequate cellularity in both groups. The sensitivity of the ERCP was 33.3 and accuracy was 46.7%. For the EUS-FNA group, the sensitivity was 92.9%, with an accuracy of 94.3%. The rate for pancreatitis was significantly higher in the ERCP group (33 vs 0%; $P < 0.01$).

Comment

The use of ERCP for the evaluation of pancreaticobiliary masses continues to wane as more data show the superiority of EUS because of its ability to provide a tissue diagnosis, more accurate locoregional staging, and a much lower incidence of pancreatitis. Wakatsuki *et al.* show that, in the case of pancreatic solid masses without a biliary stricture, EUS-FNA is superior to conventional endoscopic retrograde pancreatography with brush cytology.

With respect to pancreaticobiliary masses with bile duct stricturing, the jury is still out for ERCP with triple tissue acquisition (brush cytology, biopsy, wire-guided FNA) versus EUS-FNA. However, it seems intuitive that EUS will be superior by virtue of locoregional staging, the minimal risk of pancreatitis and the ability to obtain multiple FNA samples. We await a prospective study on this particular issue.

Transesophageal endoscopic ultrasound-guided fine-needle aspiration (EUS-FNA) and endobronchial ultrasound-guided transbronchial needle aspiration (EBUS-TBNA) biopsy: a combined approach in the evaluation of mediastinal lesions

Vilmann P, Krasnik M, Larsen SS, Jacobsen GK, Clementsen P. *Endoscopy* 2005; **37**: 833–9

BACKGROUND. With the development of EBUS-TBNA we now have the opportunity to perform fine-needle aspiration from either a transoesophageal or a transbronchial platform. Vilmann *et al.* attempted to answer the question of which method is superior in a group of 33 patients who received both procedures.

INTERPRETATION. Twenty out of 33 patients carried the diagnosis of a non-small cell lung cancer. The remaining 13 presented with a suspicious mediastinal lesion in the setting of a suspected lung neoplasm. EBUS-TBNA and EUS-FNA were unsuccessful in one patient each. The breakdown of the cytological findings is given in Table 9.2. The two sampling procedures were found to be quite complementary to each other. EBUS-TBNA detected eleven additional cancers and three more suspicious samples that were not obtained by EUS-FNA. However, EUS-FNA found twelve additional cancer diagnoses and one suspicious sample and another diagnostic benign condition (sarcoidosis) that had not been found using EBUS-TBNA. The validation of the diagnoses was made by either

Table 9.2 Cytological findings obtained by EBUS-TBNA and EUS-FNA in patients with suspected lung neoplasm

Sampling modality	No. of lesions sampled	No. of lesions demonstrating malignancy	No. of lesions demonstrating benign cytology	No. of lesions demonstrating suspicious cytology
EUS-FNA	59	26	30	3
EBUS-TBNA	60	28	28	4

Source: Vilmann *et al.* (2005).

thoracotomy or clinical follow-up. When EUS-FNA and EBUS-TBNA were combined the diagnostic accuracy was 100%.

Comment

EUS-FNA and EBUS-TBNA exhibited similar test characteristics in the diagnosis of mediastinal malignancy. The combination of the two was the most accurate diagnostic approach. Therefore, in the setting of a high index of suspicion for malignancy the combination of these two tests should be considered when either one is negative on its own.

The role of pancreatic cyst fluid molecular analysis in predicting cyst pathology

Khalid A, McGrath KM, Zahid M, *et al. Clin Gastroenterol Hepatol* 2005; **3**: 967–73

BACKGROUND. The sensitivity of cytological analysis stemming from pancreatic cyst aspiration can be challenging because of the acellular nature of the specimen. Cyst fluid carcinoembryonic antigen (CEA) levels have been found to be elevated in mucinous cystic neoplasms, but this test cannot distinguish benignity from malignancy, or quantify the malignant potential of benign cysts. Khalid *et al.* used k-ras exon-1 activation as well as analysing a panel of markers of loss of heterozygosity (LOH) to predict the biological behaviour compared with surgical histology.

INTERPRETATION. Thirty-six patients with pancreatic cysts who either underwent surgery (31 cases) or had cytologically proven malignancy via FNA samples (five cases) were included in the analysis. All samples were obtained by EUS-FNA. CEA levels, the amount of DNA in the cyst fluid and its quality (the ability to be amplified) differed significantly between benign and malignant cysts. It should be emphasized, however, that a degree of overlap was seen between the groups with benign and malignant cysts. Similarly, the number of LOH mutations was higher in the malignant group, but again there was overlap with the benign group. The sequence of mutation accumulation was different between the benign and malignant cysts. Ten out of eleven malignant cysts had acquired a k-ras mutation first, followed by allelic loss. In contrast, only two of 14 benign cysts acquired a k-ras mutation prior to allelic loss.

Comment

The most sensitive and specific indicator of malignancy was the pattern of mutation accumulation. K-ras mutation followed by allelic loss was found to have a sensitivity of 91% and a specificity of 93%. This type of analysis requires only 0.4 ml of cyst fluid for the analysis. CEA analysis could not be performed in 25% of the specimens because of lack of fluid for analysis. These findings need to be validated in a larger series before they become the basis for a standard of practice.

EUS followed by EMR for staging of high-grade dysplasia and early cancer in Barrett's esophagus

Larghi A, Lightdale CJ, Memeo L, Bhagat G, Okpara N, Rotterdam H.
Gastrointest Endosc 2005; **62**: 16–23

BACKGROUND. Accurate staging of high-grade dysplasia and early cancer in Barrett's oesophagus is crucial in the selection of patients for endoscopic or surgical therapy. EUS has been shown to be the most accurate modality for determining the depth of tumour invasion and regional lymph node metastases. However, for high-grade dysplasia and intramucosal cancer, EUS staging, even with high-frequency echoprobes, has been shown to be problematic. Larghi *et al.* employed cap endoscopic mucosal resection (EMR) following EUS staging

INTERPRETATION. A total of 48 patients were enrolled in the study. Eight patients were found to have submucosal invasion or local lymphadenopathy. Seven out of eight had their EUS staging verified following surgery, whereas one was found to be overstaged. Twenty-five patients presented with high-grade dysplasia and 23 with early carcinoma. Among the 25 patients with high-grade dysplasia and no evidence of submucosal invasion by EUS, EMR revealed disease confined to the epithelium in 19. In the remaining six patients, EMR found adenocarcinoma to the lamina propria (four patients) and to the muscularis propria (two patients). In the early cancer group, in which staging indicated confinement to the mucosa in all 15 patients, EMR confirmed intramucosal cancer in nine cases, while in six cases submucosal invasion was confirmed histologically.

Comment

Overall, EUS provided accurate staging of the depth of tumour penetration in 41/48 (85%) patients, with understaging in one and understaging that was detected by EMR in the remaining six. EMR was carried out on an outpatient basis and was not associated with complications. EMR provided accurate histological staging in these cases of superficial oesophageal malignancy. With verification of these findings by other investigators, 'staging EMR' may well become the procedure of choice in cases of superficial cancer/high-grade dysplasia in which there is no evidence of lymphadenopathy or submucosal invasion.

Ethanol lavage of pancreatic cystic lesions: initial pilot study

Gan SI, Lauwers GY, Bounds BC, Brugge WR. *Gastrointest Endosc* 2005; **61**: 746–52

BACKGROUND. Surgical resection has been the only avenue for the treatment of pancreatic cystic neoplasms. Gan *et al.* report on a series of 25 patients who underwent ethanol lavage in an attempt at definitive non-surgical therapy.

INTERPRETATION. A single-site open-label trial of EUS-guided ethanol lavage was performed. After aspiration of the cyst contents, the collapsed cyst was then lavaged with ethanol for 3–5 min. Of the 23 patients with full follow-up (1 year), eight (35%) had complete resolution of their cysts on follow-up imaging. There were no differences between the resolved and persistent cysts with respect to location, mean cyst diameter, mean cyst wall thickness, presumed diagnosis, or mean ethanol concentration. Five subjects underwent surgical resection. Histological analysis revealed epithelial ablation.

Comment

In this small dose-ranging study, EUS-guided ethanol lavage appears to have been safe and efficacious. Further work will be needed to determine the factors that are associated with successful ablation.

EUS-guided FNA of pancreatic metastases: a multicenter experience

DeWitt J, Jowell P, Leblanc J, *et al. Gastrointest Endosc* 2005; **61**(6): 689–96

BACKGROUND. Very little has been written on the EUS characteristics of pancreatic metastatic disease.

INTERPRETATION. This is a retrospective, multicentre study of 24 patients with documented metastatic lesions of the pancreas. The most common source was the kidney (ten) followed by skin (six), lung (four), colon (two), liver (one) and stomach (one). In 16 of the cases, pancreatic metastases were documented as tumour recurrence, and only in four cases was EUS-FNA used to provide the initial diagnosis. When compared with a group of 24 patients with pancreatic malignancies, there were no EUS characteristics that separated primary from metastatic disease, except for well-defined margins for the latter.

Comment

This is the largest EUS series of pancreatic metastases in the literature. The only delineating EUS feature that separates pancreatic metastases from primary pancreatic neoplasms is the propensity to have a well-defined margin.

Assessment of publication bias in the reporting of EUS performance in staging of rectal cancer

Harewood GC. *Am J Gastroentrol* 2005; **100**: 808–16

BACKGROUND. The analysis of publication bias is exceedingly uncommon in the medical literature, aside from meta-analytic studies. With the advent of new technologies, the initial publications usually involve smaller studies with positive results. Does the diagnostic advantage of newer technologies remain when larger studies are published? Harewood addresses publication bias with respect to EUS in the setting of rectal cancer staging.

INTERPRETATION. A Medline search was performed between 1985 and 2003 for all published estimates of EUS staging accuracy for rectal cancer. All studies were fully published in the English literature. Data extracted included: accuracy of EUS; year of publication; impact factor of the journal; and the type of journal (gastroenterology, surgery, etc.). Forty-one out of 202 abstracts met the inclusion criteria and included 4118 subjects. The mean T-staging and N-staging accuracy was 85.2 and 75%, respectively. Both T-staging and N-staging rates had diminished over time. Compared with the larger studies, most of the smaller studies found higher T- and N-stage accuracies. This trend led Harewood to conclude that the performance of EUS for rectal cancer staging may be overestimated in the literature because of publication bias.

Comment

It is crucial to evaluate critically a new technology and its impact on disease management. In the case of EUS staging of rectal cancer, Harewood points out the potential effect of publication bias, in that the earlier (and smaller) studies found the highest rates of T- and N-stage accuracy, whereas the more recent and larger studies found lower accuracy rates.

Endoscopic ultrasound errors in esophageal cancer

Zuccaro G, Rice TW, Vargo JJ, *et al. Am J Gastroenterol* 2005; **100**: 601–6

BACKGROUND. Most EUS staging data for oesophageal cancer involve symptomatic patients with advanced disease. Studies addressing the test characteristics of EUS in the earlier stages of oesophageal malignancy are extremely limited. Moreover, the assessment of EUS staging errors in a balanced cohort of limited/advanced oesophageal cancer is unknown.

Interpretation. A total of 266 patients underwent oesophagectomy without pre-operative chemoradiotherapy. A hundred and eight (41%) had malignancy confined to the oesophageal wall (pTis–pT2); 158 (59%) were advanced beyond the oesophageal wall (pT3, pT4, pN1 or pM1). Logistic regression analysis was performed to identify correlates of error in T classification and disease extent by using ten clinical and tumour characteristics (gender, age, dysphagia, weight loss, tumour length, location, traversability, morphology, histopathological type and histological grade). Erroneous T classification occurred in 119 (45%) of patients. When the T classification was dichotomized to confinement to the oesophageal wall (pTis–pT2) or advancement beyond the oesophageal wall (pT3, pT4), errors occurred in 42 patients (16%). EUS erroneously predicted N classification in 67 patients (25%). Logistic regression analysis indicated that weight loss and tumour length were the only clinical and tumour characteristics that were associated with EUS errors. The odds of misclassification decrease with longer tumour length and greater weight loss.

Comment

Multiple biases may influence the results of EUS classification. Errors in T classification may be much more common than previously reported. The authors found that no tumour characteristics, such as location or traversability, played a role in misclassification. Rather, tumour length and weight loss appeared to be the only factors associated with misclassification. The authors make a bold statement that where EUS is needed most to classify oesophageal cancer (when the clinical and endoscopic clues are ambiguous for disease extent), it is most likely to be in error. Perhaps for early tumours EUS followed by EMR (see the discussion of the paper by Larghi *et al.* earlier in this chapter) offers the best approach for staging accuracy.

Conclusion

Advances in EUS over the past year included some critical appraisals of its diagnostic test characteristics. We now have data suggesting that EUS is superior to ERCP in suspected acute biliary pancreatitis and in the evaluation of pancreatic masses without biliary strictures. Smaller oesophageal tumours are associated with an increased risk of staging errors. The combination of EUS followed by EMR can provide accurate pathological staging of oesophageal malignancy in some of these cases. The appearance of the k-ras oncogene in pancreatic cyst fluid may turn out to be a powerful diagnostic test in the evaluation of pancreatic cysts. In some of these patients, EUS-directed ethanol lavage may offer the hope of a non-surgical cure. Does the pancreas age? It appears that it does and we hope that it does so gracefully! These age-related EUS changes may have profound implications in the way that we diagnose chronic pancreatitis. We must always respect the evolution of technology and its shortfalls: EUS staging of rectal cancer, though a valuable diagnostic tool, may not have the highly touted test characteristics that we originally surmised. We look forward to further advances in

EUS as it solidifies its position as a potent diagnostic and therapeutic avenue for our patients.

Further reading

1. Sumiyama K, Suzuki N, Tajiri H. A linear-array free-hand 3-D endoscopic ultrasound. *Ultrasound Med Biol* 2003; **29**: 1001–6.
2. Brugge WR, Lewandrowski K, Lee-Lewandrowski E, Centeno BA, Szydlo T, Regan S, del Castillo CF, Warshaw AL. Diagnosis of pancreatic cystic neoplasm: a report of the cooperative pancreatic cyst study. *Gastroenterology* 2004; **126**: 1330–6.
3. Ahmad NA, Kochman ML, Lewis JD, Ginsberg GG. Can EUS alone differentiate between malignant and benign cystic lesions of the pancreas? *Am J Gastroenterol* 2001; **96**: 3295–300.
4. Rice TW, Blackstone EH, Adelstein DJ, Zuccaro G Jr, Vargo JJ, Goldblum JR, Rybicki LA, Murthy SC, Decamp MM. N1 esophageal carcinoma: the importance of downstaging. *J Thorac Cardiovasc Surg* 2001; **121**: 454–64.
5. Gress F, Gottlieb K, Sherman S, Lehman G. Endoscopic ultrasonography-guided fine-needle aspiration biopsy of suspected pancreatic cancer. *Ann Intern Med* 2001; **134**: 459–64.

10

Biliary endoscopy

JOHN DUMOT

Introduction

Biliary endoscopy or endoscopic retrograde cholangiopancreatography (ERCP) remains one of the most challenging endoscopic procedures performed in gastroenterology. In spite of advances in technology, ERCP continues to carry relatively high rates of the procedure-related complications of pancreatitis, bleeding and perforation compared with routine endoscopy and endoscopic ultrasonography. Advances in non-invasive imaging have reduced the overall number of purely diagnostic ERCP procedures. Numerous investigations have tried to improve the technical success and reduce the incidence of complications. Ten recent articles were selected from a Medline search for discussion in this chapter because of their contribution to the advancement of our knowledge of ERCP. Prospective controlled studies were given preference in this brief review.

Post-operative ERCP versus laparoscopic choledochotomy for clearance of selected bile duct calculi: a randomized trial

Nathanson LK, O'Rourke NA, Martin IJ, *et al. Ann Surg* 2005; **242**: 188–92

BACKGROUND. In a significant number of patients common bile duct stones will be encountered during laparoscopic cholecystectomy. In expert hands, laparoscopic extraction of the stones can be achieved via the cystic duct. These investigators performed a large multicentre trial in Australia to compare laparoscopic choledochotomy with post-operative ERCP in the clearance of bile duct stones found on intra-operative cholangiogram when the cystic duct clearance failed.

INTERPRETATION. The study concluded that most common bile duct stones can be cleared via the cystic duct (77%). The numbers of patients in the laparoscopic choledochotomy (41) and ERCP (45) groups were small. Each group required one open conversion. Eleven of 45 patients required two ERCP procedures. None of the patients in the ERCP group suffered a bile leak compared with six of those in the choledochotomy group. Four patients in the choledochotomy group required post-operative ERCP: three for leaks and one for retained stones. Overall, three patients in each group required re-operation. The rates of other complications, such as pancreatitis and sepsis, did not differ between the two groups.

Comment

This study enrolled subjects at seven metropolitan hospitals for almost 5 years. The experience of the surgeons and gastroenterologists varied, so the study is likely to be applicable in a wide range of community settings. As cholecystectomy has transitioned from an open to a laparoscopic approach, most investigations have centred on the non-invasive pre-operative detection of common bile duct stones. This prompted pre-operative clearance in as many patients as possible with choledochotomy being reserved for those failing pre-operative ERCP. These investigators have continued to push their skills to perform cholecystectomy and clearance of the bile duct as a single-stage operation, either with trans-cystic or with 'closed' choledochotomy. This study supports the technique of operative cholangiogram to define the biliary anatomy and detect common bile duct stones. The authors conclude that most common bile duct stones can be cleared via the cystic duct at the time of the cholecystectomy, the remainder being cleared by choledochotomy or ERCP. As a result of their experience, they would avoid choledochotomy in ducts less than 7 mm and those with a severely inflamed surgical field. Treatment failures in both groups suggest there is room for improvement with each approach.

Endoscopic biliary drainage by nasobiliary drain or by stent placement in patients with acute cholangitis

Sharma BC, Kumar R, Agarwal N, Sarin SK. *Endoscopy* 2005; **37**: 439–43

Background. ERCP with biliary drainage is a well-recognized therapy for acute cholangitis with fewer overall complications compared with emergency surgery or percutaneous trans-hepatic drainage. Early ERCP studies reported efficacy using nasobiliary drainage (NBD) without sphincterotomy or stone extraction. NBD allows monitoring of biliary drainage and interim cholangiogram but the catheter may be accidentally dislodged. Endoscopic plastic stents are easier to place than NBD and limited data are available to compare the two methods.

Interpretation. This study randomized 150 patients to NBD or stent placement, the groups being balanced for gender, clinical signs and cause of obstruction. The rate of successful placement was equivalent in the two groups. No immediate complications occurred in either group and all devices functioned without occlusion or migration. The treatment effect and mortality were equivalent in the two groups.

Comment

This study enrolled 150 patients over 4 years in a single-centre study. The investigators made efforts to minimize the amount of contrast injection and avoided sphincterotomy or stone extraction at the time of the initial procedure. The theoretical advantages of NBD are the possibilities for maintenance of patency with lavage, sampling bile for culture, chemical dissolution of stones and follow-up cholangiography. Disadvantages of NBD include malfunction due to kinking and dislodgement, and discomfort. These data confirm the findings of Lee *et al.*, who originally reported the comparison of NBD and stents for decompression of the biliary tree in acute cholangitis |**1**|. In general, endoscopic stent placement appears to be as effective as NBD and will probably remain our preferred method for the foreseeable future.

Pancreatic juice cytology in the diagnosis of intraductal papillary mucinous neoplasm of the pancreas: significance of sampling by peroral pancreatoscopy

Yamaguchi T, Shirai Y, Ishihara T, *et al. Cancer* 2005; **104**: 2830–6

BACKGROUND. Intraductal papillary mucinous neoplasms (IPMNs) are being found more often, either because of increased incidence or the more widespread use of cross-sectional imaging. Growth patterns are variable and the histology ranges from pre-malignant adenomatous papillary growth to invasive adenocarcinoma. Pre-operative staging is difficult with current imaging studies and routine cytology during ERCP has a low predictive value for the final histopathological diagnosis. Peroral pancreatoscopy allows a direct view of the lesions and may increase the yield of cytology over routine catheter-based sampling methods.

INTERPRETATION. The authors studied 103 consecutive patients with IPMN and compared the results of cytology obtained by pancreatoscopy and catheter methods. Specimens collected with pancreatoscopy were also influenced by ductal lavage, which is routinely employed to improve visualization. Catheter cytology specimens were influenced by secretin stimulation. Catheter cytology was also collected in 81 patients with typical pancreatic carcinoma and 78 patients with chronic pancreatitis for comparison. The sensitivity of catheter cytology was 38% for IPMN cancers and 25% for typical cancers compared with 68% for IPMN by pancreatoscopy cytology. The sensitivity rose to 80% in IPMN of the main duct by pancreatoscopy.

Comment

This is an excellent study of the pathological evaluation of patients with IPMNs using available mother–daughter endoscopic instruments. The authors were careful to characterize the IPMNs in great detail according to histopathological grading and location (region of the pancreas and main or branch duct). The cytology specimens were interpreted by cytopathologists blinded to clinical data. The implications of this study are important in patients with an indeterminate risk of advanced neoplasia. For example, an elderly patient with a benign adenomatous IPMN may choose to avoid surgical resection because the natural history of these lesions is variable and difficult to predict. If that same patient had a better pre-operative assessment with pancreatoscopy-directed cytology and an invasive cancer were identified, surgical resection could be recommended with more certainty. This study may have been more compelling if catheter-based cytology data had been available for those patients with pancreatoscopy cytology, which would allow direct comparison of sampling techniques, the patients serving as their own controls.

Single operator duodenoscope-assisted cholangioscopy is an effective alternative in the management of choledocholithiasis not removed by conventional methods, including mechanical lithotripsy

Farrell JJ, Bounds BC, Al-Shalabi S, *et al.* *Endoscopy* 2005; **37**: 542–7

Background. Peroral cholangioscopy has the limitations of requiring two operators as well as the added expense of fragile small-bore daughter cholangioscopes. The investigators described experience with a breastplate apparatus designed to hold the cholangioscope in an inverted position while the endoscopist manoeuvred the duodenoscope and electrohydraulic lithotripsy (ELH) catheter through the working channel of the cholangioscope.

Interpretation. The investigators reported the outcome of 75 patients undergoing cholangioscopy (26 with difficult common bile duct stones requiring ELH after failing routine methods [mechanical lithotripsy] and 49 patients after cholangiography) to search for the presence of occult stones or for the assessment of strictures. All patients were clear of stones and without complications.

Comment

This is a very small study with a positive outcome. The most telling statistic was found in the discussion: only one cholangioscope injury was incurred during the study period! The use of ELH in the bile duct is not unprecedented but their determination to complete the procedure may be. The number of ELH procedures per patient ranged from one ($n = 15$) to nine ($n = 1$), with a trend to a lower mean number of sessions in the second half of the study compared with the first half (1.4 sessions and 2.5 sessions, respectively). Stones located above the bifurcation, multiple stones and the presence of a stricture were factors predictive of an increased number of sessions required to clear the duct. Single-operator cholangioscopy may not follow the rule that 'two heads are better than one'.

Endoscopic drainage of pancreatic pseudocysts: long-term outcome and procedural factors associated with safe and successful treatment

Cahen D, Rauws E, Fockens P, Weverling G, Huibregtse K, Bruno M.
Endoscopy 2005; **37**: 977–83

BACKGROUND. Endoscopic drainage of pancreatic pseudocysts was described over a decade ago but not widely accepted because it entails significant risk and long-term data are lacking. No comparative trials have demonstrated superiority of surgical, percutaneous or endoscopic drainage approaches. The major advantage of endoscopic management over percutaneous drainage is the absence of an external catheter, which is a nuisance and may become dislodged or infected from skin colonization. The endoscopic approach attempts to mimic the surgical cyst–enteric anastomosis.

INTERPRETATION. This is a single-centre experience of 92 patients over a 17-year period from an endoscopic database. Ten patients were lost to follow-up. The overall success rate was 71%. One death occurred in the series, in a patient with decompensated cirrhosis 1 month after the drainage procedure. Significant morbidity that required surgical intervention occurred in eight patients and ten were managed conservatively or with endoscopic stent exchange. Of the 22 patients undergoing surgical drainage due to complications or failure of endoscopic drainage, four developed a new pseudocyst during the follow-up period. Three of these recurrent pseudocysts were drained endoscopically.

Comment

The investigators found that three factors were predictive of a more favourable outcome: (i) localization of the pseudocyst in the head of the gland; (ii) drainage duration of more than 6 weeks; and (iii) insertion of multiple prostheses. The authors also suggest that more aggressive management of complications may have improved the overall success and prevented surgery, but only three patients underwent surgery for infection—the only likely complication that may have been more aggressively treated. Avoiding straight stents may have prevented one pseudocyst perforation that required surgery. The instances when endoscopic drainage failed and then surgical drainage resulted in recurrent cyst formation that was, in turn, treated with a second attempt at endoscopic drainage suggest that both approaches have value. Individualized care of patients with pseudocysts is warranted until a comparative trial proves the superiority of one method over the other.

Effect of pre-operative biliary stenting on immediate outcome after pancreaticoduodenectomy

Jagannath P, Dhir V, Shrikhande S, Shah RC, Mullerpatan P, Mohandas KM. *Br J Surg* 2005; **92**: 356–61

BACKGROUND. Endoscopic stent placement has been implicated in post-operative complications in patients undergoing surgical resection of the pancreas. Colonization of the biliary tree during the procedure is the hypothesized cause of the poor outcome. Data from surgical series have been retrospective and difficult to interpret.

INTERPRETATION. In this observational cohort study, a detailed evaluation of 144 patients undergoing pancreaticoduodenectomy over a 10-year period is reported. Patients were grouped according to the placement of a pre-operative biliary stent ($n = 74$) or no stent ($n = 70$) placement. Intra-operative bile cultures were obtained in both groups. Bile culture growth was noted in 35 (47%) of patients with stents and 22 (31%) without stents. Bile culture growth was related to post-operative complications of bleeding, pancreatic leak, wound infection, sepsis and overall morbidity and mortality.

Comment

This is an interesting study that provides useful information regarding the effect of pre-operative biliary drainage. The investigators' use of routine intra-operative bile cultures made comparison of the outcome more reliable than in previous studies. Once the bile duct has been manipulated, bacterial colonization is believed to contaminate the operative field. This study clearly shows that nearly one in three patients without pre-operative drainage has a colonized biliary tree. Although bile culture growth was clearly related to infectious complications, non-infectious morbidity occurred with equal frequency. The investigators suggested that early intervention after complicated biliary stent placement may have contributed to the morbidity, and postponing surgery for 6 weeks may be beneficial. As the treatment of pancreatic cancer evolves, pre-operative chemoradiotherapy occurs more frequently and adequate drainage becomes an important factor. A recent report suggested placing self-expanding metallic stents before surgical resection because the larger diameter may provide better drainage without interfering with the surgical outcome |**2**|.

The impact of hands-on ERCP workshop on clinical practice

Sedlack RE, Petersen BT, Kolars JC. *Gastrointest Endosc* 2005; **61**: 67–71

BACKGROUND. Hands-on endoscopic continuing medical education workshops offer unique experiences to physicians using models or live animals in order to improve or learn new skills. There is little information regarding the impact of these workshops on physicians' practice.

INTERPRETATION. Forty-eight practising endoscopists attended a 2-day hands-on workshop on ERCP skills. Thirty-one of 48 physicians completed surveys before and 3 months after the workshop. The attendees had a wide range of expertise in performing ERCP; all were credentialled to perform ERCP in their institution and were board-certified in gastroenterology. Surveys indicated increased confidence in standard sphincterotomy, needle–knife sphincterotomy, stone extraction, mechanical lithotripsy, metal stent placement and cytology after attendance at the workshop. Physicians also reported increased application of pre-cut sphincterotomies, although the increase was not statistically significant.

Comment

This article illustrates the usefulness of hands-on workshops in the dissemination of ERCP skills. It is useful for us to understand and quantify the benefits of a short course on ERCP techniques because a significant amount of time and money is spent in preparation for and attendance at these programmes. The authors help build the confidence of the attendees as well as those intimately involved in planning and conducting these educational programmes.

Serum amylase, pancreatic stents, and pancreatitis after sphincter of Oddi manometry

Sheehan SJ, Lee JH, Wells CK, Topazian M. *Gastrointest Endosc* 2005; **62**: 260–5

BACKGROUND. ERCP-induced pancreatitis remains the most common complication in spite of numerous attempts to prevent this dreaded outcome. This study reports the authors' institution's experience with monitoring for pancreatitis after ERCP with routine serum amylase.

INTERPRETATION. Records of 88 patients undergoing sphincter of Oddi manometry (SOM) for suspected sphincter of Oddi dysfunction were reviewed and analysed. The characteristics associated with pancreatitis were a history of pancreatitis or post-ERCP pancreatitis, and pancreatic stent placement. Fifty-two of 88 patients had a pancreatic stent placed after SOM. Pancreatitis occurred in 8 of 36 (22%) patients without a stent and only 3 of 52 (6%) with a stent ($P = 0.04$). In general, elevated serum amylase was associated with pancreatitis and a normal amylase concentration was associated with no pancreatitis, but the association was not statistically significant in the group with a pancreatic stent.

Comment

Over a 5-year period, 88 of 180 patients undergoing SOM were included in this retrospective review because serum amylase measurements had been obtained 2 h after the procedure, according to the authors' clinical practice. Therefore, all patients in this case series were experiencing new or increased abdominal pain after the SOM. The investigators reported their usual practice with respect to timing sphincterotomy and pancreatic duct stent placement. It is unclear why abdominal pain 2 h after SOM would be a predictor of pancreatitis (reported to occur in 37 patients, ten [27%] of them developing pancreatitis), because the authors state in the methods section that amylase was measured 'in patients with any immediate or delayed abdominal symptoms after the procedure'. Even so, the review is useful for identifying those individuals at low risk of severe pancreatitis. In our practice, it is difficult to discharge a patient from the unit with new or worsening symptoms even with the reassurance of a 2-h amylase measurement. Their results confirmed our experience, 2 of 59 patients (3%) having normal amylase levels at 2 h but still developing pancreatitis. This study deserves confirmation in a prospective trial with a cost analysis of any change in clinical practice offered by the simple intervention of measuring serum amylase.

Oral allopurinol does not prevent the frequency or severity of post-ERCP pancreatitis

Mosler P, Sherman S, Marks J, *et al.* *Gastrointest Endosc* 2005; **62**: 245–50

BACKGROUND. Prevention of ERCP-induced pancreatitis with medical interventions has failed numerous times. Early information on steroids, biological agents and various pancreatic modulators (octreotide and somatostatin) has been promising but there have been inconsistent results in larger clinical trials. Allopurinol showed promise in an animal model in preventing ERCP-induced pancreatitis, and the proposed mechanism was scavenging of the free radicals known to be operative in acute pancreatic injury. Another clinical study demonstrated a clinical benefit, pancreatitis occurring in 3% in the allopurinol group and 18% in the placebo group [3].

INTERPRETATION. Oral allopurinol 600 mg 4 h before and 300 mg 1 h before ERCP failed to reduce the incidence of ERCP-induced pancreatitis. The randomization was balanced between treatment ($n = 355$) and placebo ($n = 346$) for all factors except prior pancreatitis, which was slightly more frequent in the placebo group. In fact, the incidence of ERCP-induced pancreatitis was higher in the treatment group (13%) than in the placebo group (12%).

Comment

Allopurinol did not reduce the rate of ERCP-induced pancreatitis in this large multicentre study with balanced groups. The main difference between the study of Katsinelos *et al.* [3] and the Mosler study is sample size: 250 and 701, respectively. Another, smaller study by Budzynska *et al.* [4] of 200 patients also noted a slightly higher rate of pancreatitis in the allopurinol group, which should put the question of allopurinol to rest. The strongest evidence to date for medical therapy in the prevention of ERCP-induced pancreatitis remains with gabexate [5,6].

Prospective, randomized controlled trial of prophylactic pancreatic stent placement for endoscopic snare excision of the duodenal ampulla

Harewood GC, Pochron NL, Gostout CJ. *Gastrointest Endosc* 2005; **62**: 367–70

BACKGROUND. Pancreatic duct stent placement has been shown to reduce the incidence of ERCP-induced pancreatitis in high-risk procedures such as pancreatic sphincterotomy and SOM. Endoscopic snare ampullectomy is usually performed for therapeutic removal of adenomatous tissues and results in significant injury to the pancreatic duct. This randomized trial was halted because of a very high rate of pancreatitis in the control group compared with the stent group.

INTERPRETATION. The trial was stopped after 19 patients had been randomized and treated: 3 of 9 (33%) patients developed pancreatitis in the control group and 0 of 10 (0%) in the stent group.

Comment

The evidence that pancreatic stents can reduce the incidence of pancreatitis after significant manipulation of the pancreatic duct continues to grow. It seems that efforts in this area should be directed to consistent stent placement with a minimum of resource use and risk. This trial was conducted over a 3-year period and involved only 19 patients, which demonstrates the difficulty in designing and conducting endoscopic research. Hopefully, the future of endoscopic research will involve more collaboration and in turn faster accumulation of knowledge that can be generalized to a broader setting.

Conclusion

The reviewed year was remarkable for several interesting and relevant controlled trials dealing with ERCP. We learned of the value of ERCP for removing common bile duct stones compared with laparoscopic choledochotomy, both of which have their failures and limitations in terms of finding skilled operators. The effectiveness of biliary stents was confirmed to be equivalent to that of the more cumbersome nasobiliary tube placement—hooray for the patients suffering the nasal passage trauma. Two expert centres demonstrated the utility of placing endoscopes into the bile duct in difficult stone cases and identifying malignant transformation of pancreatic ductal cells. Cahen and colleagues shared their success with endoscopic therapy of pancreatic pseudocysts, which looks extremely promising compared with surgical series. Jagannath and colleagues taught us more about the intricacies of bacterial colonization in patients with and without biliary drainage undergoing pancreaticoduodenectomy. We learned of the value of ERCP workshops for practising biliary endoscopists. We confirmed the practice of placing pancreatic duct stents after significant manipulation of the pancreatic duct, and maybe we can cut down on the number of patients being hospitalized for observation after ERCP based on a 2-h amylase level. And finally we acquired more evidence that pancreatic stents can reduce the incidence of pancreatitis after pancreatic duct manipulation, but medical therapy continues to lack effective and reproducible results!

References

1. Lee DW, Chan AC, Lam YH, Ng EK, Lau JY, Law BK, Lai CW, Sung JJ, Chung SC. Biliary decompression by nasobiliary catheter or biliary stent in acute suppurative cholangitis: a prospective randomized trial. *Gastrointest Endosc* 2002; **56**: 361–5.
2. Wasan SM, Ross WA, Staerkel GA, Lee JH. Use of expandable metallic biliary stents in resectable pancreatic cancer. *Am J Gastroenterol* 2005; **100**: 2056–61.
3. Katsinelos P, Kountouras J, Chatzis J, Christodoulou K, Paroutoglou G, Mimidis K, Beltsis A, Zavos C. High-dose allopurinol for prevention of post-ERCP pancreatitis: a prospective randomized double-blind controlled trial. *Gastrointest Endosc* 2005; **61**: 407–15.
4. Budzynska A, Marek T, Nowak A, Kaczor R, Nowakowska-Dulawa E. A prospective, randomized, placebo-controlled trial of prednisone and allopurinol in the prevention of ERCP-induced pancreatitis. *Endoscopy* 2001; **33**: 766–72.
5. Cavallini G, Tittobello A, Frulloni L, Masci E, Mariani A, Di Francesco V. Gabexate for the prevention of pancreatic damage related to endoscopic retrograde cholangio-pancreatography. *N Engl J Med* 1996; **335**: 919–23.
6. Masci E, Cavallini G, Mariani A, Frulloni L, Testoni PA, Curioni S, Tittobello A, Uomo G, Costamagna G, Zambelli S, Macarri G, Innocenti P, Dragonetti C; Gabexate in Digestive Endoscopy—Italian Group II. Comparison of two dosing regimes of gabexate in the prophylactics of post-ERCP pancreatitis. *Am J Gastroenterol* 2003; **98**: 2182–6.

Part IV

Hepatology and liver transplantation

11

Chronic viral hepatitis

ANNA WIECKOWSKA, NIZAR ZEIN

Introduction

Chronic viral hepatitis is the major cause of liver-related morbidity and mortality worldwide and remains a significant epidemiological and clinical problem. Its serious sequelae include cirrhosis, liver failure and hepatocellular carcinoma. Successful eradication or suppression of viral replication has been shown to lead to clinical improvement and better prognosis. The current standard of treatment for chronic hepatitis C includes a combination of pegylated interferon α (IFN-α), an immune modulator, and ribavirin, a nucleoside analogue. For chronic hepatitis B, interferon, lamivudine, adefovir or entecavir have been used. However, currently available therapies are effective only in a limited number of patients, and are unsuitable for certain patient populations because of significant side effects. Important advances have been made in recent years in the understanding and management of these diseases. This chapter reviews some publications from the past 18 months that have contributed to our understanding and treatment of chronic viral hepatitis.

Chronic hepatitis C infection

Hepatitis C virus (HCV) is the leading cause of chronic liver disease, with more than 170 million people infected worldwide. Complications include cirrhosis, hepatic decompensation and hepatocellular carcinoma. HCV is also the leading indication for liver transplantation, which has important financial implications. The current interferon-based therapies are effective in only a fraction of the population. The introduction of pegylated interferon has significantly improved the sustained viral response (SVR) rate, which is still under 50% of treated patients globally. Interferon therapies are not always tolerated by the patient because of their numerous side effects. The following articles discuss strategies to improve the efficacy and tolerability of the present regimens, introduce new antiviral agents and evaluate the long-term implications for patients with chronic HCV.

Optimization of standard therapies

Effects of adding ribavirin to interferon to treat chronic hepatitis C infection: a systematic review and meta-analysis of randomized trials

Brok J, Gluud LL, Gluud C. *Arch Intern Med* 2005; **165**: 2206–12

BACKGROUND. There has been a considerable improvement in the treatment of chronic hepatitis C in the past decade. While interferon monotherapy was associated with a SVR of about 10%, the benefit of combining pegylated interferon with ribavirin is evident, giving a SVR of more than 40%. Although combination therapy is now the standard of care for the treatment of chronic hepatitis C, its effect on clinical outcomes, such as morbidity, mortality and quality of life, is controversial. This systematic review and meta-analysis of randomized, controlled trials evaluates the beneficial and harmful effects of ribavirin plus interferon versus interferon alone for the treatment of patients with chronic hepatitis C infection.

INTERPRETATION. A total of 9991 patients from 72 trials were analysed. Treatment with ribavirin plus interferon significantly improved sustained viral clearance as well as liver histology in treatment-naive patients and non-responders. Although morbidity (cirrhosis and hepatocellular carcinoma) and mortality were significantly reduced (Fig. 11.1), the effects on quality of life were unclear. Moreover, combination therapy significantly increased the risk of haematological, dermatological, gastrointestinal and several other types of adverse events.

Comment

This large meta-analysis demonstrated that, although increasing the number of adverse events during treatment, the effect of combining ribavirin and interferon leads to improved clinical outcomes in patients with chronic hepatitis C. Although these findings seem intuitive, caution must be taken in interpreting results obtained using the meta-analysis design. Numerous biases exist, including inadequate randomization, the inter-trial variability in patient characteristics and treatment regimens, and lack of data in a large number of studies. To better understand the effect of ribavirin on treatment outcome, large, long-term randomized trials comparing combination therapy versus interferon monotherapy would be necessary. This is unlikely to happen, combination therapy being the standard of care.

Trial	Events/participants: Combination therapy	Events/participants: Monotherapy
Chemello et al., 1995	2/15	3/15
Lai et al., 1996	0/21	1/19
Davis et al., 1998	0/173	1/172
McHutchison et al., 1998	1/456	3/456
Poynard et al., 1998	1/559	0/281
Andreone et al., 1999	0/26	1/24
Pol et al., 1999	2/62	4/65
Cavaletto et al., 2000	2/50	5/50
Fried et al., 2002	0/435	2/224
de Lédinghen et al., 2002	3/229	0/92
62 trials with no events		
Total (95% CI)	11/2026	20/1398

Test for heterogeneity: $\chi^2 = 7.64$, df = 9 (P = 0.57), $I^2 = 0\%$

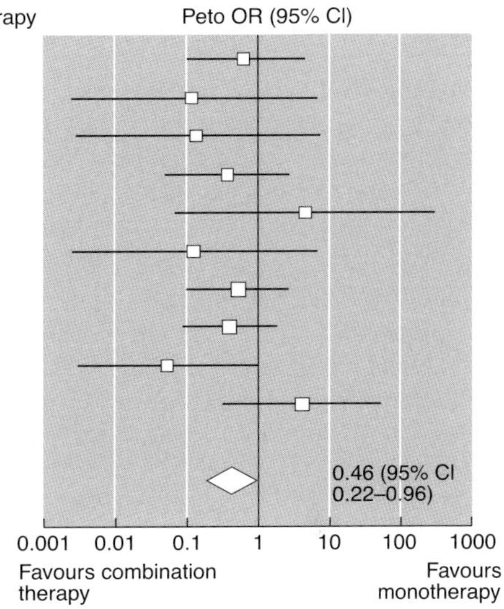

Fig. 11.1 Effect of treatment with ribavirin plus interferon versus treatment with interferon only on mortality plus morbidity in chronic hepatitis C infection. CI, confidence interval; I^2, intertrial heterogeneity; OR, odds ratio. Source: Brok *et al.* (2005).

Peginterferon alfa-2b and ribavirin for 12 versus 24 weeks in HCV genotype 2 or 3

Mangia A, Santoro R, Minerva N, *et al. N Engl J Med* 2005; **352**: 2609–17

Peginterferon-alpha-2a (40KD) and ribavirin for 16 or 24 weeks in patients with genotype 2 or 3 chronic hepatitis C

Von Wagner M, Huber M, Berg T, *et al. Gastroenterology* 2005; **129**: 522–7

Background. Hepatitis C viral kinetics demonstrates two phases of viral decline after treatment initiation: the first, rapid phase represents the interferon-dependent inhibition of virus production; the second, slower phase reflects the rate of death of infected cells. The two phases have been shown to be different for genotype 1 and genotype non-1, being much faster for the latter. Based on these data, the aim of the following two multicentre randomized controlled trials was to investigate whether shorter treatments may be effective in genotype 2 and 3 patients whose HCV RNA was undetectable at week 4.

INTERPRETATION. In the first study, Mangia *et al.* randomized patients with genotype 2 or genotype 3 to a standard-duration regimen (24 weeks, $n = 70$) or a variable-duration regimen (12 weeks [$n = 133$] if the HCV RNA was negative at 4 weeks, and 24 weeks [$n = 80$] if the HCV RNA was positive at 4 weeks). The treatment regimen included pegylated IFN-α2b (1 μg/kg) plus ribavirin (1000–1200 mg daily according to weight). There was no difference in the percentage of patients with negative RNA at 4 weeks between the standard-duration and variable-duration groups (64 and 62%, respectively). Similarly, the SVR was not different (76 and 77%, respectively). Most importantly, patients treated for 12 weeks in the variable-duration group had SVR rates similar to those of patients treated for 24 weeks, suggesting that a shorter duration of therapy may be sufficient in some patients. The overall SVR was better for genotype 2 than for genotype 3 (80 vs 66%; $P < 0.001$) independently of the duration of treatment.

The study by Von Wagner and colleagues supports these findings. Patients were treated with pegylated IFN-α2a at 180 μg/week and ribavirin 800–1200 mg/day. If HCV RNA was <600 IU/ml (rapid responders), the patients were randomized to a shorter duration of treatment (16 weeks) or the standard duration (24 weeks). Ninety-three per cent (142/153) of patients were rapid responders. SVR rates were similar for rapid responders whether treated for 16 weeks or for 24 weeks (82 and 80%, respectively), but much lower in patients whose HCV RNA was >600 IU/ml at 4 weeks (SVR = 36%). Patients with genotype 3 and a high pre-treatment viral load (>800 000 IU/ml) had lower SVR rates than those with genotype 3 and a low viral load (59 vs 85%).

Comment

These studies demonstrate that a shorter duration of treatment with pegylated interferon and weight-based ribavirin dosage is sufficient for patients with genotype 2 or 3 chronic hepatitis C who achieve a rapid virological response at week 4. However, the trials have been criticized in regard to their applicability to the US population because of a difference in patient characteristics (higher body mass index and more African-American patients in the USA compared with Europe) and the doses of medication used (higher interferon doses compared with the study by Mangia *et al.* and lower ribavirin doses recommended in the USA for genotypes 2 and 3). Moreover, caution must be taken with genotype 3 patients, who seem to have a less impressive response to therapy.

Treatment of hepatitis C in patients with advanced disease

Antiviral therapy for cirrhotic hepatitis C: association with reduced hepatocellular carcinoma development and improved survival

Shiratori Y, Ito Y, Yokosuka O, *et al.*; Tokyo-Chiba Hepatitis Research Group. *Ann Intern Med* 2005; **142**: 105–14

Treatment of advanced hepatitis C with a low accelerating dosage regimen of antiviral therapy

Everson GT, Trotter J, Forman L, *et al. Hepatology* 2005; **42**: 255–62

BACKGROUND. Cirrhotic patients with hepatitis C have a 30% risk of developing decompensated liver disease after a decade, with a risk of liver-related death of 2–6% per year. Moreover, the yearly risk of developing hepatocellular carcinoma (HCC) varies between 1 and 3% in the USA and Europe, with an even higher incidence in Japan. Hepatitis C accounts for more than 40% of liver transplantation, being the most common indication at the present time. However, viral recurrence is universal after transplantation and may progress rapidly to cirrhosis and graft loss. Eradication of the virus in patients with advanced hepatitis C is difficult, not only because of a lower SVR compared with patients with early disease, but also because of the possibility of further decompensation on therapy. The goal of the first study was to elucidate the role of antiviral therapy in the prevention of liver cancer and in potentially improving long-term survival in cirrhotic patients with HCV. The second study had the specific aim of assessing the effectiveness, tolerability and outcome of a low accelerating dose regimen (LADR) of antiviral therapy in the treatment of patients with advanced HCV infection.

INTERPRETATION. The first study, by Shiratori *et al.*, describes a prospective cohort of 345 patients with chronic hepatitis C and cirrhosis enrolled in previous trials. The mean follow-up period was 8 years. Seventy-four patients received no treatment and 271 patients received 6–9 million unites (mU) of interferon three times weekly for 26–88 weeks, from which 23% had an SVR (15% for genotype 1 and 47% for genotype non-1). Fewer treated patients developed HCC (31%, vs 47% of untreated patients) (Fig. 11.2), the annual incidence of HCC being 4–5% in treated patients compared with

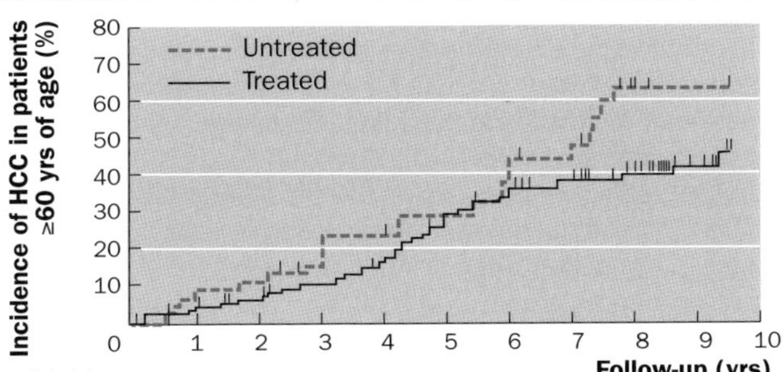

Patients at risk (n)

Treated	98	90	86	79	74	60	54	47	35	24
Untreated	44	39	38	33	30	25	19	15	6	3

Fig. 11.2 Incidence of hepatocellular carcinoma (HCC) in patients ≥60 years of age. The Kaplan–Meier method was used to gauge the cumulative incidence of HCC development in interferon-treated and untreated patients. Source: Shiratori *et al.* (2005).

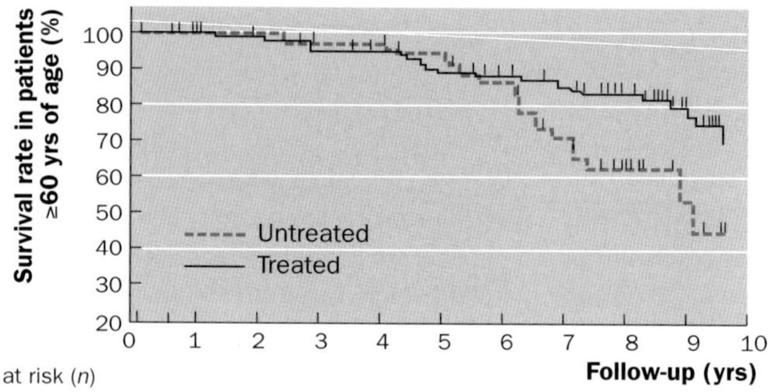

Patients at risk (*n*)										
Treated	98	94	91	87	85	77	70	65	51	32
Untreated	44	43	42	39	39	35	30	23	14	6

Fig. 11.3 Survival rate in patients ≥60 years of age. The Kaplan–Meier method was used to evaluate survival of interferon-treated and untreated patients. Source: Shiratori *et al.* (2005).

6–8% in untreated patients, and fewer of the treated patients died (17 vs 32%) (Fig. 11.3). The difference was especially evident in sustained virological responders. The study was non-randomized and patients in the untreated group were older and had higher baseline alanine aminotransferase values. However, the difference between the two groups persisted even after adjusting for age.

In the second study, 124 patients with cirrhosis (70% had genotype 1) were treated with an LADR. The LADR was defined as IFN-α 2b (1.5 mU three times weekly) or pegylated IFN-α (0.5 μg/kg/week for pegylated IFN-α2b and 90 μg/week for pegylated IFN-α2a) with or without ribavirin, with dose adjustment every 2 weeks. The mean Child–Turcotte–Pugh (CTP) score was 7.4 ± 2.3 (45% CTP A, 36% CTP B and 19% CTP C) and 63% had clinical complications of cirrhosis. The mean MELD (Model for End-stage Liver Disease) score was 11.0 ± 3.7, 73% of patients being listed before, during or after LADR. The absolute neutrophil count was >800/μl, haemoglobin >10 g/dl, and platelets >35 000/μl at initiation of treatment.

Forty-six per cent were HCV RNA-negative at the end of treatment and 24% achieved an SVR. The virological response was better in patients with genotype non-1 (SVR 50% vs 13% for those with genotype 1), in patients with less severe liver disease and those who achieved target doses and duration of therapy. Patients with genotype non-1 had a better end-of-treatment response, higher SVR rate and lower relapse rate (Fig. 11.4). Fifteen (32%) of 47 transplanted patients were rendered HCV RNA-negative at the time of transplantation and 80% of these did not experience post-transplantation recurrence of HCV.

Comment

The above studies demonstrated that a reasonable SVR can be achieved using antiviral therapy in patients with advanced HCV liver disease, and that responders experience slowing of disease progression, inhibition of HCC and prevention of the

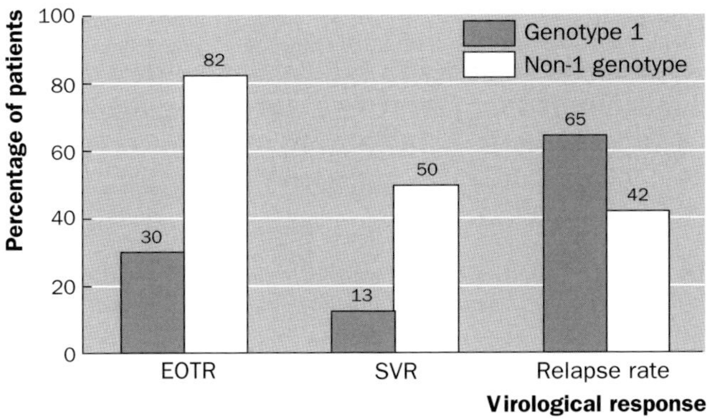

Fig. 11.4 HCV genotype was a major determinant of the virological response to LADR. Thirty per cent of patients with genotype 1 and 82% of those with non-1 genotypes had an end-of-treatment response (EOTR). Thirteen per cent of patients with genotype 1 and 50% of those with non-1 genotypes had an SVR. The relapse rate was 65% for genotype 1 and 42% for non-1 genotypes. SVR, sustained virological response; EOTR, end-of-treatment response. Source: Everson *et al.* (2005).

post-transplantation recurrence. Although the results are encouraging, caution must be exercised in treating these patients because severe serious adverse events have been observed, some contributing to mortality. This supports the AASLD (American Association for the Study of Liver Diseases) practice guidance suggesting that patients with a MELD score of 18 or less should be considered for treatment 'as long as treatment is administered by experienced clinicians, with vigilant monitoring for adverse events'.

Treatment of liver transplant recipients infected with hepatitis C

Peginterferon alfa-2a for hepatitis C after liver transplantation: two randomized, controlled trials

Chalasani N, Manzarbeitia C, Ferenci P, *et al.*; Pegasys Transplant Study Group. *Hepatology* 2005; **41**: 289–98

A randomized, open-label study to evaluate the safety and pharmacokinetics of human hepatitis C immune globulin (Civacir) in liver transplant recipients

Davis GL, Nelson DR, Terrault N, *et al.*; Collaborative Antiviral Study Group. *Liver Transpl* 2005; **11**: 941–9

BACKGROUND. Hepatitis C is currently the most common indication for orthotopic liver transplantation. However, recurrence after transplantation is universal and recent data suggest decreased long-term survival of these patients after transplantation. Moreover, accelerated recurrent hepatitis C infection after orthotopic liver transplantation may rapidly result in decompensated liver disease and cirrhosis. Efforts have been made to offer antiviral therapy to patients at risk. Treatment before orthotopic liver transplantation has been attempted in selected candidates but response rates and tolerance of current therapies are low. Treatment of recurrent hepatitis C after transplantation has been discouraging because of low SVR and feared adverse effects, including anaemia from ribavirin and rejection of the transplant. The first paper reports two randomized controlled trials, a 'prophylaxis trial' and a 'treatment trial' to evaluate the safety and efficacy of pegylated IFN-α2a alone in patients who had undergone orthotopic liver transplantation. The second paper describes a multicentre, randomized, open-label study evaluating the safety, pharmacokinetics and antiviral effects of high doses of a human hepatitis C-enriched immune globulin (HCIG, Civacir) in patients undergoing liver transplantation for chronic hepatitis C.

INTERPRETATION. Chalasani *et al.* report the results of pegylated interferon treatment for 48 weeks versus no treatment in patients transplanted for chronic hepatitis C. Fifty-four patients were included in the 'prophylactic trial', which started 3 weeks after transplantation (26 patients in the pegylated interferon group and 28 untreated patients), and 77 patients with histological evidence of hepatitis were enrolled in the 'treatment trial' (34 in the pegylated interferon group and 33 untreated patients). Although patients treated with pegylated interferon had significantly less HCV RNA, the SVR rates were low (8% in the treated prophylactic group and 12% in the treated treatment group) and not statistically different between treated and untreated patients. Three of the four patients who developed an SVR had genotype 2 or 3. Interferon therapy was shown to be relatively safe and the incidence of acute rejection was similar in the treated and untreated groups.

In the second paper, Davis *et al.* evaluated HCV treatment in patients with decompensated chronic hepatitis C at the time of (reperfusion phase) or shortly after (8–12 h) liver transplantation using an immune globulin product enriched in human hepatitis C antibody, Civavir. In this multicentre trial, a total of 18 patients were randomized to receive low-dose HCIG (75 mg/kg) or high-dose HCIG (200 mg/kg), or no treatment. A total of 17 infusions of HCIG were administered in each treated patient over 14 weeks (during and after transplantation). Although serum alanine aminotransferase levels normalized in most subjects in the high-dose group and no patient developed hepatic fibrosis, serum HCV RNA levels were not suppressed at either dose. Although infusions were generally safe and tolerated (most adverse reactions being related to the underlying illness and transplantation), the infusion rate could not be maximized because of symptoms (back pain, headache, nausea and vomiting, chills, etc.) for 18–30% of the doses.

Comment

The studies described above show two different strategies of the treatment of hepatitis C in recipients of orthotopic liver transplantation. The study from Chalasani *et al.* shows that pegylated interferon alone seems to be relatively safe even early in the post-transplantation period. However, response rates to pegylated interferon, both in the prophylactic group and in the treatment group, were quite disappointing and the histological advantage was unclear. Previous reports have suggested that using a combination of interferon and ribavirin may lead to a higher virological response. Erythropoietin administration and dose modification according to renal clearance could improve the tolerance of ribavirin, and longer-term treatment may be shown to be beneficial. The study by Davis *et al.* investigated the role of immunoglobulin administered within 12 h of liver transplantation, based on the positive experience with hepatitis B immunoglobulin and disease prevention. Although the treatment appeared safe and most of the patients had normalized liver function tests, there was no demonstrable effect of HCIG infusion on the serum HCV RNA levels, suggesting that the dose may be insufficient or the pooled antibody is ineffective in neutralizing HCV. Further studies are warranted to assess higher doses and long-term effects in modifying the natural history of the disease.

Emerging therapies

Etanercept as an adjuvant to interferon and ribavirin in treatment-naive patients with chronic hepatitis C virus infection: a phase 2 randomized, double-blind, placebo-controlled study

Zein NN; Etanercept Study Group. *J Hepatol* 2005; **42**: 315–22

Background. Given that a considerable proportion of patients with chronic HCV do not achieve an SVR after treatment with pegylated IFN-α plus ribavirin, investigators are continually searching for new and potentially more effective therapies. Tumour necrosis factor α (TNF-α), which has been shown to be increased in patients with chronic HCV, seems to be implicated in liver injury in these patients, and

the resistance to interferon therapy. Etanercept, a TNF-α antagonist, has been shown to be safe and even beneficial in patients with autoimmunity and concomitant hepatitis C. This study is a double-blind, randomized, placebo-controlled trial assessing the efficacy and safety of etanercept as adjuvant to interferon and ribavirin in treatment-naive patients with HCV.

INTERPRETATION. In this phase 2 trial, 50 subjects were randomly assigned to receive interferon and ribavirin plus etanercept or interferon and ribavirin plus placebo for 24 weeks. Patients who tested negative for HCV RNA at 24 weeks continued on interferon and ribavirin until week 48. After 24 weeks, 63% of patients (12/19) in the etanercept arm achieved undetectable HCV RNA (primary end-point) compared with 32% (8/25) in the placebo arm ($P = 0.04$), and a similar proportion had a biochemical response. An advantage in histological improvement was also observed in the etanercept group, although the number of patients in which a liver biopsy was available was limited. No major adverse events were reported, and patients receiving etanercept had lower frequencies of most adverse event categories (in particular cardiovascular, cutaneous, gastrointestinal and neurological) compared with the group receiving only interferon and ribavirin (placebo group).

Comment

This study was successful with respect to its primary end-point, as etanercept given to patients with HCV for 24 weeks as adjuvant therapy to interferon and ribavirin had beneficial effects on virological and biochemical responses at the end of the etanercept randomization period. Although the 48-week response rate and the sustained viral eradication at 72 weeks did not reach statistical significance, the authors suggest that the adjuvant etanercept therapy may have been too short, and longer studies are necessary to answer this question. Moreover, the study seems to suggest a slowing of the progression of fibrosis in patients on etanercept. This observation parallels previous reports showing that TNF-α is an important mediator in the development of fibrosis. However, conflicting data come from a recent DDW (Digestive Disease Week) report by Marrero [1] that has not confirmed significant histological improvement in chronic HCV patients (non-responders to pegylated interferon/ribavirin) subsequently treated with etanercept alone for 24 weeks. Further studies with longer follow-up are needed to confirm whether similar results will be observed with pegylated interferon plus ribavirin.

A randomized, double-blind, placebo-controlled dose-escalation trial of merimepodib (VX-497) and interferon-alpha in previously untreated patients with chronic hepatitis C

McHutchison JG, Shiffman ML, Cheung RC, *et al. Antivir Ther* 2005; **10**: 635–43

Background. Current therapies based on interferon and ribavirin for chronic HCV infection lack an adequate SVR and are associated with severe toxic effects. Ribavirin, an essential component of the treatment, is a nucleoside analogue that inhibits inosine monophosphate dehydrogenase (IMPDH), an enzyme necessary for HCV RNA and DNA synthesis. Ribavirin is, however, associated with dose-limiting haemolytic anaemia that compromises the SVR. New, safer IMPDH inhibitors are under development, one of them being merimepodib (VX-497 or MMPD), which has been shown in preliminary studies to have no effect on haemoglobin.

Interpretation. The study by McHutchinson and colleagues is a double-blind, placebo-controlled dose-escalation trial of merimepobid, a small molecule that selectively inhibits IMPDH, in combination with standard IFN-α. The objectives of the study were to evaluate the tolerability of the IFN-α/MMPD combination and to evaluate the effect on HCV RNA. Patients were randomized to IFN-α at 3 mIU three times a week, alone or in combination with 100 or 300 mg (every 8 h) of MMPD for 4 weeks ($n = 54$, all genotype 1). At the end of 4 weeks, all patients were offered 48 weeks of treatment with IFN-α plus ribavirin. The addition of merimepobid to IFN-α was well tolerated. Although the intention-to-treat analysis did not demonstrate a statistically significant difference, the per-protocol primary efficacy analysis based on treatment-compliant patients showed a greater reduction in mean HCV RNA for the combination of 100 mg MMPD plus IFN-α compared with IFN-α alone.

Comment

Although experimental studies have suggested that IMPDH inhibitors other than ribavirin have antiviral activity, this study did not demonstrate a clear benefit of adding merimepobid to interferon. Moreover, preliminary pharmacokinetic–pharmacodynamic results of the anti-HCV activity of merimepobid in combination with pegylated interferon and ribavirin have resulted in discontinuation of clinical trials. Larger, longer-duration trials involving merimepobid or other IMPDH inhibitors in conjunction with pegylated interferon (with or without ribavirin) would be required to determine whether this combination can increase the SVR rate.

Optimization of care for patients with chronic hepatitis C

Susceptibility to hepatitis A in patients with chronic liver disease due to hepatitis C virus infection: missed opportunities for vaccination

Shim M, Khaykis I, Park J, Bini EJ. *Hepatology* 2005; **42**: 688–95

BACKGROUND. Hepatitis A virus (HAV) rarely causes fulminant liver failure, the overall case fatality rate of acute HAV in the general population being 0.01–0.3%. However, it is a more significant cause of morbidity and mortality in patients with chronic liver disease because it may be associated with a high risk of liver failure and death (in more than a third of patients in some studies). Vaccination against HAV has been recommended for patients with chronic HCV infection since 1996. However, the rate of adherence to these recommendations in clinical practice is unknown. The aims of this study were to determine the frequency of HAV testing and vaccination among patients with chronic HCV infection.

INTERPRETATION. Data on 1193 patients diagnosed with chronic HCV infection were analysed retrospectively over a 1-year period. During 1646 person-years of follow-up, HAV antibody testing was performed in 640 subjects (53.6%), and 317 (49.5%) of those tested were negative for HAV antibody. Only 94 of the 1193 patients (7.9%) received the HAV vaccine, including 26.8% of the 317 susceptible patients, 0.9% of the 323 patients who were already immune to HAV, and 1.1% of the 553 subjects who were never tested. Among the 94 vaccinated patients, 45 received only one dose of the vaccine. The incidence rate of HAV was 1.82 per 1000 person-years (it occurred only in unvaccinated patients). Of the three patients who developed acute HAV infection, one died of acute liver failure.

Comment

This large retrospective study in the New York population of chronic HCV patients showed that, despite published recommendations, a substantial proportion of patients were not tested for HAV and most of the susceptible individuals were never vaccinated. The aetiology of this missed opportunity for prevention is unclear. It may have resulted from the lack of awareness of the necessity for adequate efficacy of the vaccine, or from specific patient characteristics, such as compliance with follow-up visits and social status. It has been shown that vaccination against HAV is safe and efficacious in patients with chronic liver disease. Previous studies have suggested that, even if the vaccination series has not been completed or not completed on schedule, partial protective immunity may still be conferred [2]. However, the goal should still be to aim for a full vaccination course as the immunogenicity of the vaccine in patients with chronic liver disease may be lower, especially in those with decompensated liver disease.

Chronic hepatitis B infection

One-third of the world's population has been infected with hepatitis B, including 400 million who are chronically infected. Patients with chronic infection are at high risk of developing cirrhosis and its complications. Hepatocellular carcinoma has a high incidence in this population, irrespective of cirrhosis. Vaccination of the at-risk population is the primary method of preventing infection with hepatitis B virus (HBV), and the long-term response to vaccination has been evaluated in recent studies. For patients who have chronic infection, nucleoside analogue therapy allows long-term suppression of HBV, but the development of drug resistance is a real problem. Moreover, the rate of response to therapy is low, especially if clearance of hepatitis B surface antigen (HBsAg) is used to define the optimal outcome. Trials in recent years have evaluated strategies to improve the response to therapy and minimize resistance to the present treatment regimens. New emerging drugs are also discussed in this section.

Optimization of therapy

Peginterferon Alfa-2a, lamivudine, and the combination for HBeAg-positive chronic hepatitis B

Lau GK, Piratvisuth T, Luo KX, *et al.*; Peginterferon Alfa-2a HBeAg-Positive Chronic Hepatitis B Study Group. *N Engl J Med* 2005; **352**: 2682–95

Peginterferon alfa-2a alone, lamivudine alone, and the two in combination in patients with HBeAg-negative chronic hepatitis B

Marcellin P, Lau GK, Bonino F, *et al.*; Peginterferon Alfa-2a HBeAg-Negative Chronic Hepatitis B Study Group. *N Engl J Med* 2004; **351**: 1206–17

BACKGROUND. The current regimens used for hepatitis B treatment are suboptimal with respect to the virological response and seroconversion, and involve side effects of interferon therapy and potential resistance to drugs of the nucleoside analogue family. Combination therapy with interferon plus a nucleoside analogue should conceptually be more effective than monotherapy, because of the different mechanisms of action of the two agents. Moreover, if a shorter course of therapy proves to be possible, viral resistance to the nucleoside analogue may be avoided. To date, data have been conflicting. The two large multicentre trials presented below assess the combination of pegylated interferon and lamivudine in patients positive and negative for hepatitis B envelope antigen (HBeAg).

INTERPRETATION. The first study, by Lau *et al.*, randomized 814 HBeAg-positive patients 1:1:1 to pegylated IFN-α2a (180 μg once weekly) alone, lamivudine alone

(100 mg per day) or pegylated IFN-α2a plus lamivudine for a total of 48 weeks of treatment and 24 weeks of follow-up. Most of the patients in the study were Asian (87%) and were infected with HBV genotype B or C. Pegylated IFN-α2a alone and in combination with lamivudine were better than lamivudine alone in efficacy, in HBeAg seroconversion (32 vs 19% for pegylated IFN-α2a alone [P <0.001] and 27 vs 19% [P = 0.02] for the combination treatment) (Fig. 11.5), HBV DNA suppression (32 vs 22% [P = 0.01] and 34 vs 22% [P = 0.003], respectively) and HBsAg seroconversion (16 patients in the interferon group vs 0 in the lamivudine group).

The study by Marcellin *et al.*, with an identical study design, confirms the findings of Lau *et al.* in HBeAg-negative patients. Patients on combination therapy or pegylated IFN-α2a alone had a significantly better response than patients on lamivudine alone with respect to the rate of liver function test normalization (60 vs 59 vs 44%), sustained suppression of viral DNA to below 400 copies/ml (20 vs 19 vs 7%) and loss of HBsAg (12/356 patients in the interferon group versus none treated with lamivudine alone). The addition of lamivudine to pegylated IFN-α2a did not improve the response rates.

Comment

These two large multicentre trials show that interferon offers an improvement in efficacy over lamivudine in the treatment of patients with hepatitis B. Combination therapy did not add any advantage over interferon alone. However, these results do not categorically rule out the possibility that combination therapy may provide clinically relevant benefits. In the studies discussed above, significantly fewer patients on combination therapy than on lamivudine monotherapy had mutations in the YMDD (tyrosine methionine aspartate aspartate) motif of HBV at the end of

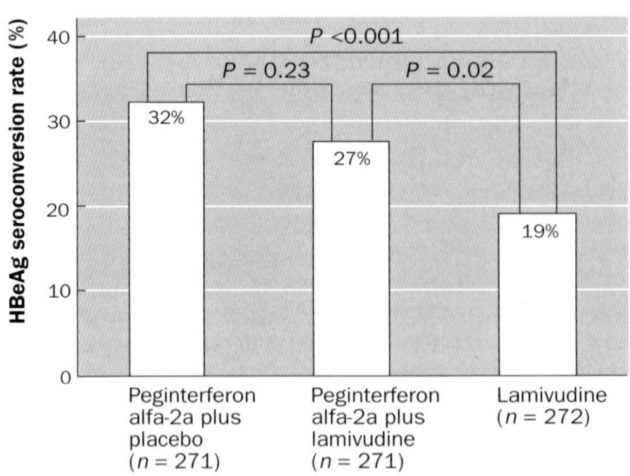

Fig. 11.5 Rates of HBeAg seroconversion after 24 weeks of follow-up. The percentage of patients with seroconversion in each group is shown at the top of the corresponding bar. Source: Lau *et al.* (2005).

the treatment, suggesting more profound suppression of HBV DNA with interferon. Moreover, a recent study from Hong Kong [3] suggests that sequential therapy may be beneficial. A higher rate of SVR (36 vs 14%) was found in HBeAg-positive patients treated with combination therapy compared with those on lamivudine alone. It was hypothesized that interferon, being given before lamivudine in the 8-week induction period, may have enhanced the immune clearance of HBV, and that adding lamivudine at a later time would have prevented re-infection of hepatocytes.

A dose-ranging study of the efficacy and tolerability of entecavir in lamivudine-refractory chronic hepatitis B patients

Chang TT, Gish RG, Hadziyannis SJ, *et al.*; BEHoLD Study Group. *Gastroenterology* 2005; **129**: 1198–209

BACKGROUND. Entecavir is a nucleoside analogue that selectively inhibits HBV replication by affecting both the priming of HBV DNA polymerase and the synthesis of the DNA strands. This drug has recently been approved by the US Food and Drug Administration for use in both HBeAg-positive and -negative patients. It has been shown to be effective in treating naive patients, but, more importantly, it seems to have good efficacy against lamivudine-resistant strains. However, the dose to be used and the tolerability of the medication in lamivudine-resistant and -refractory patients has not been clearly defined.

INTERPRETATION. In this randomized, dose-ranging phase 2 study, the efficacy and safety of entecavir in lamivudine-refractory HBeAg-positive and -negative patients were compared with those of lamivudine. A hundred and eighty-one patients who were viraemic despite lamivudine treatment for 24 or more weeks or who had documented lamivudine resistance were switched to entecavir (1.0, 0.5 or 0.1 mg daily) or continued on lamivudine (100 mg daily) for up to 76 weeks. Entecavir at a dose of 1.0 of 0.5 mg daily was well tolerated and resulted in significant reductions in HBV DNA levels and normalization of alanine aminotransferase levels compared with lamivudine treatment. One milligram of entecavir was more effective than 0.5 mg in this population.

Comment

Entecavir seems to be a potent inhibitor of HBV in lamivudine-resistant patients as its use led to a reduced viral load and normalization of liver function tests in most patients in the study. However, several questions remain unresolved, including the criteria for stopping therapy and the longevity of response. In this study, a very small proportion of HBeAg-positive patients achieved a serological response (HBeAg loss), the usual criterion for stopping the therapy in that population. However, an encouraging proportion of both HBeAg-positive and -negative patients achieved protocol-defined complete response and sustained response, based on decreases in HBV DNA and alanine aminotransferase. Entecavir resistance also needs to be assessed more closely over longer treatment periods in future studies.

Prevention of complications in hepatitis B

Lamivudine for patients with chronic hepatitis B and advanced liver disease

Liaw YF, Sung JJ, Chow WC, *et al.*; Cirrhosis Asian Lamivudine Multicentre Study Group. *N Engl J Med* 2004; **351**: 1521–31

Background. There are more than 450 million HBV carriers worldwide and HBV-related liver disease accounts for about 1.2 million deaths per year throughout the world. The suppression of HBV has been shown to improve liver histology and liver function and to markedly reduce future complications, including liver decompensation and hepatocellular carcinoma. In patients with more advanced liver disease, interferon therapy may not be applicable because of severe side effects. Lamivudine has been shown to be beneficial and relatively safe in this population; however, its effectiveness in preventing disease progression in patients with chronic hepatitis B and advanced fibrosis or cirrhosis is unknown. The following multicentre trial evaluated this question in a large HBV population.

Interpretation. Long-term virological and clinical responses were assessed in patients with chronic HBV and histologically confirmed cirrhosis or advanced fibrosis who were assigned randomly to receive lamivudine 100 mg per day ($n = 436$) or placebo ($n = 215$). The study was stopped prematurely (after a median duration of treatment of 32.4 months instead of a planned 5 years) because of a significant reduction in disease progression in the treatment group compared with the placebo group. A statistically significant lower number of patients on lamivudine, compared with placebo, had an increase in Child–Pugh score (3.4 vs 8.8%, respectively; $P = 0.02$) and in hepatocellular carcinoma development (3.9 vs 7.4%, respectively; $P = 0.047$).

Comment

This well-designed study clearly showed that continuous treatment with lamivudine delays clinical progression in patients with chronic hepatitis B and advanced fibrosis or cirrhosis by significantly reducing the incidence of hepatic decompensation and the risk of hepatocellular carcinoma. However, one argument against long-term treatment with nucleoside analogues is the emergence of viral resistance, and potential viral breakthrough and liver decompensation. Liaw and colleagues addressed this issue by confirming that genotypic resistance YMDD mutations developed in 49% of the patients treated with lamivudine for a median period of 32 months. Sixty-two per cent of patients with a YMDD mutation had a viral breakthrough compared with only 5% of those without the mutation, and the Child–Pugh score was more likely to increase in these patients compared with patients without a mutation who were receiving lamivudine. However, there was still a significant benefit compared with patients receiving placebo. Different strategies, one of them being the addition of adefovir, have been shown to be beneficial in preventing the development or suppressing the replication of YMDD mutants and may add to the long-term advantage of the treatment.

Hepatitis B vaccination

Antibody levels and protection after hepatitis B vaccination: results of a 15-year follow-up

McMahon BJ, Bruden DL, Petersen KM, *et al. Ann Intern Med* 2005; **142**: 333–41

Waning immunity to plasma-derived hepatitis B vaccine and the need for boosters 15 years after neonatal vaccination

Lu CY, Chiang BL, Chi WK, *et al. Hepatology* 2004; **40**: 1415–20

BACKGROUND. It has been shown that universal vaccination of infants and children against hepatitis B results in lower prevalence of hepatitis B and its complications [4]. It is thought that, despite the decrease in hepatitis B surface antibody over time, the immunity is maintained by memory B lymphocytes. Information on the duration of the protection afforded by hepatitis B vaccination is limited. The following two studies try to answer this question by evaluating a longer duration of protection and assessing indications for boosters.

INTERPRETATION. The study by McMahon *et al.* reports a cohort of 1578 Alaskan natives vaccinated for hepatitis B in the early 1980s with plasma-derived vaccine. Eight hundred and forty-one patients (53%) were tested at 15 years of follow-up. Among these, 84% continued to have anti-hepatitis B surface antigen (anti-HBs) present 15 years after vaccination; 66% had anti-HBs levels of 10 mIU/ml or greater. Initial high anti-HBs levels, older age at vaccination and male sex were associated with higher titres at long-term follow-up. Over the 15-year follow-up, 16 patients had definitive breakthrough infections, but only six had positive DNA; one of these remained positive over a 3-year period. All the breakthrough infections were asymptomatic and most occurred in patients who did not respond to the vaccination initially.

The second study, from Taiwan, assessed the duration of protection following neonatal immunization with hepatitis B vaccine and indications for booster immunization. Anti-HBs was measured in two groups of 15-year-old children who received neonatal immunization. The first group included 78 children born to HBsAg- and HBeAg-positive mothers and had developed protective levels of anti-HBs (≥10 mIU/ml) after neonatal immunization. The second group consisted of 113 healthy children whose anti-HBs titres after neonatal immunization were unknown. Anti-HBs was undetectable in a significant proportion of both groups (29.9% in those born to HBsAg-positive mothers compared with 62.4% in healthy children; $P = 0.001$). In both groups, a single booster increased the serological response to the vaccine in most patients, although the increase in anti-HBs titres was blunted in children with low pre-booster anti-HBs titres. The authors suggest that the anti-HBs status should be determined 10–15 years after receiving the hepatitis B vaccine, and that boosters should be given to prevent breakthrough infections at later age.

Comment

These two studies suggest that initial vaccination offers protection against HBV for at least 15 years, giving a low number of breakthrough infections. However, anti-HBs titres seem to wane with time. The study by McMahon *et al.* reveals that patients vaccinated at a younger age (especially 0.5–4 years of age) have a faster decline in anti-HBs, and the study by Lu *et al.* shows a high rate of undetectable or low titres 15 years after neonatal vaccination. The question persists of whether their waning immunity makes these patients vulnerable to acquisition of the infection during their adolescent years and whether boosters are necessary, as memory immunity may play a protective role even later in life. Further monitoring is needed to assess the duration of protection after 15 years of follow-up. Moreover, the long-term immunogenicity of the new recombinant hepatitis B vaccine compared with the plasma-derived vaccine needs to be assessed.

Conclusion

The past 18 months have been rich in literature describing the optimization of treatment in viral hepatitis C and B. In hepatitis C, shortening the treatment duration in patients with favourable genotypes has been suggested, and treatment strategies for patients with recurrent hepatitis C after liver transplantation have been evaluated. As standard therapy with interferon and ribavirin has important side effects and limited efficacy, new and encouraging therapies are under investigation. Similarly, in the hepatitis B literature the improvement of treatment efficacy is the goal, as therapies based on lamivudine result in very low seroconversion rates. Although combination therapies with interferon and lamivudine have not produced encouraging results, newer therapies are flourishing. Deeper understanding of the pathogenesis of viral hepatitis infection through basic research and multicentre efforts to apply these findings to clinical practice should be of great assistance in making future advances in viral hepatitis.

References

1. Marrero RJ, Sobhonslidsuk A, Mendez P, Torres M, Bejarano P, O'Brien C, Schiff ER. *A Pilot Study of Etanercept Treatment for Inhibition of Fibrotic Progression in Chronic Hepatitis C Infection*. Chicago, IL: Abstract S1557. DDW 2005.
2. Centers for Disease Control and Prevention. Protection against viral hepatitis: recommendations of the Immunization Practices Advisory Committee (ACIP). *MMWR Recomm Rep* 1990; **39**: 126.
3. Chan HL, Leung NW, Hui AY, Wong VW, Liew CT, Chim AM, Chan FK, Hung LC, Lee YT, Tam JS, Lam CW, Sung JJ. A randomized controlled trial of combination therapy for chronic hepatitis B: comparing interferon-α2b and lamivudine with lamivudine alone. *Ann Intern Med* 2005; **142**: 240–50.
4. Chang MH, Chen CJ, Lai MS, Hsu HM, Wu TC, Kong MS, Liang DC, Shau WY, Chen DS. Universal hepatitis B vaccination in Taiwan and the incidence of hepatocellular carcinoma in children. Taiwan Childhood Hepatoma Study Group. *N Engl J Med* 1997; **336**: 1855–9.

12

Cholestatic liver diseases

DAVID BARNES

Introduction

Cholestatic liver diseases include a wide variety of disorders, including diseases of the intrahepatic and extrahepatic biliary tree. The following group of articles reveals the newest information on two of the most common cholestatic liver diseases, primary biliary cirrhosis and primary sclerosing cholangitis. There is also new information on intrahepatic cholestasis of pregnancy and biliary atresia.

Primary biliary cirrhosis

The effect of ursodeoxycholic acid therapy of the natural course of primary biliary cirrhosis

Corprechot C, Carrat F, Bahr A, Chretein Y, Poupon R-E, Poupon R.
Gastroenterology 2005; **128**: 297–303

BACKGROUND. Primary biliary cirrhosis (PBC) is a chronic cholestatic liver disease which progresses to cirrhosis in 10–15 years. Multiple randomized trials, analysis using pooled trial data and long-term observational studies have shown that ursodeoxycholic acid (UDCA) improves the results of liver biochemical studies, delays histological progression and prolongs survival. Two recent meta-analyses have questioned the long-term benefits of UDCA [1,2]. The present study used a multistate modelling approach (Markov model) using histological stage, death and orthotopic liver transplantation as end-points to compare survival in the study population with the expected survival in a control population and the survival predicted by the Mayo survival model of PBC.

INTERPRETATION. The study demonstrated that the survival rate of patients with early PBC (Stages 1 and 2) was similar to that of a control population and was better than the spontaneous survival rate predicted by the Mayo model. The probability of death or liver transplantation remained significantly increased in patients who initiated treatment at a late histological stage (Stage 3 or 4).

Comment

Primary biliary cirrhosis is a cholestatic autoimmune liver disease which usually progresses to biliary cirrhosis and liver failure. UDCA is the only drug currently approved in the USA for patients with PBC but data supporting its use are mixed. Several clinical trials have shown that UDCA decreases histological progression and prolongs survival. However, two meta-analyses do not support its use.

The relative rarity of the disease and the long natural history make it difficult to carry out long-term randomized controlled trials to demonstrate the efficacy of a particular treatment.

To compensate for the difficulty of conducting long-term clinical trials, the authors used a multistate modelling approach (Markov model) which can be used to analyse incomplete disease history data and individual patient data using only a portion of the patient's lifetime. The patient population consisted of 262 patients with PBC who received 13–15 mg/kg UDCA daily for a mean of 8 years. The main end-points used in the Markov model included histological stage progression (Stages 1–4), death, and orthotopic liver transplantation. In this model, all patients that are at a given stage at a given time are considered to have the same prognosis, which allows for the use of incomplete observations. The survival of the treated patients was compared with (i) the expected survival of the French population matched for age and sex, and (ii) the survival predicted by the updated Mayo model |**3**|.

The mean follow-up of the 262 patients in the study was 8 years. There were 394 paired biopsy specimens for analysis. Forty-five patients developed cirrhosis, 16 patients died and 20 patients underwent orthotopic liver transplantation. The overall survival rates were 92% at 10 years and 82% at 20 years. Survival without liver transplantation was 84 and 66% at 10 and 20 years respectively. These rates were slightly lower than those of the age- and sex-matched controlled population (relative risk [RR] 1.4; $P = 0.1$). Survival surpassed that predicted by the Mayo model (RR 0.5; $P < 0.01$). Importantly, in patients with early-stage disease (Stage 1–2), the survival without orthotopic liver transplantation was not different from that of the control population (RR 0.8; $P = 0.5$). Survival was significantly prolonged compared with the spontaneous survival rate without orthotopic liver transplantation predicted by the Mayo model (RR 0.2; $P < 0.001$). In patients with late-stage disease (Stage 3–4), survival without orthotopic liver transplantation was less than that of the control population (RR 2.2; $P < 0.5$) and was similar to the survival predicted by the Mayo model ($P = 0.5$). In patients with Stage 4 PBC (cirrhosis) the predicted survival rate without orthotopic liver transplantation was 57 and at 39% at 10 and 20 years, respectively, which was a 4-fold decrease compared with the control population ($P < 0.05$).

In summary, using a Markov model, the authors demonstrated that treatment with UDCA normalizes the survival rate in patients with PBC when it is given at an early stage of the disease. The authors acknowledge a decrease in the efficacy of UDCA at advanced histological stages and point out the need for other therapeutic options in this patient population.

Budesonide combined with UDCA to improve liver histology in primary biliary cirrhosis: a three-year randomized trial

Rautiainen H, Karkkainen P, Karvonen A-L, *et al. Hepatology* 2005; **41**: 747–52

BACKGROUND. PBC is a chronic cholestatic liver disease with autoimmune characteristics. UDCA is the only currently approved treatment in the USA for PBC but its effect on liver histology and disease progression remains uncertain. The addition of prednisolone to UDCA has been shown to improve liver histology in PBC but is associated with serious side effects. The purpose of this study was to determine whether budesonide, a glucocorticoid with a high first-pass metabolism in the liver, is useful in treating PBC when added to UDCA.

INTERPRETATION. Budesonide combined with UDCA improved liver histology compared with UDCA alone but was associated with mild systemic glucocorticoid side effects.

Comment

Ursodeoxycholic acid is the only currently approved treatment in the USA for PBC. Its benefits in decreasing the progression of the liver disease and improving survival are controversial. For this reason, additional treatment options are felt to be necessary. Given the immune-mediated nature of PBC, immunosuppressive medications may have a role in treatment. Prednisolone combined with UDCA has been shown to improve liver histology but is associated with serious side effects [4]. Budesonide is a non-halogenated glucocorticoid which is absorbed in the small intestine. Ninety per cent of an oral dose is metabolized during the first pass in the liver in healthy people. Its metabolites, including 16α-hydroxyhydroxyprednisolone and 16β-hydroxybudesonide, have markedly less glucocorticoid activity. In addition, the glucocorticoid receptor binding activity of budesonide is 10–20 times higher than that of prednisolone and therefore budesonide may have a proportionally greater effect on liver inflammation. The pharmacodynamics of budesonide in patients with early-stage PBC is similar to that in healthy volunteers, but there is an increased risk of corticosteroid side effects in patients with cirrhosis, probably as a result of the shunting of portal blood flow away from the liver. A previous study using budesonide (9 mg) in combination with UDCA 10–15 mg/kg/day demonstrated improved liver histology and biochemistry compared with UDCA alone in a 2-year trial, and glucocorticoid side effects were minimal [5]. An additional trial using budesonide 9 mg combined with UDCA in a subgroup of patients with a suboptimal response to UDCA showed improvements in bilirubin and alkaline phosphatase, but at the expense of worsening osteoporosis and hyperglycaemia [6].

The present study was a 3-year prospective, randomized controlled trial comparing the effect of a lower dose of budesonide (6 mg/day) and UDCA

15 mg/kg/day compared with UDCA alone on liver histology and liver function tests in non-cirrhotic patients with PBC.

Seventy-seven patients with PBC Stage 1–3 (pre-cirrhotic) were randomized to UDCA 15 mg/kg/day and budesonide 6 mg/day (41 patients) or UDCA 15 mg/kg/day (36 patients). Liver biopsies were performed at the beginning and at the end of the study. Liver function tests, glucose and cortisol values were measured every 4 months. In addition, serum pamino-terminal propeptide of type III procollagen (S-PIIINP) was used as a serum marker of fibrosis and urinary N-telopeptide collagen was used as a marker of bone resorption.

Serum levels of alkaline phosphatase, ALT (commonly used alanine aminotransferase) and GGT (gamma-glutamyltranspeptidase) improved in both groups. The bilirubin level remained stable in the combination treatment group but rose in the group receiving UDCA alone, although the mean bilirubin level remained within normal limits in both groups. Serum PIIINP decreased significantly in the combination treatment group. Urinary N-telopeptide collagen showed no difference between groups. A comparison of liver histology after 36 months of therapy revealed significant differences between groups in stage ($P = 0.009$) and fibrosis ($P = 0.0009$) in favour of the combination treatment group. There was a 22% improvement in stage in the combination treatment group and a 20% deterioration in the group receiving UDCA alone ($P = 0.07$). Fibrosis decreased by 25% in the combination treatment group ($P = 0.08$) but increased by 70% in the group receiving UDCA alone ($P = 0.005$). Inflammation decreased in both groups, by 34% in the combination treatment group ($P = 0.02$) and 10% in the group receiving UDCA alone (difference not significant). One patient stopped budesonide therapy because of steroid-related side effects. One patient had low cortisol levels, which normalized after the budesonide was reduced to 3 mg/day. Glucocorticoid-related side effects were reported in seven patients and included bruises, thinning of the skin, ache, nausea, hirsutism and some weight gain. None of the side effects was severe and none required a change in treatment or dose. The mean level of plasma cortisol decreased after 2 years in the combination treatment group, demonstrating a slight systemic effect of budesonide.

The investigators point out that PBC can be a progressive disease despite UDCA therapy, only a minority of patients having a complete response to treatment. Combination treatment to prevent progressive disease is needed and the combination of UDCA and budesonide in non-cirrhotic patients might be beneficial. The authors felt, however, that the systemic glucocorticoid side effects may carry an unnecessary risk of diabetes and osteoporosis during long-term use in asymptomatic patients with early-stage disease. Longer-term studies using the combination of budesonide and UDCA are warranted to confirm its safety and assess its effect on survival before it should be routinely used in the management of PBC.

A randomized, controlled crossover trial of ondansetron in patients with primary biliary cirrhosis and fatigue

Theal JJ, Toosi MN, Girlan L, *et al. Hepatology* 2005; **41**: 1305–12

BACKGROUND. Fatigue is a common symptom in PBC and affects the quality of life of most patients. There is no known treatment for fatigue; the pathogenesis is unclear but may be centrally mediated. There is evidence in animals and humans that the serotonin-1a receptor may mediate fatigue [7,8]. The purpose of this study was to study the effect of ondansetron, a serotonin receptor antagonist, on fatigue in patients with PBC.

INTERPRETATION. Administration of ondansetron in patients with PBC did not provide significant fatigue reduction compared with a placebo.

Comment

Fatigue is a common and well-recognized symptom of PBC and has a major impact on the quality of life. Previous clinical trials have shown that drugs, including UDCA, cyclosporin, thalidomide and antioxidants, do not provide relief of fatigue. Given the evidence that fatigue in PBC may be centrally mediated and related to serotonin activity, the authors hypothesized that ondansetron, a serotonin receptor antagonist, would successfully reduce fatigue in PBC.

In this randomized, crossover trial, patients with PBC received active medication in one trial period and were crossed over to receive placebo in the other trial period. In this manner, patients served as their own controls. The two trial periods were 4 weeks in duration and separated by a minimum of a 1-week washout period. Patients received either ondansetron 4 mg by mouth three times a day or an identical placebo tablet. Fatigue was assessed in each subject with the Fatigue Severity Score (FSS) and the Fatigue Impact Scale (FIS), both of which have been validated previously in PBC. The Walter-Reed Performance Assessment Battery (PAB), which requires an instructional session to practice cognitive tasks before the trial, was also used.

Sixty patients from three centres were randomized to placebo in the first trial period and ondansetron in the second trial period (group 1) or ondansetron then placebo (group 2); 54 of the patients completed both phases of the study. When combining the data from periods 1 and 2, the primary outcome, FSS, decreased significantly when patients were taking ondansetron versus placebo ($P = 0.025$) but the responses in periods 1 and 2 were not equal. For this reason, each trial period was analysed separately, and it was found that in period 1 there was no difference in FSS and FIS between the ondansetron and the placebo group, the two groups having equal decreases in fatigue scores. In period 2, however, there were significant improvements in FSS and FIS in the ondansetron group versus the placebo group. Performance in the Walter-Reed PAB improved in all subjects during period 1 but was unchanged in period 2. Two major side effects were noted in the study, including constipation and headache. Headaches occurred at equal frequencies in the ondansetron and placebo groups but constipation was much more likely to occur with ondansetron. Constipation was noted in 90% of patients taking active medication in period 1 and 63% of those taking it in period 2 versus 22 and 13% in patients taking placebo in periods 1 and 2, respectively.

Although ondansetron apparently provided relief of fatigue in the second period of the study, the authors felt that ondansetron-induced constipation was a likely cause of subject unblinding in period 2.

Patients were warned of potential side effects of treatment, including constipation, and by period 2 they were able to observe a change in constipation and determine which treatment they were taking. This 'sequence effect' due to the crossover design could result in changes in their perception of fatigue, resulting in unreliable reporting. Further analysis of the data indicated additional confounding effects. A carry-over effect was noted, as patients in both groups did not return to their original baseline FSS after period 1 had been completed. For these reasons, the authors discarded data from the second part of the trial and drew conclusions only from the findings from period 1, which indicated that there was no significant difference in the reduction of fatigue when ondansetron was compared with placebo. The authors therefore concluded that ondansetron did not improve fatigue significantly in patients with PBC.

Methotrexate (MTX) plus ursodeoxycholic acid (UDCA) in the treatment of primary biliary cirrhosis

Combes B, Emerson SS, Flye NL, *et al.* *Hepatology* 2005; **42**: 1184–93

BACKGROUND. PBC is a chronic, progressive cholestatic liver disease. UDCA has been shown to improve laboratory test results and liver histology in some trials but its effect on improvement in survival is controversial. Liver disease tends to progress despite UDCA therapy. Uncontrolled trials have suggested that oral pulse treatment with methotrexate may prove useful in the treatment of pre-cirrhotic PBC. The purpose of this trial was to compare the effect of methotrexate plus UDCA with that of UDCA alone on the course of PBC.

INTERPRETATION. This study showed that the combination of methotrexate and UDCA did not improve the clinical course of PBC treated with UDCA alone.

Comment

PBC is a slowly progressive cholestatic liver disease. UDCA has been shown in numerous clinical trials to provide improvement in liver enzyme measurements and histology. PBC often progresses despite UDCA therapy and novel treatments are needed to arrest the progression of the disease completely. Methotrexate has anti-inflammatory and immunosuppressive properties and an uncontrolled trial has suggested that it may be helpful in the management of PBC [9]. In this randomized controlled trial, 265 patients with PBC were randomized to receive either UDCA plus methotrexate (132 patients) or UDCA plus placebo (133 patients). The patients had no symptoms of hepatic decompensation, such as ascites, variceal bleeding or encephalopathy. Randomization was stratified based on the histological stage of disease, approximately half the patients having Stage 1 or 2 and half having Stage 3 or 4. The dose of methotrexate was 15 mg per 1.73 m^2 body surface area with a maximum dose of 20 mg per week.

The primary measure of treatment outcome was liver transplant-free survival. Secondary end-points included time to clinical decompensation (development of ascites, encephalopathy, variceal bleeding, transplant or death), a doubling of serum bilirubin to 2.5 mg/dl or greater, a fall in serum albumin to 2.5 g/dl or less, or histological progression by at least two stages or to cirrhosis.

The mean duration of treatment in the study was 7.6 years (range 4.6–8.8 years). There were no differences between the two groups in transplant-free survival. A total of 14 and 16 liver transplants or deaths were observed in the methotrexate and placebo groups respectively. In addition, there was no difference between the two groups in the rate of clinical deterioration or histological progression of disease. The trial was stopped early by the National Institutes of Health (USA) on the advice of the Data Safety Monitoring Board for reasons of futility. The authors concluded that methotrexate added to UDCA did not provide a clinically important beneficial effect in PBC on transplant-free survival, time to clinical deterioration or time to subclinical progression. There was no beneficial effect of methotrexate on histological stage.

This study is persuasive evidence that methotrexate added to UDCA is not beneficial to patients with PBC. The trial contained a large number of patients and was conducted over a long period of time and showed no beneficial effect of methotrexate on survival, disease progression or hepatic histology.

Alendronate improves bone mineral density in primary biliary cirrhosis: a randomized placebo-controlled trial

Zein CO, Jorgensen RA, Clarke B, *et al. Hepatology* 2005; **42**: 762–71

BACKGROUND. PBC is associated with accelerated bone loss and the development of osteoporosis. Bisphosphonates have been shown to be effective in treating post-menopausal osteoporosis. The purpose of this study was to compare the effects of treatment using the bisphosphonate alendronate with placebo treatment on bone mineral density and bone turnover in patients with bone loss associated with PBC.

INTERPRETATION. Alendronate significantly improved bone mineral density in patients with PBC-related bone loss when compared with a placebo.

Comment

PBC, a chronic cholestatic liver disease, is associated with accelerated bone loss that often results in osteoporosis and its complications, such as compression fractures and long bone fractures. The bone loss has been attributed to decreased osteoblast activity and increased bone resorption [**10–12**]. Bisphosphonates have been shown to be effective in treating post-menopausal osteoporosis by inhibiting osteoclast-mediated bone resorption. The purpose of this study was to test the efficacy of alendronate versus placebo in the treatment of patients with PBC who had already begun to develop bone loss.

Patients were selected for the study if they had a well-established diagnosis of PBC, an estimated survival of more than 80% at 2 years, and no known oesophageal varices. To be eligible for the study, patients had to have pre-existing bone loss, as evidenced by a lumbar spine bone mineral density (BMD) t-score below –1.5. The study was a double-blind, randomized, placebo-controlled trial using alendronate 70 mg or placebo given by mouth once per week for 1 year. BMD was calculated before entry into the study and after 1 year of treatment, with measurements at the lumbar spine (L2–L4) and proximal femur. Lateral thoracic and lumbar spine X-rays were taken before entry and at 1 year to look for evidence of new compression fractures or worsening of previously noted compression fractures. Biochemical markers of bone turnover were also measured, including serum osteocalcin and urinary amino telopeptide of type I collagen of organic bone matrix (NTx) at the beginning of the study and at 1 year.

Thirty-four patients were enrolled in the trial; 17 were randomized to receive alendronate 70 mg once weekly and 17 patients were randomized to the placebo group. After 1 year there was a significant improvement in both lumbar spine and proximal femur BMD in the alendronate group compared with placebo.

There was no significant difference in the number of compression fractures seen between patients who received alendronate and those who received placebo (1 of 14 alendronate patients versus 0 of 13 placebo patients; $P = 0.3$) Evidence of worsening of pre-existing compression fractures was seen in one of four patients receiving placebo (25%) and none of eight patients receiving alendronate ($P = 0.14$). One patient in the placebo group experienced a hip fracture during the study. There were statistical differences in each of the two measurements of bone turnover between the alendronate and placebo groups. Osteocalcin levels decreased significantly in the alendronate group compared with the group receiving placebo, suggesting a decrease in bone turnover in the alendronate treatment group. Urinary NTx decreased by 6.5% in the alendronate group but increased by 21.1% in the placebo group, indicating increased bone resorption in the patients treated with placebo. The BMD changes seen in both groups were not related to oestrogen therapy. Gastrointestinal side effects were reported in equal numbers in the alendronate and placebo groups. Four patients underwent endoscopy during the study because of gastrointestinal symptoms; three of these studies were negative but one patient had gastritis with antral erosions. He was also noted to have anaemia (haemoglobin 7.9 g/dl); the authors believed that the episode of anaemia was due to injury of the gastric mucosa by alendronate. There was no evidence of hepatic toxicity associated with the use of alendronate.

Despite its small size, this study demonstrated that alendronate improves BMD in patients with PBC who have begun to develop bone loss. The safety profile of alendronate seemed acceptable, although one patient developed gastric erosions and associated anaemia attributed to the use of alendronate. The authors were careful to exclude patients from the study who had pre-existing oesophageal varices, because of the known potential for alendronate to cause oesophagitis. The authors felt that larger studies were needed to evaluate safety. However, it is certainly encouraging that treatment is available to prevent the often severe consequences of osteoporosis in this patient population.

Risk factors and comorbidities in primary biliary cirrhosis: a controlled interview-based study of 1032 patients

Gershwin MP, Selmi C, Worman HJ, *et al.*; USA PBC Epidemiology Group. *Hepatology* 2005; **42**: 1194–202

BACKGROUND. PBC is liver disease characterized by immune destruction of the small intrahepatic bile ducts. Although the aetiology is unknown, it is classified as an autoimmune disease, given the female predominance, the increased incidence in first-degree relatives and its association with other autoimmune diseases. Environmental factors may also play a role in the induction of PBC in people who are genetically susceptible. In this study, 1032 patients with PBC and 1041 controls were administered a questionnaire eliciting social, demographic, personal and medical histories and seeking risk factors and comorbidities associated with PBC.

INTREPRETATION. Environmental factors, such as cigarette smoking and the use of certain cosmetic products, and infectious agents acquired through urinary tract infections may play a role in inducing PBC in patients with genetic susceptibility.

Comment

PBC is classified as an autoimmune disease. There is a female predominance and PBC is associated with other autoimmune diseases. The factors inducing PBC in genetically susceptible individuals are unclear but exposure to household chemicals and certain bacteria have been implicated [13,14].

In this study, a large group of patients from 23 referral centres across the USA and a control group matched for sex, age, race and geographic location were included. All patients and controls were administered a telephone questionnaire which was derived from standardized questions from the US National Health and Nutrition Examination Survey (NHANES III). The questionnaire contained over 180 questions and 300 subquestions concerning demographics, lifestyle, and medical reproductive and occupational histories.

The study included 1032 patients with PBC and 1041 controls. In a multivariable analysis, a family history of PBC, other autoimmune diseases (systemic lupus erythematosus or Sjögren syndrome) and a history of urinary tract infections were significantly associated with PBC. In addition, a history of cigarette smoking, the use of nail polish and a history of hormone replacement therapy were also significantly associated with the development of PBC. Never having been pregnant was protective.

The aetiology of PBC remains unclear but there is emerging evidence that environmental factors may play a causative role in people with a genetic predisposition. The findings from this large case–control study support the previous studies which propose that a family history of PBC, the occurrence of multiple autoimmune diseases, cigarette smoking and a history of urinary tract infection are all risk factors for acquiring PBC. The authors also found that additional environmental factors, such as the use of certain cosmetic products, may predispose to the development of PBC.

By focusing on the risk factors identified in the study, it is hoped that the interaction between genetic predisposition and environmental factors will elucidate the exact pathogenesis of PBC more clearly.

Primary sclerosing cholangitis

High-dose ursodeoxycholic acid in primary sclerosing cholangitis: a 5-year multicenter, randomized, controlled study

Olsson R, Boberg KM, De Muckadell OS, *et al. Gastroenterology* 2005; **129**: 1464–72

BACKGROUND. There is no proven medical treatment to slow the progression of primary sclerosing cholangitis (PSC). Uncontrolled trials and pilot studies have suggested that high-dose UDCA (20–30 mg/kg/day) may slow the progression of the disease. The purpose of this study was to determine the effects of high-dose UDCA on survival, symptoms, biochemical changes and quality of life in patients with PSC.

INTREPRETATION. The authors found no statistically significant improvements in the incidence of death or liver transplantation in patients receiving high-dose UDCA versus those receiving a placebo. There were no differences between the treatment and control groups in symptoms, quality of life or medication side effects.

Comment

PSC is a chronic cholestatic liver disease characterized by inflammation and scarring of the intra- and extrahepatic bile ducts. It is a slowly progressive disease and leads to biliary cirrhosis after 10–15 years. No medical treatment has been shown to be beneficial in slowing the progression of the disease. UDCA has been shown to be beneficial in the treatment of PBC, another cholestatic liver disease. UDCA has several properties, including stimulation of bile secretion, reducing the aberrant expression of HLA class I molecules on hepatocytes, and protection of the cell membranes of biliary epithelial cells. A previous randomized controlled trial of UDCA at a dose of 13–15 mg/kg/day in PSC demonstrated no significant effect on survival over the 2 years of the study [15]. Preliminary data from subsequent studies suggest that high-dose UDCA may be beneficial. A small, randomized trial with 26 patients using UDCA at 20 mg/kg/day demonstrated possible benefit in cholangiographic appearance and fibrosis [16]. Another study of 30 patients treated with UDCA 25–30 mg/kg/day demonstrated improvement in the Mayo risk score after 1 year of treatment compared with a control group from a previous randomized controlled trial [17]. This improvement translated into significantly better survival at 4 years in the high-dose UDCA group.

In the present study, 219 people were randomized to receive either UDCA at a dose of 17–23 mg/kg/day or an identical placebo for 5 years. The primary end-point of the study was death or liver transplantation. Secondary end-points included changes in the frequency of PSC-associated symptoms (itching, right upper quadrant abdominal pain, fever and jaundice), changes in quality of life and changes in laboratory test results.

The authors estimated that 346 patients were needed to detect a difference in the primary end-point but they were only able to enrol slightly more than 60% of their target.

The end-point of death or liver transplantation occurred in 7.2% of patients in the UDCA group versus 10.9% of patients in the placebo group ($P = 0.368$). The authors point out that there was a positive trend in favour of UDCA treatment when measuring the occurrence of liver transplantation as a single end-point (5.2% in the UDCA group vs 7.9% in the placebo group; 98% confidence interval –10.4 to 4.6%). There was no difference between the two groups in the incidence of cholangiocarcinoma, although two of the three patients in the UDCA-treated group who developed cholangiocarcinoma did so within the first 5 months of the study, whereas all four of the patients in the placebo-treated group developed cholangiocarcinoma after 1 year. The incidences of pruritus and abdominal pain decreased during the study and did not differ between the two groups, and there was no change in the incidence of fever in either group. Quality of life scores were constant during the study, with no differences between the two groups. Alkaline phosphatase and aminotransferase levels tended to decrease in the UDCA-treated group during the first 6 months, but this decrease was not statistically significant. The reported side effects were the same in each group.

The authors concluded that there were no statistically significant benefits in treating PSC with UDCA at a dose of 20 mg/kg/day. However, they did note a tendency towards improved survival in the UDCA group. Because the study was underpopulated on the basis of the initial assumptions, a small advantage of UDCA treatment could not be excluded, but the authors felt that the practical clinical utility of UDCA in slowing disease progression in PSC was limited.

The true benefit of high-dose UDCA in slowing the progression of PSC remains unclear. To date, this is the largest study, with the longest follow-up, with UDCA. The study was under-enrolled and therefore a small clinical benefit may have been masked. An even higher dose of UDCA (25–30 mg/kg/day) may ultimately provide some clinical benefit but we will have to wait for a large, randomized, controlled trial to establish this.

Clinical course and outcome of autoimmune hepatitis/primary sclerosing cholangitis overlap syndrome

Floreani I, Rizzotto ER, Ferrara F, *et al. Am J Gastroenterol* 2005; **100**: 1516–22

BACKGROUND. There are three immune-mediated liver diseases: autoimmune hepatitis (AIH), PBC and PSC. Some patients have features of more than one autoimmune liver disease. For example, AIH together with PBC is frequently reported in adult patients. AIH/PSC overlap, while relatively common in children, has been reported only rarely in adults. The purpose of this study was to assess the natural history of AIH/PSC overlap syndrome compared with a group of patients with PSC alone.

INTERPRETATION. Adult patients with AIH/PSC overlap tend to be younger at the time of diagnosis than patients with PSC alone. Patients with overlap were diagnosed initially as having AIH and were subsequently found to have overlapping AIH/PSC. They tended to respond to immunosuppression and UDCA therapy and had a better survival than patients with PSC alone.

Comment

PBC, AIH and PSC are all immune-mediated liver diseases. Occasionally features of these diseases overlap, resulting in what have been termed 'overlap syndromes'. Most commonly seen are AIH/PBC overlap in adults and AIH/PSC in children. An AIH/PSC overlap has been reported uncommonly in adults. The purpose of this study was to evaluate the natural history and outcome of a group of adults with AIH/PSC overlap syndrome, comparing the findings with those in a group of patients with PSC alone.

AIH/PSC overlap was defined by the following criteria: (i) a total aggregate AIH score greater than 15 using the revised scoring system for AIH based on the International Autoimmune Hepatitis Group [18]; (ii) antinuclear antibody or anti-smooth muscle antibodies at a titre ≥40; and (iii) histology revealing piecemeal necrosis, rosetting of lymphocytes, and moderate or severe periportal or periseptal lobular inflammation.

A possible association with inflammatory bowel disease was assessed in each case. Patients with AIH/PSC overlap were treated with azathioprine and prednisolone. These two medications were tapered to a maintenance dose of 10–15 mg/day and 50–75 mg/day respectively. The diagnosis of PSC was based on cholangiographic criteria. Liver biopsy was obtained in most patients. All patients had regular biochemical and clinical follow-up.

Seven patients met the criteria for AIH/PSC overlap syndrome and their clinical course was compared with that of 34 patients with PSC alone. The mean follow-up was 93.3 ± 65.9 months in the AIH/PSC overlap group and 98.1 ± 65.9 months in the PSC alone group. AIH/PSC overlap patients were all initially diagnosed as having AIH and subsequently became resistant to immune suppression, which led to further diagnostic testing; this included an endoscopic retrograde cholangiopancreatography (ERCP), which revealed the classic bile duct changes of PSC. The mean time from the initial diagnosis of AIH to the discovery of AIH/PSC overlap syndrome was 17 months. Patients with the overlap syndrome were younger (21.4 ± 5 vs 32.3 ± 10.2 years; $P < 0.01$). Levels of transaminases and immunoglobulin G were significantly higher in the overlap group. Inflammatory bowel disease was more common in the group with PSC only ($P < 0.05$). Only one patient at the time of diagnosis of the overlap syndrome had cirrhosis on biopsy. Once the diagnosis of overlap syndrome was made, patients received immune suppression in addition to UDCA, which led to a significant reduction in aspartate aminotransferase (AST) over 5 years of treatment ($P < 0.05$). A decrease in ALT was seen but was not statistically significant. Alkaline phosphatase did not change significantly. Over time, the Mayo PSC prognostic score remained stable in the overlap group but progressed steadily in the PSC group. Seven patients underwent orthotopic liver transplantation: six in the PSC group and one in the overlap group. There were five case of cholangiocarcinoma, all of which occurred in the PSC group. In addition, there were five extrahepatic malignancies, all of which occurred in the PSC group. Nine patients died, all in the PSC group: eight from neoplasms and one from cardiac arrest.

In summary, this study of AIH/PSC overlap was small because of the uncommon incidence of the condition in adults, but several disease characteristics emerged from the study. Patients with AIH/PSC overlap tend to present at a younger age than patients with typical PSC. They respond to immune suppression with improvement in liver enzymes. When compared with patients with typical PSC, they have a markedly better long-term survival rate.

Intrahepatic cholestasis of pregnancy

Efficacy and safety of ursodeoxycholic acid versus cholestyramine in intrahepatic cholestasis of pregnancy

Kondrackiene J, Beuers U, Cupcinskas L. *Gastroenterology* 2005; **129**: 894–901

BACKGROUND. Intrahepatic cholestasis of pregnancy (ICP) is a liver disease of unclear aetiology, characterized by pruritus and elevated serum bile acids, starting in the second or third trimester of pregnancy and persisting until delivery. The maternal prognosis is good but the morbidity of pruritus can be considerable. Fetal complications, such as pre-term delivery, fetal distress and intrauterine fetal deaths, have been reported. The aim of this study was to assess the efficacy of UDCA versus cholestyramine in treating ICP.

INTERPRETATION. UDCA is safe and more effective than cholestyramine in treating ICP.

Comment

The aetiology of ICP is unknown but may be related to hormone-triggered dysfunction of hepatocyte canalicular bile salt transporters. Numerous treatments have been tried without showing clear efficacy, including antihistamines, benzodiazepine, phenobarbital, anion exchange resins, S-adenosyl methionine and cholestyramine. UDCA may have a role in treating ICP as it stimulates biliary secretion of endogenous bile acids and protects the cell membranes of biliary epithelial cells. Two small randomized trials with UDCA did not demonstrate efficacy with this treatment, but both trials contained only eight patients in each group [**19,20**]. The aim of this study was to assess the efficacy and safety of UDCA in ICP.

The diagnosis of ICP was defined as pruritus starting in the second or third trimester of pregnancy associated with elevation of at least one of the following laboratory tests: alanine aminotransferase, aspartame aminotransferase and fasting serum bile acids. The primary end-point of the study was a reduction in the severity of pruritus by more than 50% after 14 days of treatment. Secondary end-points were the outcome of pregnancy (term of delivery, Apgar score, and status of the newborn infant), reduction in serum bile acids and aminotransferase levels, and drug safety. Pruritus was assessed by self-report using a scale of 0–4. Patients were randomized to receive either UDCA 8–10 mg/kg/body weight per day or cholestyramine 8 g/day for 14 days.

Eighty-four patients were enrolled in the study between 25 and 35 weeks of gestation, equal numbers of patients receiving UDCA and cholestyramine. Treatment was started at a median time of onset of 35 weeks. Ten patients in the

UDCA group and four in the cholestyramine group withdrew or violated the study protocol. After 4 days of treatment, the pruritus score was significantly lower in patients receiving UDCA compared with those receiving cholestyramine, and this difference persisted for the 14 days of the study. Reduction of the pruritus score by more than 50% was seen in 67% of the patients treated with UDCA versus 19% of those treated with cholestyramine ($P = 0.0021$). No stillbirths occurred in either group. The Apgar score at 1 min was similar in the two treatment groups but was significantly higher at 5 min in the UDCA-treated group (9.4 ± 0.05 vs 8.7 ± 0.06; $P < 0.5$). Delivery occurred significantly closer to term in patients receiving UDCA compared with those receiving cholestyramine (38.7 ± 1.7 and 37.4 ± 1.5 weeks respectively; $P < 0.05$). Serological evaluation revealed significantly reduced serum aminotransferase levels and endogenous bile acid levels in the group receiving UDCA, although serum bilirubin GGT and alkaline phosphatase levels did not change. Cholestyramine did not result in a change in serum aminotransferase or endogenous bile acid levels, and serum bilirubin and alkaline phosphatase increased significantly.

The findings of this study strongly suggest that treatment of ICP with UDCA for 14 days is superior to treatment with cholestyramine for the relief of pruritus, improvement of serum liver tests and delivery at or near term. These results suggest that UDCA should be the first-line therapy for ICP.

Biliary atresia

Outcome in adulthood of biliary atresia: a study of 63 patients who survived for over 20 years with their native liver

Lykavieris P, Chardot C, Sokhn M, Gauthier F, Valayer J, Bernard O. *Hepatology* 2005; **41**: 356–71

BACKGROUND. Biliary atresia is a congenital disorder characterized by complete obstruction of some or all of the extrahepatic biliary tree, with associated abnormalities of the intrahepatic bile ducts. If not treated, the disease leads to death within the first 3 years of life. Treatment consists of the Kasai operation designed to restore bile flow, and liver transplantation if the Kasai procedure is unsuccessful or if there is subsequent development of cirrhosis and liver failure. The purpose of this study was to report the status of the liver disease and general condition of patients with biliary atresia who have undergone the Kasai operation and survived without needing liver transplantation for at least 20 years.

INTERPRETATION. Long-term follow-up of patients who underwent the Kasai procedure for biliary atresia revealed that 18% avoided liver transplantation, but even upon reaching adulthood most had significant liver disease and required lifelong follow-up.

Comment

Biliary atresia is a congenital condition characterized by complete obstruction of some or all of the extrahepatic bile duct. There are also associated abnormalities of the intrahepatic duct. The Kasai operation re-establishes bile drainage and improves the prognosis but liver transplantation is often necessary if the Kasai operation does not restore significant bile flow or if the patient later develops jaundice or the complications of portal hypertension. The purpose of this study was to assess the clinical status of patients who had undergone the Kasai operation and survived without liver transplantation into adulthood (20 years of age).

In this retrospective study, 271 children were identified who had undergone the Kasai operation for biliary atresia between 1968 and 1983. One hundred and seventy-five patients died (most of them before liver transplantation was available), 32 underwent liver transplantation before the age of 20, and 63 (23%) survived with their native liver for at least 20 years and were the subject of this report. Two patients died of liver failure at ages 24 and 30 years. Ten patients underwent liver transplantation between 20 and 28 years of age. Twenty-year survival was significantly better in children who had incomplete resection of their extrahepatic tree. Patients who underwent hepatic portocholecystostomy had a 35% survival rate and those with cystojejunostomy had a 40% survival rate, whereas those who underwent hepatic portoenterostomy had a 19% survival rate. Twenty-year survival was also better in children who underwent the operation before the age of 90 days. Adult height was equal to or greater than the mean of the general population in 49 patients except for three girls who had other severe medical illnesses. All females had their menstrual period between age 12 and 15 years. All male patients had normal puberty. Histological, clinical and/or ultrasound evidence of cirrhosis was found in all but two patients. No patient developed hepatocellular carcinoma. Among the 63 survivors there was evidence of portal hypertension in 44, 20 of whom had gastrointestinal bleeding; in 13 of the 20 this was treated successfully with surgical portosystemic shunts, and the remaining seven patients underwent endoscopic therapy or β-blockade. One patient developed hepatopulmonary syndrome at age 24. Nineteen patients had at least one episode of acute bacterial cholangitis which responded to antibiotics. Quality of life information was available in 52 patients, 38 of whom were considered to be leading a normal life. Seven female patients had delivered nine children and three male patients had fathered two children apiece. Fifty-one patients were currently alive with their native liver; four of the 51 were awaiting liver transplantation. Therefore, out of the initial cohort of 271 patients, survival without immediate need for liver transplantation was estimated at 17%. Of this group, 21 of the 271 had abnormal serum bilirubin levels and only five (2%) of the total group had normal transaminases and GGT, no signs of portal hypertension and no cholangitis.

In summary, except for a very small minority of patients, the Kasai operation does not appear to be a permanent cure for biliary atresia. Hepatic complications were present in the vast majority of patients who survived into adulthood. The authors stressed that lifelong follow-up is essential if complications of biliary cirrhosis that necessitate liver transplantation are to be detected.

Conclusion

It is evident that progress is being made in the pathogenesis, treatment and management of complications of PBC. There is mounting evidence that environmental factors play a role in the genesis of PBC in genetically susceptible individuals. The utility of UDCA in PBC, especially if started early in the course of the disease, continues to gain support. On the other hand, methotrexate does not appear to have a role in treating PBC and ondansetron does not seem to have a role in alleviating PBC-associated fatigue. The bisphosphonate alendronate improves bone mineral density in PBC and its routine use should decrease the bone complications previously encountered in this disease. The use of high-dose UDCA in treating PSC remains controversial. Previous evidence has suggested that it slows the progression of the disease but a randomized controlled trial showed no beneficial effect of UDCA on survival or the prevention of cholangiocarcinoma in a 5-year multicentre trial. The clinical course and outcome of AIH/PSC overlap syndrome have been clarified. It seems to have a better prognosis then PSC alone. A large trial demonstrated the utility of UDCA in intrahepatic cholestasis of pregnancy. Finally, a long-term study of patients who had biliary atresia and who had previously undergone the Kasai operation revealed that only a small number of patients reached adulthood without the need for liver transplantation. Those who do survive for over 20 years will continue to require life-long care.

References

1. Goulis J, Leandro G, Burroughs AK. Randomized controlled trials of ursodeoxycholic acid therapy for primary biliary cirrhosis: a meta-analysis. *Lancet* 1999; **354**: 1053–60.
2. Gluud C, Christensen E. Ursodeoxycholic acid (UDCA) in primary biliary cirrhosis (PBC)—a Cochrane hepato-biliary systemic review. *J Hepatol* 1999; **30**(Suppl 1): 83.
3. Lindor K, Therneau T. Survival in ursodeoxycholic acid-treated patients with primary biliary cirrhosis. *Gastroenterology* 1996; **111**: 1782–3.
4. Leuschner M, Guldutuna S, You T, Hubner K, Bhatti S, Leuschner U. Ursodeoxycholic acid and prednisolone versus ursodeoxycholic acid and placebo in the treatment of early stages of primary biliary cirrhosis. *J Hepatol* 1996; **25**: 49–57.

5. Leuschner M, Maier K-P, Schlichting J, Strahl S, Herrmann G, Dahm HH, Ackermann H, Happ J, Leuschner U. Oral budesonide and ursodeoxycholic acid for treatment of primary biliary cirrhosis: results of a prospective double-blind trial. *Gastroenterology* 1999; **117**: 918–25.
6. Angulo P, Jorgensen RA, Keach JC, Dickson ER, Smith C, Lindor KD. Oral budesonide in the treatment of patients with primary biliary cirrhosis with a suboptimal response to ursodeoxycholic acid. *Hepatology* 2000; **31**: 318–23.
7. Swain MG, Maric M. Improvement in cholestasis-associated fatigue with serotonin receptor agonist using a novel rat model of fatigue assessment. *Hepatology* 1997; **25**: 291–4.
8. Wilson WM, Maughan RJ. Evidence for a possible role of 5-HT in the genesis of fatigue in men: administration of paroxetine, a 5-HT re-uptake inhibitor, reduces the capacity to perform prolonged exercise. *Exp Physiol* 1992; **77**: 921–4.
9. Kaplan MM, Knox TA. Treatment of primary biliary cirrhosis with low-dose weekly methotrexate. *Gastroenterology* 1991; **101**: 1332–8.
10. Hodgson SF, Dickson ER, Wahner HW, Johnson KA, Mann KG, Riggs BL. Bone loss and reduced osteoblast function in primary biliary cirrhosis. *Ann Intern Med* 1985; **103**: 855–60.
11. Pereira SP, Bray GP, Pitt PI, Li F, Moniz C, Williams R. Non-invasive assessment of bone density in primary biliary cirrhosis. *Eur J Gastroenterol Hepatol* 1999; **11**: 323–8.
12. Crosbie OM, Freaney R, McKenna MJ, Hegarty JE. Bone density, vitamin D status, and disordered bone remodeling in end-stage chronic liver disease. *Calcif Tissue Int* 1999; **64**: 295–300.
13. Long SA, Quan C, Van de Water J, Nantz MH, Kurth MJ, Barsky D, Colvin ME, Lam KS, Coppel RL, Ansari A, Gershwin ME. Immunoreactivity of organic mimeotopes of the E2 component of pyruvate dehydrogenase: connecting xenobiotics with primary biliary cirrhosis. *J Immunol* 2001; **167**: 2956–63.
14. Selmi C, Gershwin ME. Bacteria and human autoimmunity: the case of primary biliary cirrhosis. *Curr Opin Rheumatol* 2004; **16**: 406–10.
15. Lindor K. Ursodiol for primary sclerosing cholangitis. Mayo primary sclerosing cholangitis–ursodeoxycholic acid study group. *N Engl J Med* 1997; **336**: 691–5.
16. Mitchell SA, Bansi DS, Hunt N, von Bergmann K, Fleming KA, Chapman RW. A preliminary trial of high-dose ursodeoxycholic acid in primary sclerosing cholangitis. *Gastroenterology* 2001; **121**: 900–7.
17. Harnois DM, Angulo P, Jorgensen RA, LaRusso NF, Lindor KD. High-dose ursodeoxycholic acid as a therapy for patients with primary sclerosing cholangitis. *Am J Gastroenterol* 2001: **96**: 1558–62.
18. Alvarez F, Berg PA, Bianchi FB, Bianchi L, Burroughs AK, Cancado EL, Chapman RW, Cooksley WG, Czaja AJ, Desmet VJ, Donaldson PT, Eddleston AL, Fainboim L, Heathcote J, Homberg JC, Hoofnagle JH, Kakumu S, Krawitt EL, Mackay IR, MacSween RN, Maddrey WC, Manns MP, McFarlane IG, Meyer zum Buschenfelde KH, Zeniya M, *et al.* International Autoimmune Hepatitis Group Report: review of criteria for diagnosis of autoimmune hepatitis. *J Hepatol* 1999; **31**: 929–38.
19. Diaferia A, Nicastri PL, Tartagni M, Loizzi P, Iacovizzi C, Di Leo A. Ursodeoxycholic acid therapy in pregnant women with cholestasis. *Int J Gynecol Obst* 1996; **52**: 133–40.

20. Palma J, Reyes H, Ribalta J, Hernandez I, Sandoval L, Almuna R, Liepins J, Lira F, Sedano M, Silva O, Toha D, Silva JJ. Ursodeoxycholic acid in the treatment of cholestasis of pregnancy: a randomized, double-blind study controlled with placebo. *J Hepatol* 1997; **27**: 1022–8.

13

Fatty liver disease

WILLIAM CAREY

Introduction

Non-alcoholic fatty liver disease (NAFLD) has become the most common cause of chronically abnormal liver test results. It is a major contributor to cirrhosis and a frequent cause of liver transplantation, and has assumed the mantle of the most important liver disease in many parts of the developed world. It is estimated that NAFLD is present in one-third of the general population. NAFLD is currently considered to have two major subtypes. Steatosis is defined as the presence of fat, mainly macrovesicular, within hepatocytes. Experimental steatosis is completely reversible, and is not associated with fibrosis, cirrhosis or liver failure. Steatohepatitis, often referred to as non-alcoholic steatohepatitis (NASH) when seen in the non-alcoholic, on the other hand, is an aggressive disease characterized by varying degrees of inflammation (usually involving polymorphonuclear cells), hepatic damage characterized by Mallory bodies, and by fibrosis, often leading to cirrhosis. This sharply bifurcated classification ignores the fact that the liver lesion in some patients with the changes of NAFLD may change from steatosis to NASH and back again.

Many lines of research indicate that insulin resistance plays a central role in hepatic steatosis. Insulin resistance leads to hyperinsulinaemia, and a cascade of alterations in hepatic lipid management ensues. Progression to steatohepatitis from steatosis is thought to represent the result of a 'second hit' to the liver that may occur in some individuals with steatosis. NASH is estimated to occur in 3% of the US population. The nature of the second hit has been a matter of intense investigation. It elicits an inflammatory response, activation of stellate cells, and eventual fibrosis. Oxidative stress and the release of tumour necrosis factor and other proinflammatory cytokines appear to play a major role. Other cytokines, especially those of the adipocytokine class, may play a protective role in liver injury from steatosis, so it is more accurate to say that the amount of stellate cell activation represents the balance between protective and injurious cytokines.

The natural history of non-alcoholic fatty liver disease: a population-based cohort study

Adams LA, Lymp JF, St Sauver J, *et al. Gastroenterology* 2005; **129**: 113–21

BACKGROUND. The very high and increasing prevalences of obesity and metabolic syndrome, which are important precursors of NAFLD, indicate a concordantly high prevalence of fatty liver disease. Some studies indicate that up to 34% of the US population may have NAFLD. The natural history of NAFLD is poorly documented, yet is a subject of critical interest. Most studies exhibit considerable selection bias. This study used a community-based epidemiological database to quantify the disease burden posed by NAFLD compared with the general state-wide population in Olmstead County (Minnesota) over a period of up to 16 years.

INTERPRETATION. The survival rate of those with NAFLD was lower than the expected survival rate of the general population. Higher mortality was associated with greater age, impaired glucose metabolism and the presence of cirrhosis. Liver disease was the third leading cause of death in those with NAFLD, but the 13th leading cause of death in the general population from the same state.

Comment

A total of 435 NAFLD patients were identified. Only a modest increase in mortality was seen compared with the general population in the county. Only 3% of those without apparent cirrhosis at the time of entry were known to have developed cirrhosis and 3.1% developed a liver-related complication. This figure probably underestimates the true frequency of cirrhosis, as only 65 patients underwent a liver biopsy. Although the survival rate was significantly lower in NAFLD patients, no difference was observed before 6 years, and by 10 years the absolute difference in survival was 10% (77% for NAFLD patients vs 87% for the general population). The cause of death in NAFLD patients was most often extrahepatic malignancy (28%) or ischaemic heart disease (25%) rather than being liver-related (13%). It is noteworthy that only 0.5% of NAFLD patients developed hepatocellular carcinoma over 16 years. Selection bias may have affected the findings. Because of the distinctive employment opportunities in Rochester, Minnesota, residents of Olmstead County may not reflect the population of the state as a whole. It would be interesting to compare NAFLD and non-NAFLD patients from the same county. Overall, this study puts the disease burden of NAFLD in perspective. Most patients with NAFLD do not have cirrhosis or progress to it. NAFLD appears to confer a small but measurable risk of increased mortality after 10 years. The primary associations with increased mortality are higher age, impaired glucose metabolism, and cirrhosis at baseline. Therapeutic interventions for NAFLD need to be chosen with this low risk in mind.

Under diagnosis of pediatric obesity and under screening or fatty liver disease and metabolic syndrome by pediatricians and pediatric sub specialists

Riley MR, Bass NM, Rosenthal P, Merriman RB. *J Pediatrics* 2005; **147**: 839–42

BACKGROUND. Obesity is a public health problem and is not restricted to adults. The consequences of obesity and metabolic syndrome are problems that are also seen in children. The purpose of this investigation was to determine how often general paediatricians, paediatric endocrinologists and paediatric gastroenterologists diagnose children as overweight and how often interventions are provided, including nutritional counselling and screening for NAFLD and metabolic syndrome.

INTERPRETATION. Nearly one-third of the 2256 visits reviewed were by overweight children. In only one-third of these visits was a diagnosis of overweight recorded, and counselling was infrequent. Specific attention should be given to the provision of diagnosis and intervention for overweight children.

Comment

There is no question that obesity among children is becoming more prevalent and that adequate recognition and counselling are important. This study may not provide an entirely accurate picture of the extent to which healthcare workers are aware of obesity in children. Short, focused visits make record-keeping, and therefore retrospective chart reviews, subject to misinformation. This study should serve as a wake-up call for physicians who see children to be vigilant and proactive when dealing with obesity, regardless of the age of the patient. Children under 5 were particularly unlikely to be assigned a diagnosis; diagnosis of overweight and nutritional counselling was less likely to occur during visits to gastroenterologists. In only 22% of visits was a diagnosis assigned, and counselling was offered in 13%. Endocrinologists did moderately better than gastroenterologists; screening for metabolic syndrome was recorded in 34% of visits. Not surprisingly, gastroenterologists were most likely to screen for NAFLD. Body mass index (BMI) calculation in children is somewhat more complex than in adults. The Centers for Disease Control (CDC) website provides the following information on this subject. After BMI is calculated for children and for teenagers, the BMI number is plotted on the CDC BMI-for-age growth charts (for either girls or boys) to obtain a percentile ranking. The percentile indicates the relative position of the child's BMI number among children of the same sex and age. The growth charts show the weight status categories used with children and teenagers (underweight, normal weight, at risk of being overweight, and overweight).

BMI-for-age weight status categories and the corresponding percentiles are shown in Table 13.1.

Table 13.1 BMI-for-age weight status categories and the corresponding percentiles

Weight status category	Percentile range
Underweight	Less than the 5th percentile
Normal weight	From the 5th percentile to the 85th percentile
At risk of overweight	From the 85th to less than the 95th percentile
Overweight	Equal to or greater than the 95th percentile

The CDC and the American Academy of Pediatrics (AAP) recommend the use of the BMI to screen for overweight in children, beginning at 2 years old.

A BMI percentile calculator is available at http://apps.nccd.cdc.gov/dnpabmi/Calculator.aspx.

Decreased serum adiponectin: an early event in pediatric non-alcoholic fatty liver disease

Louthran MV, Barve S, McClain CJ, Joshi-Barve S. *J Pediatr* 2005; **147**: 835–8

Background. This study was designed to explore the relationship between a number of cytokines and measures of obesity and NAFLD in children.

Interpretation. Serum adiponectin is reduced in children with NAFLD. Proinflammatory cytokines (levels or activity of tumour necrosis factor α, interleukin-6 and interleukin-8) were not elevated in obese children. This suggests that the suppression of 'good' cytokines rather than the elevation of activity of 'bad' cytokines is related to the development of NAFLD in children.

Comment

Adiponectin is a member of the class of adipose tissue-derived secretory proteins, called adipocytokines. Adiponectin can directly increase the transport, oxidation and dissipation of fatty acids in skeletal muscle, reducing the levels of intramyocellular lipids and thus improving insulin signalling. The protein can also increase the sensitivity of hepatocytes to insulin, either through a direct action or indirectly by lowering the circulating concentrations of lipids as a result of its action on muscle. Obesity and especially visceral fat impair adipocytokine secretion, resulting in the promotion of hypertension, impaired fibrinolysis, and insulin resistance. In morbidly obese adults, an inverse relationship between serum adiponectin levels and alanine transaminase (ALT), a commonly used liver test, has been demonstrated (Fig. 13.1).

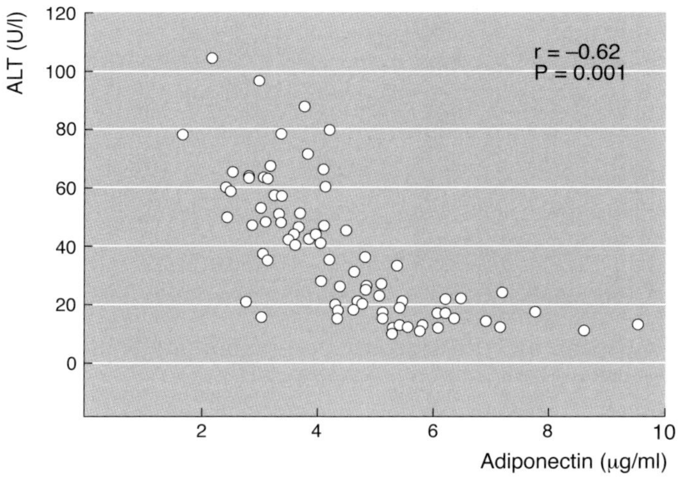

Fig. 13.1 Relationship between plasma levels of adiponectin and ALT in 90 morbidly obese Chinese individuals (45 males and 45 females). *r*, Spearman correlation coefficient. Source: Louthran *et al.* (2005).

Hydroxylation and glycosylation of the four conserved lysine residues in the collagenous domain of adiponectin: potential role in the modulation of its insulin-sensitizing activity

Wang Y, Xu A, Knight C, Xu LY, Cooper GJ. *J Biol Chem* 2002; **277**: 19521–9

This study extends observations previously made in adults to obese children with NAFLD. It increases the web of evidence that alterations in adipocytokines are relevant to NAFLD.

Is adiponectin level a predictor of non-alcoholic fatty liver disease in non-diabetic male patients?

Sargin H, Sargin M, Gozu H, *et al. World J Gastroenterol* 2005; **11**: 5874–7

BACKGROUND. Adiponectin is a hepatic insulin sensitizer and also an inhibitor of tumour necrosis factor. Previous studies indicated decreased levels of adiponectin in adults with NAFLD. This study looked specifically at adiponectin levels in non-diabetic adult men.

INTERPRETATION. A statistically significant inverse relationship exists between adiponectin levels and BMI, pro-insulin, aspartate transaminase (AST), a commonly used liver test, ALT and gamma-glutamyl-transpeptidase (GGT), another commonly used liver test in NAFLD patients. Low adiponectin levels might be a predictor of NAFLD in male diabetics.

Comment

This study confirms the general concept that obesity is associated with impaired secretion of adiponectin, and that it correlates with ALT elevations. The study sheds no light on the possible interaction between adiponectin and the more serious form of liver disease, NASH.

Relation between elevated serum alanine aminotransferase and metabolic syndrome in Korean adolescents

Park HS, Han JH, Choi KM, Kim SM. *Am J Clin Nutr* 2005; **82**: 1046–51

BACKGROUND. Around the world, concern about NAFLD is increasing. Unexplained elevations in aminotransferase concentrations have been strongly associated with adiposity and thus may represent NAFLD. Studies in many ethnic groups and all age groups are required to validate the association between NAFLD and metabolic syndrome. This study looked at the relationship of ALT elevations with the metabolic syndrome in a group of Korean adolescents.

INTERPRETATION. Data were obtained from 1594 subjects aged 10–19 from the Korean National Health and Nutrition Examination Survey 1998, a cross-sectional health survey of a nationally representative sample of non-institutionalized civilian South Koreans. BMI, waist circumference, blood pressure, fasting glucose, lipid profiles and serum ALT were measured. The prevalence of elevated ALT (>40 U/l) was 3.6% in boys and 2.8% in girls. The prevalence of metabolic syndrome was 3.3% in both boys and girls. The components of the metabolic syndrome were significantly worse in the group with elevated ALT concentrations than in the group with normal ALT concentrations. The odds ratios [OR] (95% confidence interval [CI]) for elevated ALT were 6.6 (3.7–11.8), 2.3 (1.2–4.6) and 3.0 (1.6–5.8) in the adolescents with abdominal obesity, high triacylglycerol concentrations, and low high-density lipoprotein cholesterol concentrations respectively. The OR for elevated ALT were 1.5 (95% CI 0.7–3.1), 2.6 (1.1–6.2) and 6.2 (2.3–16.8) in the adolescents with one, two and three risk factors (metabolic syndrome) respectively.

Comment

This study validates findings in other ethnic groups. It takes advantage of the excellent health records in Korea and the data obtained solidify the relationship between metabolic syndrome and NAFLD. As in many cohort studies, only non-invasive tests were used, and in this study ultrasonography was not employed. This limitation does not detract from the important observations about the frequency of unexplained ALT elevations (2.8–3.6%) in otherwise healthy Korean adolescents. A very similar incidence of metabolic syndrome (3.3%) and the statistical association of the two highlight once again the association of these two disorders. This study provides an underestimate of the frequency of ALT perturbations caused by metabolic syndrome. By using an ALT upper limit of normal of 40 U/l, the study ignores recent data suggesting that such values are too high. Indeed, a recent study suggests that upper limit values of 19 U/l for women and 30 U/l for men should be considered normal |**1**|.

Adipokines in NASH: post-prandial lipid metabolism as a link between adiponectin and liver disease

Musso G, Gambino R, Durazzo M, *et al. Hepatology* 2005; **42**: 1175–83

Background. Adipocytokines are associated with obesity and with NAFLD. The relationships of adipocytokines and obesity with the severe liver disease NASH are incompletely elucidated. Circulating levels of four adipocytokines (adiponectin, tumour necrosis factor α, leptin and resistin) and the post-prandial lipid and adiponectin responses to an oral fat load were assessed in 25 non-obese, non-diabetic patients with biopsy-proven NASH and correlated with metabolic indices and liver histology.

Interpretation. Hypoadiponectinaemia is present before overt diabetes and obesity appear and correlates with the severity of liver histology in NASH. Impaired post-prandial lipid metabolism may be an additional mechanism linking hypoadiponectinaemia with NASH and posing a higher cardiovascular risk in these subjects. The mechanism(s) underlying these differences are unknown, but the type of dietary fat seems to play a role. These findings may have important pathogenic and therapeutic implications in both liver and metabolic disease.

Comment

Circulating adiponectin was lower in patients with NASH compared with controls and on multiple regression analysis correlated negatively with liver steatosis, necroinflammation (OR 5.0; $P = 0.009$), and fibrosis (OR 8.0; $P = 0.003$). The magnitude of post-prandial lipaemia was significantly higher in NASH than in controls and was related to fasting adiponectin ($\beta = -0.78$; $P = 0.00003$). Controls showed a significant increase in serum adiponectin in response to the fat load, whereas patients with NASH showed a slight decrease. The post-prandial free fatty acid response correlated inversely with the adiponectin response in both groups and independently predicted the severity of liver steatosis in NASH ($\beta = 0.51$; $P = 0.031$). This study provides more solid evidence that suppression of adiponectin is important in the evolution of NASH and related complications.

Hyperinsulinemia predicts hepatic fat content in healthy individuals with normal transaminase concentrations

Ardigo D, Numeroso F, Valtuena S, *et al. Metabolism* 2005; **54**: 1566–70

Background. Insulin resistance (IR) in patients with NAFLD has been documented. Does IR predict fatty liver when the ALT is normal? This study explores IR in healthy volunteers with normal ALT values and correlates this with hepatic fat content as estimated by ultrasonography of the liver.

Interpretation. Insulin resistance results in the need for a higher insulin level to maintain blood glucose in a normal range. This state has been referred to as compensatory hyperinsulinaemia (CH). IR is a feature of metabolic syndrome, and is also frequently seen in fatty liver disease. Fasting plasma insulin (FPI) concentration has been used as a surrogate marker for IR. In this study, FPI predicted hepatic fat content and ALT in healthy volunteers with normal transaminase concentrations, independently of the other anthropometric and metabolic variables measured.

Comment

Hepatic fat content was quantified by ultrasonography in 69 healthy individuals (30 men, 39 women) without known risk factors for liver disease and with plasma ALT concentrations of less than 30 U/l. The experimental variables quantified included BMI, waist circumference, systolic and diastolic blood pressures, and fasting plasma glucose, FPI and lipid concentrations. Subjects were classified as having no (55%), mild (27%) or moderate to severe (18%) hepatic steatosis on the basis of the ultrasonography results.

Statistically significant correlations existed between liver fat content and ALT, BMI, waist circumference, systolic blood pressure, diastolic blood pressure and levels of fasting plasma glucose, fasting insulin, triglycerides and high-density lipoprotein cholesterol. Multivariate general discriminant analysis and multiple linear regression analysis indicated that fasting insulin concentration was the only independent predictor (P <0.001) of both liver fat content and ALT concentration. Fasting plasma insulin predicts hepatic fat content and ALT in healthy volunteers with normal transaminase concentrations, independently of the other anthropometric and metabolic variables measured.

The metabolic syndrome as a predictor of non-alcoholic fatty liver disease

Hamaguchi M, Kojima T, Takeda N, *et al. Ann Intern Med* 2005; **143**: 722–8

Background. The association between metabolic syndrome and NAFLD is well established. Less clear is the temporal relationship: does metabolic syndrome precede

NAFLD? This investigation explores the longitudinal association between these entities in a prospective observational study in Japan, using ultrasonography as the measure of NAFLD, in individuals enrolled in a medical check-up programme in a general hospital.

INTERPRETATION. Over 4400 apparently healthy Japanese men and women were studied. The presence of metabolic syndrome at the time of entry into the database was a strong predictor of the subsequent development of NAFLD.

Comment

Metabolic syndrome is characterized by a group of metabolic risk factors in an individual, including abdominal obesity, dyslipidaemia, hypertension, insulin resistance or glucose intolerance, and the prothrombotic state or proinflammatory states. Many criteria have been proposed. The American Heart Association and the National Heart, Lung, and Blood Institute recommend that the metabolic syndrome be identified as the presence of three or more of these components:

- Elevated waist circumference:
  Men: ≥40 inches (102 cm)
  Women: ≥35 inches (88 cm)
- Elevated triglycerides: ≥150 mg/dl
- Reduced high-density lipoprotein ('good') cholesterol:
  Men: <40 mg/dl
  Women: <50 mg/dl
- Elevated blood pressure:
  ≥130/85 mmHg
- Elevated fasting glucose:
  ≥100 mg/dl

This study of the association between metabolic syndrome and NAFLD is important. Although limited by a relatively short period of follow-up, it yields important findings. At baseline 18% of the participants appeared to have had NAFLD. An additional 10% of the 3147 participants who did not have NAFLD at the outset and who completed a second examination acquired this condition. It is equally important that regression occurred in 16% of those who had it at the outset. The most powerful predictor of development of NAFLD was the presence of metabolic syndrome. The presence of metabolic syndrome was associated with a decreased likelihood of regression of NAFLD. This study provides important information about the temporal dynamics of NAFLD and provides further evidence that metabolic syndrome (and by implication insulin resistance) is a precursor condition for the development of NAFLD. The applicability of these findings to non-Japanese patients requires confirmation, although there is no reason to believe different findings will apply to less homogeneous populations. The use of ultrasonography as a marker of NAFLD has inherent limitations, although for population-based studies it seems an appropriate tool. No information about the relative risks of simple steatosis and NASH is provided by this study.

Insulin resistance impairs sustained response rate to peginterferon plus ribavirin in chronic hepatitis C patients

Romero-Gomez M, Del Mar Viloria M, Andrade RJ, *et al. Gastroenterology* 2005; **128**: 636–41

BACKGROUND. NAFLD may be present in individuals infected with hepatitis C virus (HCV). Fat and/or NASH may influence the response to antiviral therapy. Insulin resistance, the background on which NAFLD occurs, may, by itself or mediated by hepatic steatosis, influence the outcome of treatment. This study evaluated the effect of IR and viral factors on the sustained virological response (SVR) in patients with chronic hepatitis C treated with peginterferon plus ribavirin.

INTERPRETATION. The insulin resistance index, the viral genotype and fibrosis were independently related to the SVR to treatment.

Comment

This well-powered study (159 patients) measured IR by means of the homeostasis model assessment (HOMA), a well-established method that uses the following formula:

$$\text{HOMA} = \text{insulin concentration} \times \text{fasting glucose concentration} / 22.5$$

Higher HOMA values indicate higher degrees of IR. HOMA scores were associated with a lower likelihood of SVR in genotype 1 HCV (OR 2.43 [CI 1.41–4.20]). Those with genotype 1 HCV and a HOMA score of <2 had a 61% SVR, compared with a 20% SVR if the HOMA was >4. The association of higher HOMA score and poor response to treatment was about the same degree as the association between increasing levels of hepatic fibrosis and poor response. Necroinflammatory activity and steatosis were not associated with the likelihood of an SVR. These findings are important in understanding factors that influence the treatment response. It appears that IR rather than NAFLD is a negative predictor of an SVR in hepatitis C.

IR also appears to be related to the progression of fibrosis in HCV infection [2]. This effect is apparently independent of HCV genotype. IR is seen more often in Asians, which may explain a lower response rate to anti-HCV treatment in Asians than in Caucasians.

Impact of liver steatosis on virologic response in [corrected] Italian patients with chronic hepatitis C treated with peg-interferon alpha-2b plus ribavarin

Fabris P, Floreani A, Carlotto A, *et al. Aliment Pharmacol Ther* 2005; **21**: 1173–8

BACKGROUND. The relationship of steatosis to the HCV treatment response remains incompletely characterized. The aim of this study was to evaluate the impact of liver steatosis in patients treated for chronic hepatitis C infection with combination therapy.

INTERPRETATION. Only low-grade liver steatosis negatively affects the outcome of combination therapy with peginterferon α2b plus ribavirin, and severe steatosis (which is virus-related in most cases) has no impact on the virological response.

Comment

Patients often have more than one liver problem. Interactions between them may influence the rate of progression of liver disease and may influence the response to therapy. Hepatic steatosis is particularly complicated because it may result from either host factors (insulin resistance, metabolic syndrome) or exogenous factors. Hepatitis C genotype 3 is particularly likely to elicit steatosis, yet is one of the easier HCV genotypes to treat. In this study the investigators found that most of the patients with significant steatosis had HCV genotype 2 or 3. In this context, steatosis was not associated with lowered response rates. On the other hand, low-grade steatosis (seen predominately in infection with HCV genotype 1) was independently associated with a lower response rate. In summary, it seems likely that steatosis associated with genotype 2 or 3 HCV does not result in lower rates of response to therapy. Whether or not non-viral causes of steatosis are associated with lower response rates to therapy remains to be shown. The study by Romero-Gomez and colleagues (discussed above) also suggests that steatosis does not influence the response rate.

Conclusion

The year 2005 was a year of consolidation of information about NAFLD. The generally benign nature of NAFLD has been confirmed. No major breakthroughs were recognized, but considerable new documentation is now available about the robustness of the relationship between insulin resistance and NAFLD in many different ethnic groups and in all age groups. The new information about the interplay of NAFLD, insulin resistance and responsiveness to antiviral treatment in those with hepatitis C represents a significant advance.

References

1. Prati D, Taioli E, Zanella A, Della Torre E, Butelli S, Del Vecchio E, Vianello L, Zanuso F, Mozzi F, Milani S, Conte D, Colombo M, Sirchia G. Updated definitions of healthy ranges for serum alanine aminotransferase levels. *Ann Intern Med* 2002; **137**: 1–10.
2. D'Souza R, Sabin CA, Foster GR. Insulin resistance plays a significant role in liver fibrosis in chronic hepatitis C and in the response to antiviral therapy. *Am J Gastroenterol* 2005; **100**: 1509–15.

Further reading

1. Schaffler A, Scholmerich J, Buchler C. Mechanism of disease: adipocytokines and visceral adipose tissue—emerging role in non-alcoholic fatty liver disease. *Nat Clin Pract Gastroenterol Hepatol* 2005; **2**: 273–80.
2. Bugianesi E, McCullough AJ, Marchesini G. Insulin resistance: a metabolic pathway to chronic liver disease. *Hepatology* 2005; **42**: 987–1000.

14

Update on portal hypertension

ROBERT O'SHEA, MARGARET KINNARD

Introduction

The development of symptomatic portal hypertension represents a major transition point in the natural history of cirrhosis, with a progressive risk of development of complications of end-stage liver disease. These complications are fairly common; natural history studies indicate that more than 60% of patients will develop ascites, of whom 5–10% will eventually become refractory. In addition, more than 50% will develop oesophageal varices; of these, between 25 and 40% may progress to bleeding. Each episode of gastrointestinal bleeding is associated with substantial morbidity and mortality. Early detection and more effective management of cirrhosis and portal hypertension remains an important goal, in order to intervene and possibly alter a patient's clinical course.

This chapter will present a survey of the recently published literature in portal hypertension.

Beta blockers to prevent gastroesophageal varices in patients with cirrhosis

Groszmann RJ, Garcia-Tsao G, Bosch J, *et al.*; Portal Hypertension Collaborative Group. *N Engl J Med* 2005; **353**: 2254–61

BACKGROUND. Oesophageal variceal bleeding remains one of the most dangerous manifestations of portal hypertension. Since the original study of the use of β-blockers to prevent variceal bleeding [1], multiple further studies have been done to test the utility of β-blockers in both primary and secondary prophylaxis of variceal bleeding. Unfortunately, no treatment has been perfect and there have been substantial rates of breakthrough bleeding.

INTERPRETATION. This study was designed not to test the utility of β-blockers in preventing bleeding or rebleeding, but rather to test whether their use may decrease the rate of development of varices—a sort of a 'pre-primary' prophylaxis. Patients with cirrhosis and documented portal hypertension (defined as a hepatic venous pressure gradient of >6 mmHg) who had no evidence of oesophageal or gastric varices on upper endoscopy and no previous evidence of decompensation (ascites, liver cancer, splenic or portal vein thrombosis, or a life expectancy of less than 1 year) were considered for inclusion. The sample size was calculated to detect an absolute difference of 20% (or a relative difference of 40%) in outcomes. A total of 213 of 290 patients with large varices screened over a 6-year period were treated with increasing doses of timolol, until the resting heart rate decreased by 25%, fell below 55 beats/min, or the maximum dose was achieved. Patients were stratified according to the cause of liver disease (alcoholic vs viral/other) and followed at 3-month intervals, along with annual oesophagogastroduodenoscopies (EGDs) and measurements of the hepatic venous pressure gradient (HVPG). End-points were the development of varices and clinical outcomes, including variceal or portal hypertensive bleeding, the development of complications of cirrhosis (ascites, hepatic encephalopathy), the need for liver transplant, or death.

Eighty-four patients in total developed varices or variceal bleeding; however, no statistically significant differences in outcome rates between the timolol group and the placebo group were noted. Baseline values of HVPG and aspartate aminotransferase were independent predictors in a multivariate Cox analysis in the subgroup of patients who developed varices or bleeding. Haemodynamic studies during the period of follow-up showed an average drop of 17% in the HVPG in the timolol group; however, the HVPG overall did not differ substantially in the patients who underwent repeated measurements at 1 year: 72/108 (66%) in the timolol group and 82/105 (78%) in the placebo group. In the subgroups of patients who did achieve a significant reduction (defined as >10%), however, there was a substantial protective effect (Fig. 14.1). The authors recommend the approach of measuring baseline HVPG, and suggest that a value of 10 mmHg or greater may strongly predict the rate of oesophageal bleeding.

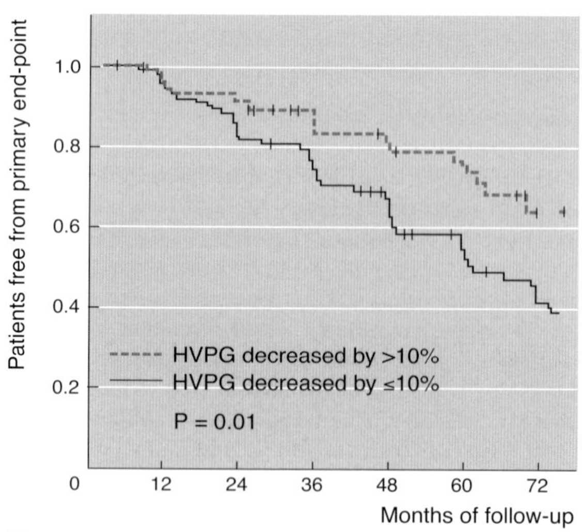

Number at risk							
HVPG decreased by >10%	69	66	62	51	35	30	16
HVPG decreased by ≤10%	85	81	68	59	41	30	20

Fig. 14.1 Probability of remaining free from developing varices or bleeding, according to change in HVPG at one year. Source: Groszmann *et al.* (2005).

Comment

In an accompanying editorial, Mukherjee and Sorrell emphasize several features of this study that deserve mention [2]. They point out that 14 patients of the alcoholic group had been abstinent for less than 1 month and that five had evidence of alcoholic hepatitis. As portal hypertension is influenced by inflammation, the inclusion of these patients may have prejudiced the study by including patients who were likely to improve. This non-differential misclassification would not have affected the outcome, just the ability to detect a true difference (inflating the beta or type II error).

In addition, the definition of an increased HVPG they used (>6 mmHg) may have been too stringent as the likelihood of developing varices may increase only after a specific threshold in pressure is reached. By including patients with such early disease, the ability to detect a difference in the two groups may have been substantially weakened.

The 95% confidence interval of the relative risk of any possible protective effect of β-blockers includes the value 1 (reflecting the overall non-significant *P*-value for the study). Therefore, given that the 95% confidence interval for these results ranges from 0.68 to 1.33, these data are also compatible with a decrease in the true relative risk of as much as 32% (reflecting a significant protective effect).

Although the authors, using an intention-to-treat approach, were obliged to conclude that β-blockers were not effective, the subgroup analyses they provide deserve closer scrutiny. In most of the studies that retested HVPG in patients treated with β-blockers, only a percentage of those treated developed a substantial decrease in HVPG, complete protection from variceal (re)bleeding being seen only in those who achieved an HVPG of less than 12 mmHg. Given this, it would seem eminently reasonable that the benefits of β-blockers in 'pre-primary' prophylaxis may only extend to those with sizeable decreases in HVPG. Although 20 patients on timolol (18% of the total) did experience significant adverse events, the possibility that early use of β-blockers may prevent the development of varices deserves further study.

Ligation versus propranolol for the primary prophylaxis of variceal bleeding in cirrhosis

Schepke M, Kleber G, Nürnberg D, *et al.*; German Study Group for the Primary Prophylaxis of Variceal Bleeding. *Hepatology* 2004; **40**: 65–72

BACKGROUND. Although the use of β-blockers is the standard of care for prophylaxis against oesophageal variceal bleeding, multiple studies have shown a high rate of intolerance due to haemodynamic or other adverse events. Moreover, although decreased, the absolute risk of bleeding – despite therapy – remains substantial. Thus, several other strategies, including endoscopic therapy, have been attempted.

INTERPRETATION. Schepke *et al.* studied patients with Child class A/B cirrhosis and at least two oesophageal varices with a diameter greater than 5 mm, but no previous bleeding related to portal hypertension, previous transjugular intrahepatic portosystemic shunt (TIPS), serious comorbidities, or contraindications to β-blockers. A total of 152 patients were ultimately randomized, 75 to variceal band ligation and 77 to propranolol. Variceal band ligation was performed weekly until eradication, at 3 months, after which serial endoscopies were then done at 6-month intervals. Propranolol was given at 40 mg twice daily and the dose was increased until there was a 20% decrease in resting heart rate or until side effects. Patients were then followed at 6-month intervals for a minimum of 2 years for clinical outcomes and possible treatment complications. Study end-points were gastrointestinal bleeding from portal hypertension (from oesophageal varices seen on endoscopy or clinically), and death. Patients were treated for bleeding on a standardized protocol, including an EGD within 6 h, octreotide or terlipressin, and supportive therapy. The sample size was estimated to detect a 50% difference in bleeding rates, decreasing the absolute risk from 20 to 10%, and with power to do one interim analysis. After the interim analysis failed to find any difference, however, the trial was stopped early. Patients were followed for a mean of 34.4 months (ranging from 1 week to 6 years). No significant differences were found between the two groups at baseline. The mean dose of propranolol was 77.3 mg. A 20% decrease in resting heart rate was seen in 79% of treated patients, with (just) over half achieving a 25% reduction in heart rate. However, 53 of the 77 patients (69%) developed side effects, and in twelve patients (16%) treatment had to be stopped. Another seven patients (25% of the total) stopped treatment because of non-compliance.

Varices were eradicated in 69 of the 75 patients (92%) randomized to variceal band ligation in two or three sessions. At a mean of 11.2 months after eradication, 60% of varices recurred, requiring a further one or two sessions. Large varices were seen in only eleven patients (15%). Three patients developed severe bleeding thought to be related to ligation ulcers; two died from severe bleeding, and the third required injection with cyanbucrylate. Overall, as shown in Table 14.1, no significant differences in primary outcomes were seen between the two treatment arms. Possible predictors of bleeding on multivariate analysis included bilirubin and creatinine, while increasing age and prothrombin time were predictive of dying.

Table 14.1 Outcomes and treatment tolerability

	Variceal band ligation, *n* (%)	**Propranolol, *n* (%)**
Variceal bleeding	19 (25.3)	22 (28.6)
Overall mortality	34 (45.3)	33 (42.9)
Bleeding-related deaths	9 (12)	8 (10.4)

Source: Schepke *et al.* (2004).

Comment

This study is one of several trials comparing endoscopic variceal ligation (EVL) with β-blockers for primary prophylaxis from variceal bleeding, and, as has been seen in a meta-analysis that incorporated this study [3], no clear difference in mortality could be shown when comparing patients randomized to each of the two treatment arms. Unlike the results of that combined study, however, no difference in the prevention of bleeding was seen in the banding group. Although there was no significant difference in outcome between patients treated with β-blockers and those who underwent EVL, the costs of the two regimens differed greatly. Given this difference, therefore, the authors' conclusion that β-blockers should be the front line of therapy seems reasonable. A substantial percentage of patients, however, did not tolerate β-blockers or had contraindications to their use; for this group EVL remains a reasonable option.

A question in this study is the extent of the adverse events related to variceal banding ulceration. This outcome seemed to be out of proportion to what other authors have reported (for example, in the same meta-analysis no other fatal bleeding from ligation ulcers was seen). As the overall results of this study are clearly sensitive to this rate, the question of whether a different protocol to prevent post-banding ulceration might have changed the overall risk benefit ratio remains an open one.

Endoscopic variceal ligation plus propranolol versus endoscopic variceal ligation alone in primary prophylaxis of variceal bleeding

Sarin SK, Wadhawan M, Agarwal SR, Tyagi P, Sharma BC. *Am J Gastroenterol* 2005; **100**: 797–804

BACKGROUND. The natural extension of the question of the optimal use of medical or endoscopic therapy in primary prophylaxis, given their seeming equivalence, is whether combination therapy (adding a β-blocker to endoscopic treatment) might further decrease bleeding rates. This study attempted to answer that question.

INTERPRETATION. One hundred and forty-four patients among 1000 patients with portal hypertension screened were found to have endoscopically high-risk varices (grade 3–4 with red colour signs), and were randomized to either EVL alone or to EVL with propranolol. The sample size was arrived at by estimating an absolute risk reduction in bleeding rates over 2 years of 15%, with a relative decrease of 75%. Baseline characteristics of the two study groups were well matched (Table 14.2): approximately 90% of patients had decompensated liver disease (Child B or C cirrhosis). Patients began treatment within 24 h of initial endoscopy. The EVL protocol involved placing as many bands as possible (range 2–8) at 2-week intervals until obliteration. Usually, this was accomplished in two to five sessions (mean 3.36) over approximately 2 months, with repeat EGD then done monthly for 3 months then at 3-month intervals.

Propranolol was dosed according to the effect on heart rate, targeting a 25% decrease in resting heart rate, a baseline heart rate of 55, or until systolic blood pressure dropped below 90 mmHg. Mean propranolol doses were 95.6 mg (94.7 mg in cirrhotics and 104 mg in non-cirrhotics), which resulted in a significant accompanying decrease in heart rate (of 26%, from 82.6 ± 6.7 to 61.3 ± 3.7) within 10 days of beginning

Table 14.2 Patient characteristics

Characteristic	Total (%) (*n* = 144)	EVL + propranolol (%) (*n* = 72)	EVL alone (%) (*n* = 72)	*P*-value
Age (mean ± SD)	42.4 ± 15	42.5 ± 15.1	42.4 ± 14.9	0.99
Male	113 (78.5)	55 (76.4)	58 (80.5)	0.52
Female	30 (21.5)	16 (23.6)	14 (19.5)	
Cirrhosis	127 (88.2)	64 (88.9)	63 (87.5)	0.8
Alcoholic cirrhosis	40 (31.5)	21 (32.8)	19 (30.1)	
Non-alcoholic	87 (68.5)	43 (67.2)	44 (69.9)	
Non-cirrhotic	17 (11.9)	8 (11.1)	9 (12.5)	
CTP score				
(mean ± SD)	8 ± 1.9	8.1 ± 1.9	7.9 ± 2.0	0.72
Child A	33 (22.9)	18 (25)	15 (20.8)	
Child B	73 (50.7)	35 (48.6)	38 (52.7)	
Child C	38 (26.4)	19 (26.4)	19 (26.4)	
Grade III EV	108 (75)	52 (72.2)	56 (77.7)	0.44
Grade IV EV	36 (25)	20 (27.7)	16 (22.2)	

CTP, Child–Turcotte–Pugh; EV, oesophageal varices.
Source: Sarin *et al.* (2005).

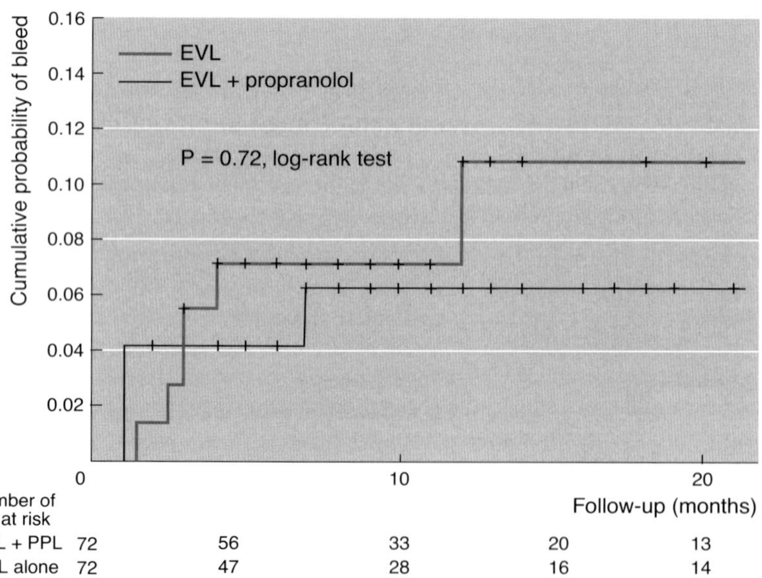

Fig. 14.2 Kaplan–Meier plot showing the actuarial probability of upper gastrointestinal bleed in patients on a combination of EVL and propranolol or EVL alone ($P = 0.72$). Source: Sarin *et al.* (2005).

treatment. Patients were followed for a mean of approximately 1 year. A total of eleven patients developed oesophageal variceal bleeding: five in the EVL and propranolol combination arm, and six who had EVL alone. All of these episodes occurred before variceal eradication. No differences were noted between the two groups, or, in subgroup analysis, among patients with differing levels of severity as measured by the Child–Turcotte–Pugh (CTP) score (Fig. 14.2). Similarly, there were no substantial differences in death rates between the two groups, although there was an increasing risk of mortality with increasing severity of liver disease. There was a 20-month survival rate of 100% in Child class A patients, but only 69% in patients with Child C cirrhosis. Combining EVL and β-blockers led to a reduction of almost 40% in the recurrence rate of oesophageal varices. Predictably, β-blocker use was associated with adverse effects: 16 patients (22%) had significant side effects and in six of these therapy had to be discontinued. Overall, the authors conclude that the two interventions are clinically equivalent and suggest that the addition of β-blockers can decrease the rate of variceal re-formation after eradication.

Comment

In an accompanying editorial, Drs Chalasani and Boyer suggested that not repeating EVL after initial eradication and following the patients for a longer period might have resulted in the detection of a difference between the two therapies |**4**|. Clearly, however, short-term outcomes are not materially affected by the addition of medical to endoscopic therapy.

Randomized study comparing banding and propranolol to prevent initial variceal hemorrhage in cirrhotics with high-risk esophageal varices

Jutabha R, Jensen DM, Martin P, Savides T, Han SH, Gornbein J.
Gastroenterology 2005; **128**: 870–81

BACKGROUND. This paper presents the results of a randomized clinical trial comparing two strategies of primary prophylaxis – EVL using a multiband ligator versus β blockade – in patients with cirrhosis and high-risk varices.

INTERPRETATION. Sixty-two patients (of 269 patients screened) were randomized in a blocked design to either EVL or long-acting propranolol. The sample size was calculated to detect an absolute decrease in the risk of oesophageal variceal bleeding of 15% (decreasing the risk from 19 to 4%) or a relative risk reduction of almost 80%. Propranolol was administered up to a maximum dose of 400 mg daily or until a 25% reduction in heart rate was achieved. Patients were treated with a mean propranolol dose of 86.9 mg. Almost all patients achieved a 25% reduction in resting heart rate; however, two developed severe hypotension and first-degree heart block.

Endoscopic variceal ligation was done using a multiband ligator device targeting the largest varices at the gastro-oesophageal junction, and banding upwards in a spiral fashion every 1–2 cm. Follow-up EVL was done at 4-week intervals until obliteration, followed by EGD half-yearly for 1 year then annually up to 5 years. In the endoscopy group, an average of five to six bands were placed initially, with progressively fewer over the ensuing three or four sessions. Patients were followed for an average of 18 months; 71% (22/31) experienced eradication of all varices. Of nine patients who underwent liver transplantation prior to completing the eradication protocol, a total of five developed recurrent oesophageal varices on surveillance EGD, and were rebanded.

The study was stopped after interim analysis showed a significant difference in the failure rate (bleeding from oesophageal varices or portal hypertensive gastropathy, or severe complications of treatment) between the two arms: 6/31 failed treatments in the propranolol arm compared with 0/31 in the EVL arm.

Specific results of this composite end-point are listed in Table 14.3.

Comment

The authors estimated the costs of the two approaches and found no significant differences between them once the differing clinical outcomes had been taken into account. The predominant costs of the endoscopic treatment approach were related to the hospitalization costs of patients with bleeding. The costs of the two approaches compared in this study may be somewhat difficult to interpret, given the availability of liver transplantation, and the sizeable percentage of patients who required liver transplantation.

The authors could not rationalize the increase in mortality seen in the β-blocker group, but speculated that the explanation for this may have been an inadequate HVPG/haemodynamic response to β-blockers, which essentially would fail to protect patients from portal hypertensive bleeding, yet leave them at a higher risk of β-blocker side effects.

Furthermore, they raised the possibility that the aetiology of liver disease may influence the response to β-blockers, and that this population, with a relatively low proportion of patients with alcoholic liver disease, may have been unusual. Overall, they concluded that β-blockers offered inferior protection from variceal bleeding.

The third gas: H_2S regulates perfusion pressure in both the isolated and perfused normal rat liver and in cirrhosis

Fiorucci S, Antonelli A, Mencarelli A, *et al. Hepatology* 2005; **42**: 539–48

BACKGROUND. Portal hypertension is ultimately the result of an essential imbalance in the opposing forces of vascular flow and resistance. Although traditionally considered fixed, it has become increasingly clear that even resistance to flow in the liver may be a dynamic function, with inflow mediated partly by the contraction of hepatic stellate cells. These, in turn, are affected by a number of endogenous vasoconstrictors and vasodilators, perhaps most notably nitric oxide. However, multiple other possible mediators of vascular tone have since been studied. A very recent addition has been the recognition of a possible role of the gaseous vasodilator H_2S, generated from the conversion of homocysteine to cystathionine by cystathionine β-synthase (CBS), which, in turn, is converted to L-cystine and 2-ketobutyrate by cystathionine γ-lyase (CSE) (Fig. 14.3).

Table 14.3 Study outcomes

Outcome	Number with event (%) Propranolol	Banding	*P*-value*	Difference	95% CI for true difference*
	(*n* = 31)	(*n* = 31)			
Treatment failure	6 (19.4)	0 (0)	0.0098	19.4%	6.4 to 37.2%
Variceal bleeding	4 (12.9)	0 (0)	0.0443	12.9%	0.8 to 29.0%
Severe adverse event	2 (6.5)	0 (0)	0.2062	6.5%	–5.2 to 21.0%
Liver transplantation	8 (25.8)	9 (29.0)	0.8654	–3.2%	–26 to 19.8%
Bleed-related mortality	2 (6.5)	0 (0)	0.2062	6.5%	–5.2 to 21%
Overall mortality	4 (12.9)	0 (0)	0.0443	12.9%	0.8 to 29%
ICU hospital days†	2.6 ± 1.3	0.4 ± 0.3	0.1044	2.2	–0.47 to 3.1%
Non-ICU hospital days†	4.0 ± 1.6	2.0 ± 0.9	0.2803	2.0	–1.67 to 5.7%

ICU, intensive care unit.
**P*-values and 95% confidence intervals (CI) of differences were calculated by using binomial methods (StatXact, version 5).
†Mean ± SE.
Source: Jutabha *et al.* (2005).

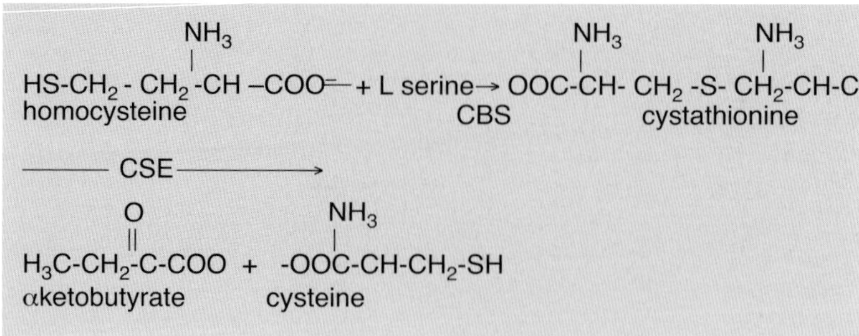

Fig. 14.3 Metabolism of homocysteine. Source: Stipanuk and Beck (1982) [5].

Interpretation. Fiorucci and colleagues investigated the role of H_2S in cirrhotic animals, based on earlier work demonstrating abnormal L-cysteine metabolism in cirrhosis and experimental data on the role of H_2S in portal hypertension. Bile duct-ligated rats and rats exposed to carbon tetrachloride were chosen as the experimental models of cirrhosis and were compared with controls. Rats were injected daily with intraperitoneal NaHS, L-cysteine, or placebo. Hepatic vascular responses in an isolated perfused rat liver model were then assessed, testing the effects of H_2S, NaHS or L-cysteine along with norepinephrine (noradrenalin), and comparing the responses in each case. In a second set of experiments, specific inhibitors of adenosine triphosphate-dependent potassium channels (K_{ATP}) and of CSE were added. Quantitative reverse transcription–polymerase chain reaction (PCR) was done to measure levels of the enzymes CSE and CSB. Lastly, hepatic stellate cells, hepatocytes and sinusoidal endothelial cells were isolated in cultures and exposed to H_2S and L-cysteine before testing for the ability to contract. CSE and CBS were present and catalytically active in rat livers, producing H_2S in response to L-cysteine in hepatocytes but not in sinusoidal endothelial cells or hepatic stellate cells. Perfusing the liver with norepinephrine – with and without H_2S or L-cysteine, the H_2S precursor – yielded the curves shown in Fig. 14.4a.

Adding a K_{ATP} channel blocker to the perfusate demonstrated reversal of the H_2S-mediated vasodilation (Fig. 14.4). The effect of H_2S on vascular resistance was not affected by nitric oxide. In rats with cirrhosis, a dose-dependent effect on perfusion pressure with norepinephrine was also seen, but the cirrhotic livers appeared to be more sensitive to its effects, with maximal vasoconstriction seen at lower doses. Adding H_2S decreased this effect, but, in contrast to the results obtained with normal livers, adding L-cysteine did not change the perfusion pressure (Fig. 14.5). Quantitative PCR to measure the amount of CSE and CBS in rats with cirrhosis showed a decrease in CSE mRNA of more than 50%. Lastly, after adding H_2S to stellate cells a reduction greater than 20% in contraction compared with controls was noted. However, there was a lack of response to L-cysteine, implying the inability to metabolize L-cysteine based on decreased expression or activity of CSE.

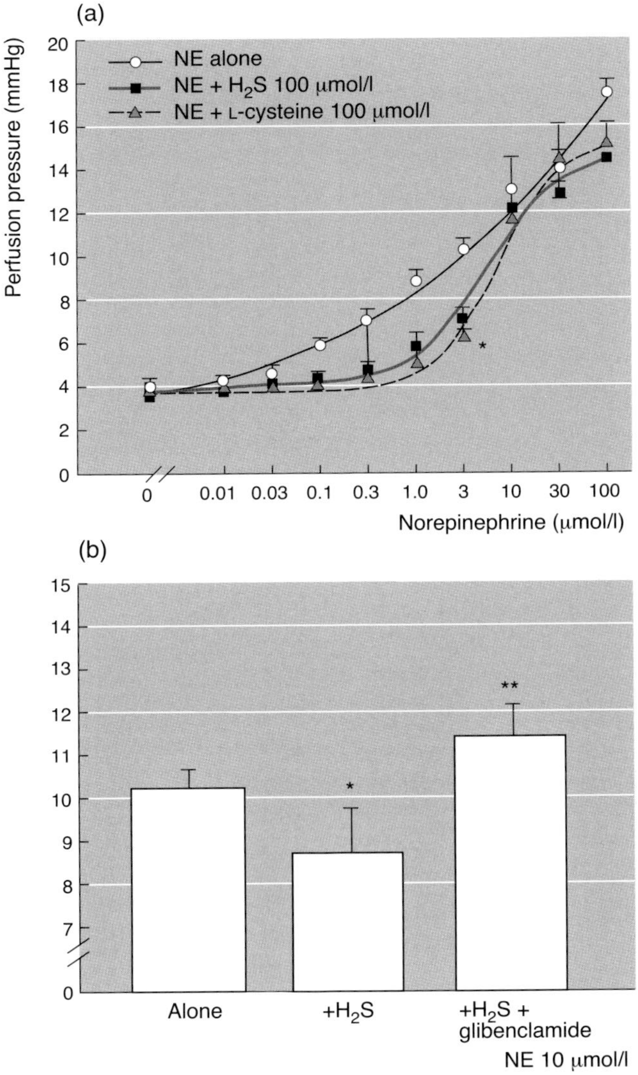

Fig. 14.4 H_2S modulates intrahepatic resistance in normal rats. (a) Effects of H_2S on norepinephrine (NE)-induced contraction in livers. Perfusing the liver with both NaHS or L-cysteine (1 mmol/l) significantly attenuated the response to NE at any concentration increment of vasoconstrictor tested. Livers were first perfused with NaHS and L-cysteine for 20 min, and then NE was added to the perfusion medium. Data are mean ± SE of seven livers. *P <0.05 for NE and NaHS or L-cysteine versus NE alone. (b) Effect of glibenclamide (a K_{ATP} channel blocker) on the H_2S-induced vasodilation. Glibenclamide (1 mmol/l) attenuated the vasorelaxation induced by H_2S in NE-treated rats. Data are mean ± SE of six livers. *P <0.05 versus NE plus NaHS. **P <0.05, H_2S + glibenclamide versus H_2S alone. K_{ATP}, adenosine triphosphate-sensitive potassium. Source: Fiorucci *et al.* (2005).

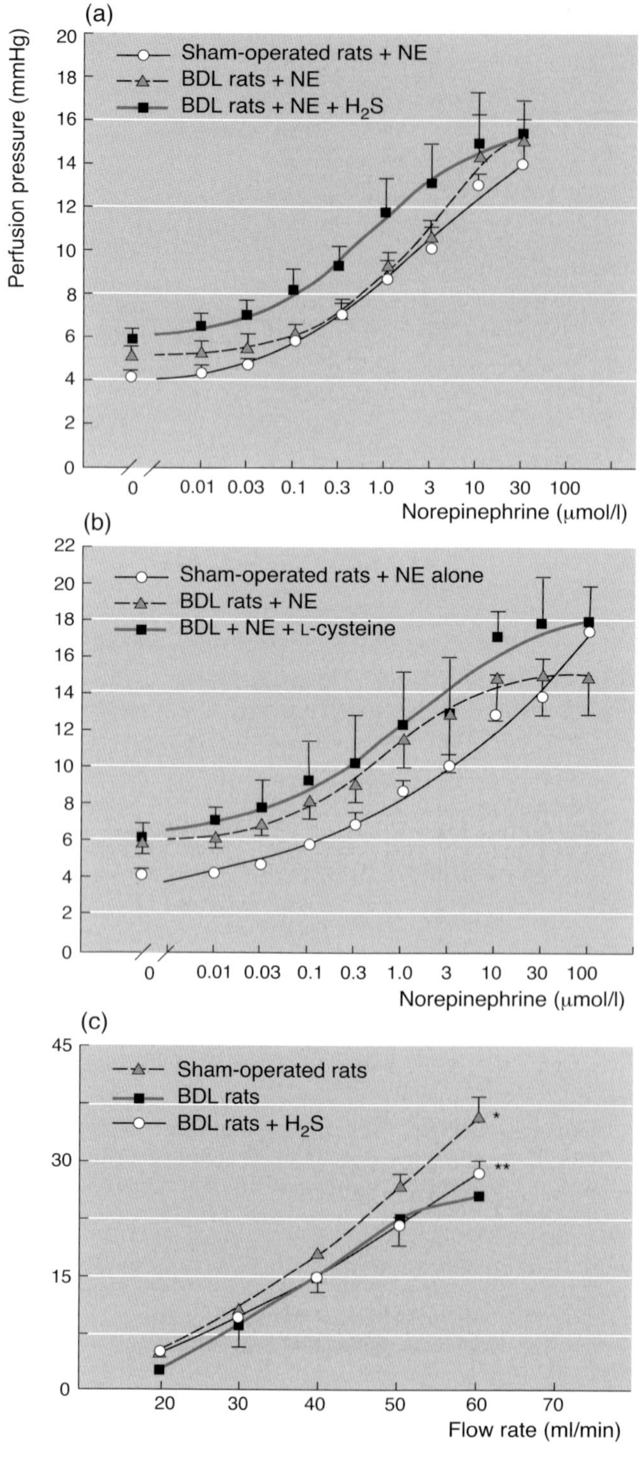
(a)
Perfusion pressure (mmHg)
Sham-operated rats + NE
BDL rats + NE
BDL rats + NE + H2S
0 0.01 0.03 0.1 0.3 1.0 3 10 30 100
Norepinephrine (μmol/l)
(b)
Sham-operated rats + NE alone
BDL rats + NE
BDL + NE + L-cysteine
0 0.01 0.03 0.1 0.3 1.0 3 10 30 100
Norepinephrine (μmol/l)
(c)
Sham-operated rats
BDL rats
BDL rats + H2S
20 30 40 50 60 70
Flow rate (ml/min)

Comment

Overall, this elegant series of studies has defined an important and independent role for H_2S in mediating hepatic vascular resistance and given some proof of a mechanism, i.e. an effect on K_{ATP} channels. Moreover, the impact of cirrhosis may be mediated by decreased synthesis and/or function of the enzymes responsible for the metabolism of L-cysteine, CBS and, perhaps more importantly, CSE, which has been localized to hepatic stellate cells. H_2S may therefore be an important target for future therapies.

Renal failure in patients with cirrhosis and sepsis unrelated to spontaneous bacterial peritonitis: value of MELD score

Terra C, Guevara M, Torre A, *et al. Gastroenterology* 2005; **129**: 1944–53

BACKGROUND. Acute renal failure in patients with cirrhosis is a very poor prognostic sign. This has been shown in a number of studies, and its importance is emphasized by its inclusion in the Model for End-stage Liver Disease (MELD) score, which is used to stratify the severity of illness in patients with cirrhosis awaiting liver transplantation. This is true in all forms of renal failure, including hepatorenal syndrome, and so the prevention of acute renal failure takes on additional importance in patients with end-stage liver disease.

Previous studies have shown that volume expansion in cirrhotics with spontaneous bacterial peritonitis (SBP), using albumin infusion, may prevent the development of hepatorenal syndrome. This study was designed to evaluate the characteristics and natural history of patients with cirrhosis who developed sepsis unrelated to SBP, in terms of renal function.

INTERPRETATION. One hundred and six patients with cirrhosis and sepsis (unrelated to SBP) admitted to a single hospital in Barcelona over an 18-month period were compared with 100 cirrhotics admitted over the same period with other complications of liver disease (gastrointestinal bleeding, ascites and hepatic encephalopathy [HE]). The

Fig. 14.5 (opposite) Effects of exogenous H_2S on pre-contracted rat liver with cirrhosis. (a) The addition of H_2S to the perfusate reduces the hyper-response of livers with cirrhosis to norepinephrine (NE). Data are mean ± SE for six rats. $*P < 0.05$ for bile duct-ligated rats + NE versus sham rats + NE. (b) Cysteine failed to reverse vasoconstriction caused by NE in rats in cirrhosis. Data are mean ± SE of six livers. $*P > 0.05$ versus NE. (c) Vasodilating effects of H_2S in the liver with cirrhosis. Bile duct-ligated rats were treated with NaHS (56 μmol/kg) intraperitoneally for 5 days, and then the isolated livers were perfused with NaHS 1 mmol/l for 20 min before determining the high-flow-rate pressure–response curve ($n = 6$; $*P < 0.05$ versus sham-operated rats; $**H_2S$ versus bile duct-ligated rats). (c) H_2S exerts a vasodilatory effect on livers with cirrhosis. Rats with cirrhosis (4 weeks after bile duct ligation) were treated with NaHS (56 μmol/kg) intraperitoneally for 5 days, and then the isolated livers were perfused with NaHS 1 mmol/l for 20 min before determining the high-flow-rate pressure–response curve ($n = 6$; $P < 0.05$ versus bile duct-ligated rats). Source: Fiorucci *et al.* (2005).

primary outcome of interest was survival 3 months after hospitalization. The diagnosis of infection/sepsis was based on culture results and standard criteria. If no cultures were positive, the diagnosis was predominantly clinical. Renal function was assessed with serum creatinine, renal failure being defined as a serum creatinine concentration greater than 1.5 mg/dl or a 50% increase in serum creatinine.

Serum levels of catecholamines, as well as plasma renin activity, aldosterone, arginine vasopressin, endothelin and atrial natriuretic peptide were tested. In a subset of ten patients, renal vascular resistance was estimated by measuring the renal resistive index by Doppler ultrasound. At baseline, patients admitted with sepsis had markers for more advanced liver disease, with higher Child–Turcotte–Pugh and MELD scores, more frequent hepatic encephalopathy and lower serum albumin and sodium levels. Baseline creatinine concentration was also higher (1.3 ± 0.7 vs 1.0 ± 0.5 mg/dl) compared with controls. Approximately 60% of patients with sepsis had either pneumonia or a urinary tract infection as the source. The remainder had a variety of other aetiologies. Renal failure was diagnosed in 29/106 patients with sepsis, and was present at the time of original presentation in 20% of all patients with sepsis; the remaining patients developed renal failure over the next 14 days. In comparison, renal failure was present in six of the 100 controls at admission and developed in an additional two during hospitalization. Haemodynamic characteristics of the patients with renal failure and controls are compared in Table 14.4.

Overall, renal failure was reversible in 22/29 patients with sepsis versus 5/8 patients without infection. Of the seven septic patients with irreversible renal failure, six ultimately died of infection and multi-organ failure. Of 106 patients, 29 (27%) with sepsis died during follow-up compared with 6/100 (6%) controls. The development of renal failure was strongly correlated with the overall risk of death. Sixty per cent of the patients

Table 14.4 Characteristics of renal function and systemic haemodynamics in patients with cirrhosis and sepsis with and without renal failure

Parameter	Renal failure (n = 29)	No renal failure (n = 77)	P-value
Renal function			
Serum creatinine (mg/dl)	2.4 ± 0.8	1 ± 0.3	0.0001
Blood urea nitrogen (mg/dl)	52 ± 15	20 ± 13	0.002
Creatinine clearance (ml/min)	26 ± 15	68 ± 39	0.0001
Renal resistive index	0.83 ± 0.09	NA	–
Serum sodium (mEq/l)	128 ± 6	134 ± 5	0.03
Serum potassium (mEq/l)	4.6 ± 1	4 ± 0.6	0.005
Serum osmolality (mosm/kg)	295 ± 16	NA	–
Urine volume (ml/day)	900 ± 450	1650 ± 900	0.001
Urine sodium (mEq/l)	18 ± 16	43 ± 36	0.01
Urine osmolality (mosm/kg)	342 ± 73	NA	–
Proteinuria (mg/day)	167 ± 157	217 ± 202	0.2
β_2-microglobulin (μg/g/creatinine)	100 ± 66	NA	–

Source: Terra *et al.* (2005).

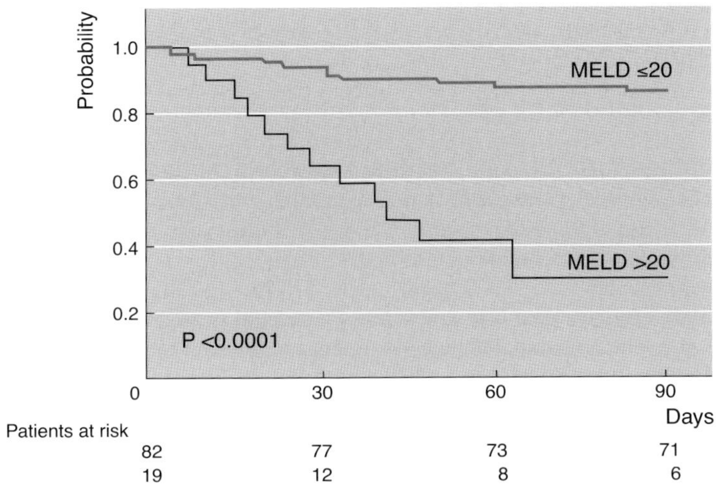

Fig. 14.6 Probability of survival of patients with cirrhosis and sepsis divided according to the MELD score obtained at diagnosis of sepsis. Patients with tumours ($n = 5$) who died during the 3-month follow-up period were excluded from the analysis. Source: Terra *et al.* (2005).

who developed acute renal failure died during follow-up, versus 13% of those who did not. This included 100% (7/7) of those who developed irreversible acute renal failure versus 12/22 (55%) of those with reversible renal failure.

In multivariable analysis, the MELD score at diagnosis was highly predictive of 3-month survival. Using a cut-off score of 20 yielded an area under the receiver operating characteristic curve of 0.83 (Fig. 14.6).

Comment

These data suggest that acute renal failure in patients with sepsis and cirrhosis is characterized by physiology of the hepatorenal syndrome (HRS) type, including severe renal vasoconstriction with preservation of tubular function. Patients with irreversible renal failure tended to have lower creatinine clearances at the time of initial diagnosis and higher levels of renal counter-regulatory hormones, including plasma renin activity, norepinephrine, vasopressin, and endothelin.

These data emphasize again the importance of renal function in determining the survival of patients with cirrhosis. The authors speculate that the pathophysiology of the acute renal failure seen in patients with cirrhosis and sepsis unrelated to SBP may be very similar to the mechanisms that precipitate HRS, a clinical scenario also associated with an intense intrinsic pre-renal vasoconstriction. Given the effects on renal function that have already been shown in treating patients with SBP with intravenous albumin to prevent HRS, the authors speculate that similar trials should be considered in patients with sepsis and cirrhosis before the development of acute renal failure.

Recombinant factor VIIa for upper gastrointestinal bleeding in patients with cirrhosis: a randomized, double blind trial

Bosch J, Thabut D, Bendtsen F, *et al.*; European Study Group on rFVIIa in UGI Haemorrhage. *Gastroenterology* 2004; **127**: 1123–30

BACKGROUND. Refractory variceal bleeding is usually thought of as disease of haemodynamics, e.g. portal pressure, inflow and resistance, dictated by vasodilatation and vasoconstriction. From a clinical perspective, however, variceal bleeding is also a function of deranged clotting ability, a result of the simultaneous decrease in the production of clotting factors from a failing liver and the consumption of factors as part of the hypercoaguable state of cirrhosis and the acute bleeding process.

INTERPRETATION. This study was a multicentre randomized clinical trial in patients who had upper gastrointestinal tract bleeding that was thought to be variceal and were able to receive treatment within 6 h and undergo EGD within 12 h of admission. Patients were recruited from 26 European hospitals. The study was designed to have the power to detect a 50% decrease (i.e. from 30% to 15%) in the rate of treatment failure, as defined by the inability to control bleeding within 24 h, failure to prevent rebleeding over the next 5 days, or death within 5 days. One hundred and twenty-one patients (of 258 patients screened) were randomized to either placebo or treatment with recombinant factor VIIa (rFVIIa), given initially before the first endoscopy and again 2, 4, 6, 12, 18, 24 and 30 h later. Patients were treated with sclerotherapy or EVL, and vasoactive drugs (terlipressin, octreotide or somatostatin), and transfused to maintain the haematocrit between 25 and 30%.

Results of endoscopic findings are given in Table 14.5. Overall, no statistically significant difference was seen when comparing the results of therapy based on the composite end-point or on outcomes of any of the three components.

Comment

Although no overall effect was proven, several trends were seen in subgroup analyses that perhaps warrant further study. Secondary analyses suggested that patients who were more ill may potentially benefit more from factor VIIa, with Child B and C patients with variceal bleeding significantly less likely to stop bleeding, to rebleed or not have control of bleeding within 24 h.

Some reluctance to accept conclusions from subgroup analyses is sensible, although there is a rationale for these conclusions. The original sample size and power calculations had estimated 120 patients in each group, probably based on the assumption that the majority of patients in the study would have had variceal

Table 14.5 Findings at first endoscopy and characteristics of therapy

	Placebo (*n* = 121)	Recombinant factor VIIa (*n* = 121)
Source of bleeding		
Oesophageal varices	77 (64%)	68 (56%)
Gastric varices	5 (4%)	11 (9%)
Gastric ulcer	9 (7%)	12 (10%)
Mallory Weiss tear	5 (4%)	12 (10%)
Portal hypertensive gastropathy	10 (8%)	5 (4%)
Other	12 (10%)	7 (6%)
Unknown	3 (2%)	6 (5%)
Type of bleeding		
Spurting	20 (17%)	16 (13%)
Oozing	50 (41%)	51 (42%)
No active bleeding	51 (42%)	54 (45%)
Type of endoscopic therapy		
Sclerotherapy and banding	3 (2%)	3 (2%)
Sclerotherapy only	37 (31%)	37 (31%)
Banding only	40 (33%)	32 (26%)
None	39 (32%)	46 (38%)
Vasoactive therapy		
Octreotide	25 (21%)	29 (24%)
Somatostatin	34 (28%)	33 (27%)
Terlipressin	13 (11%)	7 (6%)
More than one vasoactive drug	35 (29%)	32 (26%)
No vasoactive therapy	14 (12%)	20 (17%)
Proton pump inhibitor therapy	104 (86%)	109 (90%)

Data refer to number and percentage of patients.
Source: Bosch *et al.* (2004).

Table 14.6 Results of therapy

	Placebo	Recombinant factor VIIa	*P*-value
Composite (all patients)	19/119 (16%)	16/118 (14%)	0.72
Child B/C variceal bleeding	15/164 (23%)	5/62 (8%)	0.03
24-h failure (all patients)	10/119 (8%)	6/120 (5%)	0.31
Child B/C variceal bleeding	7/63 (11%)	0/62 (0%)	0.01
Prevention of rebleed (all patients)	10/116 (9%)	9/116 (8%)	1.0
Child B/C variceal bleeding	8/61 (13%)	3/62 (5%)	0.13
Mortality (5 days)	4/119 (3%)	7/118 (6%)	0.38

Source: Bosch *et al.* (2004).

bleeding, which was not the case. In fact, 30% of the patients bled from non-variceal sources and almost half of the patients had no evidence of acute bleeding at the time of initial endoscopy.

The other issue that remains unresolved after this study relates to the safety of this drug. Although no significant differences were noted in overall rates of thromboembolic events, three events in the group treated with rFVIIa were serious: one patient developed a clot in a central catheter and two patients suffered cerebrovascular accidents.

Overall, this study raises the possibility of another weapon in the armamentarium to treat patients with acute, active variceal bleeding. However, the adoption of treatment with rFVIIa without further study, which has been advocated, is probably not advisable. Definitive data will probably emerge from the current clinical trial in Asia and Europe that is testing the utility of rFVIIa in actively bleeding cirrhotics.

Influence of portal hypertension and its early decompression by TIPS placement on the outcome of variceal bleeding

Monescillo A, Martinez-Lagares F, Ruiz-del-Arbol L, *et al. Hepatology* 2004; **40**: 793–801

BACKGROUND. TIPS has become a mainstay of management for patients with end-stage liver disease, largely replacing the use of surgical shunts in patients with variceal bleeding, as well as for certain elective conditions, such as refractory ascites. However, when TIPS should be employed even in this situation is not completely clear. Early rebleeding rates and patient mortality depend on the severity of the underlying liver disease, but can be of the order of 20–40%. Standard treatment options to prevent rebleeding typically include medications to decrease portal pressure, with the use of non-selective β-blockers, along with endoscopic therapy. Unfortunately, pharmacological therapy is often of limited utility in patients with advanced liver disease, as these agents can reduce systemic blood pressure.

INTERPRETATION. This study compared the outcomes of patients randomized to TIPS versus standard therapy, based on the degree of elevation of the HVPG. Patients hospitalized with evidence of cirrhosis and endoscopically proven variceal bleeding were evaluated (Fig. 14.7). The estimated sample size was based on an estimated 70% reduction in the risk of bleeding in patients receiving TIPS for oesophageal variceal bleeding. A total of 116 patients were included.

Patients were initially treated with somatostatin, urgent endoscopy, and sclerotherapy, before undergoing measurement of HVPG. Patients were divided into low- and high-risk groups based on the HVPG (less than and greater than 20 mmHg respectively); mean HVPG was 16.1 in the low-risk group and 24 in the high-risk group. High-risk patients were then randomized to TIPS within 24 h or medical therapy with β-blockers, along with follow-up EVL if β-blockers could not be used. The portal pressure in the early TIPS group decreased on average from 24.1 to 8.2 mmHg. Statistically significant differences were seen between high-risk and low-risk patients in the severity of illness measures, including the CTP score, prothrombin time and bilirubin level, as well as the percentage

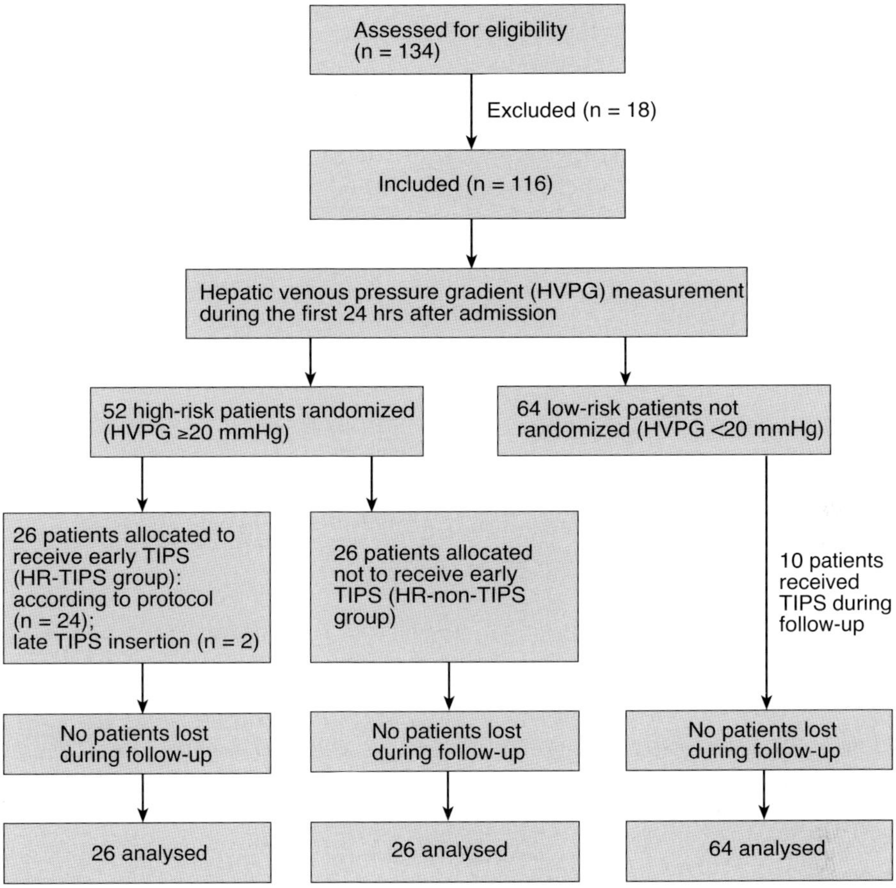

Fig. 14.7 Flow chart of the different periods of study. Source: Monescillo *et al.* (2004).

of patients actively bleeding at the time of endoscopy (Table 14.7). An HVPG greater than 20 was associated with a 7-fold higher risk of bleeding than an HVPG less than 20 mmHg. Using an HVPG of 20 as a threshold for predicting treatment failure yielded 62% sensitivity and 81% specificity, with positive and negative predictive values of 50 and 87% respectively.

Although HVPG was not statistically significantly better in predicting treatment failure compared with the CTP score, it was better in predicting mortality (Fig. 14.8).

Further predictors of mortality at 6 weeks and 1 year in multivariate analysis included the CTP score (a measure of disease severity), along with treatment failure or the inability to control acute bleeding for acute mortality, and the creatinine level and the development of other complications for 1-year mortality (Table 14.8).

Table 14.7 Results of treatment and complications during the first week of admission

Results	**Low-risk (*n* = 64)**	**High-risk, TIPS (*n* = 26)**	**High-risk, non-TIPS (*n* = 26)**
Failure of treatment, *n* (%)	8 (12%)	3 (12%)	13 (50%)*
Acute failure, *n* (%)	1 (1%)	2 (8%)	10 (38%)*
Early rebleeding, *n* (%)	7 (11%)	1 (4%)	3 (12%)
CTP class A/B/C, *n*	1/4/3	0/1/2	0/4/9
In-hospital mortality, *n* (%)	3 (5%)	3 (11%)	10 (38%)**
6-week mortality, *n* (%)	3 (5%)†	5 (17%)	10 (38%)
CTP class, A/B/C, *n*	0/1/2	1/1/3	0/3/7
Units of blood, *n* (range)	2.2 ± 2.3 (0–11)†	3.1 ± 2.6 (0–13)	3.6 ± 2.4 (0–10)
Intensive care unit, *n* (%)	2 (3%)‡	5 (19%)	4 (16%)
Complications, *n* (%)	22 (34%)§	18 (69%)	16 (61%)
Hepatic encephalopathy, *n* (%)	4 (6%)§	8 (31%)	9 (35%)
Infections, *n* (%)	10 (16%)¶	11 (42%)	9 (35%)

CTP, Child–Turcotte–Pugh.
**P* <0.01 versus high-risk-TIPS and low-risk groups.
***P* <0.02 versus high-risk-TIPS and low-risk groups.
†*P* = 0.02 versus high-risk non-TIPS group.
‡*P* <0.01 versus high-risk non-TIPS group.
§*P* <0.01 versus high-risk-TIPS group.
¶*P* <0.05 versus high-risk-TIPS group.

Table 14.8 Univariate and multivariate analysis for treatment failure and 6-week and 1-year survival

Variables	**Univariate analysis**	**Multivariate analysis**	
	***P*-value**	**Hazard rates; 95% confidence interval**	***P*-value**
6-week survival			
HVPG	<0.0001	1.360; 1.189–1.555	0.0001
Active bleeding at endoscopy	0.05	0.129; 0.035–0.473	0.002
CTP score	0.003	1.467; 1.113–1.935	0.007
Treatment failure	<0.0001		
1-year survival			
HVPG	<0.0001	1.356; 1.205–1.480	0.0001
Creatinine	0.006	10.843; 4.110–28.605	0.0001
CTP score	<0.0001	1.332; 1.127–1.574	0.001
Development of any complication†	<0.05	2.763; 1.275–3.982	0.03

CTP, Child–Turcotte–Pugh.
Source: Monescillo *et al.* (2004).

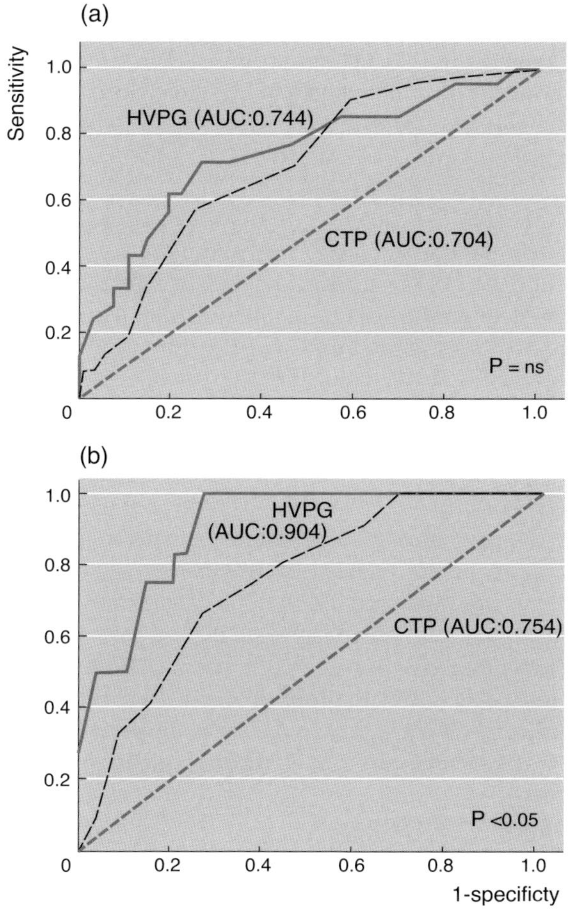

Fig. 14.8 (a) Receiver operating characteristic curve analysing the HVPG and the Child–Turcotte–Pugh score in predicting treatment failure. (b) Receiver operating characteristic curve analysing the HVPG and the Child–Turcotte–Pugh score value in predicting 6-week mortality. Source: Monescillo *et al.* (2004).

The authors conclude that early HVPG measurement is useful in predicting the outcome of bleeding, and that physicians should consider modifying practice guidelines to include this measurement in the management of patients with portal hypertensive bleeding.

Comment

A large body of work exists correlating selected cut-off points of the HVPG with the likelihood of variceal bleeding. Most recommendations suggest almost complete protection from variceal rebleeding in patients with a final post-TIPS HVPG of less than 12 mmHg [6]. Further, earlier studies have measured HVPG in a small cohort of patients and have suggested that a baseline gradient of 16–20 mmHg may portend a higher risk of bleeding or death [7]. Current recommendations from the American Association for the Study of Liver Disease (AASLD) practice guidelines are not to place a TIPS in patients who have never bled or in patients who have only bled once, reserving its use for patients who have rebled despite pharmacological and endoscopic treatment [8].

Before adopting these recommendations, however, it is important to consider the prognostic and therapeutic data that this approach yields. As other studies have shown, the degree of elevation of the HVPG yields independent information in addition to the CTP score in predicting outcomes in this population. As useful as this is in predicting at least short-term outcomes, whether the expense and potential risk of an invasive approach is justified in estimating 6-week mortality is questionable.

Placement of the TIPS clearly had a substantial impact on rebleeding, which probably accounts for the bulk of its protective effectiveness in decreasing mortality. Five patients in the high-risk non-TIPS group died of hypotensive shock or complications despite aggressive measures to stabilize them. Surprisingly, there was no increase in the rate of development of hepatic encephalopathy, which is usually seen in 10–44% of patients who undergo TIPS. If encephalopathy were a more important issue in this study, the cost–benefit ratio of TIPS in this situation might have been significantly different.

Overall, TIPS seems to be a more potent way to protect patients from the risk of rebleeding, and, by guiding therapy by measurement of the HVPG, especially high-risk patients might be targeted. Whether the costs are worth the benefits, however, remains an open question.

Diagnosis of cirrhosis by transient elastography (FibroScan®): a prospective study

Foucher J, Chanteloup E, Vergniol J, *et al. Gut* 2006; **55**: 403–8

BACKGROUND. Because of the costs, risks and low patient acceptance of liver biopsy, the gold standard for the diagnosis and staging of severity of liver diseases, the non-invasive diagnosis of cirrhosis has become the focus of a large number of investigators over the last decade. These alternative approaches have included the use of biochemical and/or radiological markers, usually including panels of laboratory studies measuring markers of collagen synthesis or lysis. In addition to studies attempting to stage the extent of fibrosis in patients (usually with alcohol or hepatitis C-related liver injury), a number of investigators have tried to further predict the presence of portal hypertension and in particular the presence of oesophageal varices based on non-invasive markers. This is important, as most guidelines recommend screening endoscopy for patients with cirrhosis, and although varices are common, some patients are clearly at a lower risk than others. The majority of these studies have focused on the degree of thrombocytopenia or on the size of the spleen or splenic

Table 14.9 Characteristics of patients at the time of the FibroScan®

	All patients	**Patients with liver biopsy**	**F3F4 fibrosis patients**
	(*n* = 711)	**(*n* = 354)**	**(*n* = 144)**
Males (%)*	403 (57)	206 (58)	102 (71)
Age (years)	52 (13)	50 (13)	53 (12)
Body mass index (kg/m^2)	24.2 (4.2)	24.5 (4.3)	25.2 (4.3)
AST (IU/l)	59.5 (86.1)	71.3 (110.5)	94.7 (138.7)
ALT (IU/l)	79.2 (108.3)	82.7 (106.6)	108.1 (119.1)
GGT (IU/l)	136 (245)	159 (229)	206 (272)
Total bilirubin (mmol/l)	16.9 (31.5)	19.7 (37.3)	27.3 (44)
Platelet count (×10^9/l)	209 (87)	213 (91)	165 (83)
Prothrombin time (%)	90 (14)	89 (15)	82 (17)
Factor V (%)	88.6 (18.5)	92.5 (15)	80.5 (20.5)
Albumin (g/l)	38.5 (5.6)	38.5 (5.2)	36.1 (6.3)
α-fetoprotein (ng/ml)	49 (456)	31 (105)	54 (270)
Fibrosis score (%)*			
No or mild fibrosis		111 (31)	
Moderate fibrosis		99 (28)	
Severe fibrosis		49 (14)	
Cirrhosis		95 (27)	
Past history of ascites*			18 (13)
Past history of bleeding varices*			14 (10)
Hepatocellular carcinoma*			19 (13)
Oesophageal varices stage 2/3*			42 (29)
US splenomegaly*			48 (33)

Results are given as mean (SD) or **n* (%).
ALT, alanine aminotransferase; AST, aspartate aminotransferase; GGT, γ-glutamyl-transpeptidase; US, ultrasonographic.
Source: Foucher *et al.* (2006).

outflow. However, many of these studies derived a prognostic index but failed to validate their results in a separate data set, usually leading to inflated and overly optimistic estimates of its sensitivity and other test characteristics.

Interpretation. Foucher *et al.* studied the use of transient elastography (FibroScan®), providing a measure of liver stiffness in 758 patients with chronic liver disease (without ascites), and correlated the findings with liver histology as well as the presence of oesophageal varices on endoscopy (Table 14.9).

Liver stiffness increased progressively with each fibrosis stage (Fig. 14.9) and was significantly correlated with clinical and biochemical features of cirrhosis and its complications (e.g. previous variceal bleeding, ascites or liver cancer), as well as varices on endoscopy and laboratory values (Table 14.10).

Choosing different cut-off values to maximize utility, the test characteristics of elastography for detection of complications of cirrhosis were defined (Table 14.11).

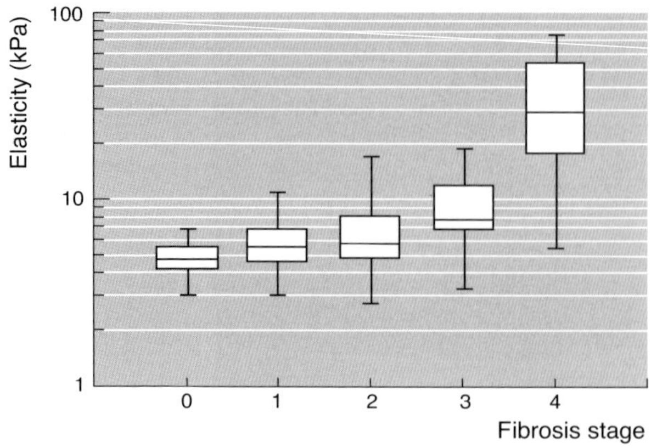

Fig. 14.9 Liver stiffness values for each fibrosis stage (0–4). The vertical axis is a logarithmic scale. The top and bottom of the boxes are the first and third quartiles. The length of the box represents interquartile ranges, within which are located 50% of the values. The lines through the middle of the boxes represent median values. Source: Foucher *et al.* (2006).

Table 14.10 Correlations between transient elastography and biochemical, clinical and ultrasonographic features

	All patients			F3F4 fibrosis patients		
	n	r	*P*-value	*n*	r	*P*-value
AST	678	0.480	<0.0001	141	0.194	0.02
ALT	698	0.216	<0.0001	141	–0.296	0.004
GGT	688	0.426	<0.0001	141	0.356	<0.0001
Total bilirubin	666	0.448	<0.0001	141	0.544	<0.0001
Platelet count	686	–0.427	<0.0001	140	–0.459	<0.0001
Prothrombin time	617	–0.500	<0.0001	137	–0.703	<0.0001
Factor V	222	–0.516	<0.0001	74	–0.659	<0.0001
Albumin	481	–0.370	<0.0001	109	–0.620	<0.0001
α-fetoprotein	355	0.451	<0.0001	94	0.153	ns
Child-Pugh score				144	0.590	<0.0001
Past history of ascites				144	0.447	<0.0001
Oesophageal varices				85	0.492	<0.0001
Oesophageal varices stage 2 or 3				85	0.370	0.0005
Past history of bleeding varices				144	0.387	<0.0001
Hepatocellular carcinoma				144	0.252	0.002
US splenomegaly				133	0.493	<0.0001

ALT, alanine aminotransferase; AST, aspartate aminotransferase; GGT, γ-glutamyl-transpeptidase; US, ultrasonographic; *n*, number of patients with a correct value.
Source: Foucher *et al.* (2006).

Table 14.11 Diagnostic accuracy of liver stiffness for complications of cirrhosis (144 patients with F3F4 fibrosis).

	AUROC (95% CI)	Cut-off (kPa)	PPV	NPV	Sensitivity	Specificity
Oesophageal varices Stage 2 or 3	0.73 (0.60–0.82)	27.5	45	90	88	53
Child-Pugh A vs Child-Pugh BC*	0.90 (0.82–0.93)	37.5	48	95	79	82
Past history of ascites	0.89 (0.81–0.94)	49.1	43	95	67	87
Hepatocellular carcinoma	0.71 (0.58–0.81)	53.7	30	90	37	87
Past history of variceal bleeding	0.88 (0.77–0.94)	62.7	47	95	57	93

AUROC, area under the ROC curve; CI, confidence interval; PPV, positive predictive value; NPV, negative predictive value.
*F3 patients were classified as Child-Pugh A.
Source: Foucher *et al.* (2006).

Comment

The authors conclude from their data that FibroScan may be an ideal method to measure the degree of hepatic fibrosis non-invasively as well as to predict the development of complications of cirrhosis, including portal hypertension.

Although it is premature to incorporate FibroScan into general practice, the results of this study are very interesting. Further long-term cohort studies will be necessary to define the best role of FibroScan in this regard.

Use of a mixed endothelin receptor antagonist in portopulmonary hypertension: a safe and effective therapy?

Kuntzen C, Gulberg V, Gerbes AL. *Gastroenterology* 2005; **128**: 164–8

BACKGROUND. Portopulmonary hypertension is a severe complication of cirrhosis and is present in 6–16% of patients with cirrhosis and refractory ascites. Survival is very poor, averaging 15 months after diagnosis in the absence of transplantation. Patients who are diagnosed or transplanted late in their course, when pulmonary artery pressures exceed a mean of 40 mmHg, will probably not survive transplantation. The aetiology is unknown but is thought to relate to vasoactive substances that, by virtue of the development of collateral vessels or poor hepatic function, are channelled into the pulmonary circuit. Although the aetiology of primary pulmonary hypertension is also poorly understood, several studies have posited a role for endothelin 1, which has been found to be elevated in animal and human studies. Trials of vasoactive substances, in particular bosentan, a specific antagonist of endothelin 1, have shown promise in primary pulmonary hypertension.

Interpretation. This paper is a case report of a 48-year-old patient with Laennec's cirrhosis (Child B), who had refractory ascites, progressive shortness of breath and spontaneous bacterial peritonitis. Evaluation included a negative V/Q scan and a computed tomography scan of the chest, but an electrocardiogram with a right axis deviation, incomplete right bundle branch block, and evidence of right ventricular hypertrophy. Chest X-ray had shown enlarged main and hilar pulmonary arteries; the echocardiogram showed a dilated right ventricle, right atrium, severe tricuspid

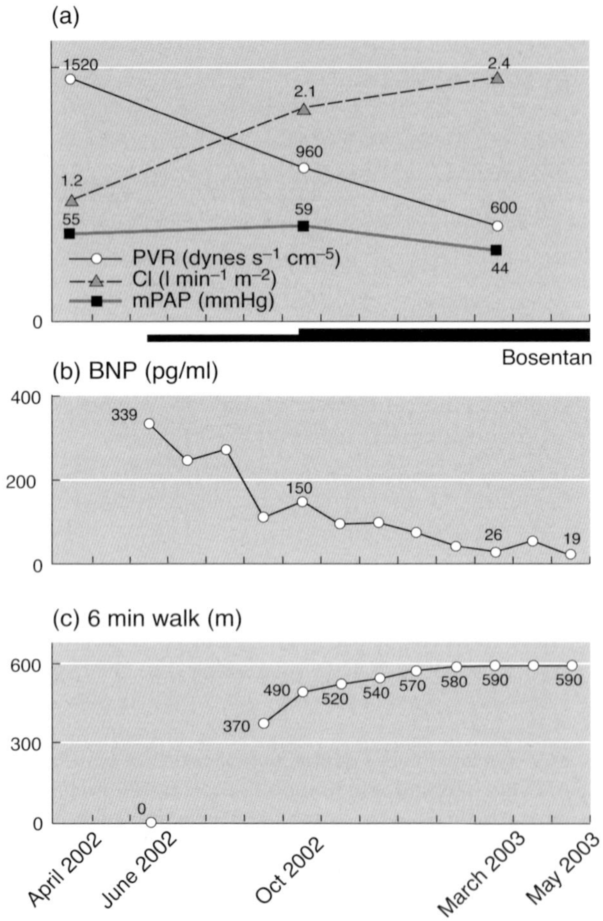

Fig. 14.10 Time course of cardiopulmonary function parameters obtained before and during bosentan therapy. Therapy was started in June 2002 with 62.5 mg twice daily. The dose was doubled in October 2002 (month 5) and was subsequently kept constant. (a) Cardiac catheterization. PVR, pulmonary vascular resistance; CI, cardiac index; mPAP, mean pulmonary artery pressure. (b) Plasma B type natriuretic peptide (BNP) concentration (normal range <18 pg/ml). (c) Six-minute walk test was performed under standardized conditions. Source: Foucher *et al.* (2006).

regurgitation with a gradient of 86 mmHg, and mild pulmonic valve insufficiency. Right heart catheterization revealed a mean pulmonary artery pressure of 55 mmHg, a pulmonary capillary wedge pressure of 10 mmHg, a pulmonary vascular resistance of 1520 dyne $s^{-1}cm^{-5}$ and a cardiac index of 1.2 l min^{-1} m^{-2}. A transthoracic echocardiogram showed no evidence of left ventricular dysfunction or valvular disease. No effect on pulmonary vascular resistance was seen with inhaled oxygen or nitric oxide, but a trial of iloprost (a prostacyclin analogue) led to a 35% reduction in vascular resistance. Serological studies to exclude possible secondary causes of pulmonary hypertension were unremarkable; negative results included antinuclear antibodies (ANA), antineutrophil cytoplasmic antibodies (ANCA) and HIV antibodies.

Because of ongoing symptoms and relative contraindications to the use of prostacyclin analogues, a trial of bosentan was begun, with a dose of 62.5 mg orally twice daily for 4 months and subsequently a dose of 125 mg orally twice daily (Fig. 14.10).

Symptomatically, the patient improved dramatically on low doses over as little as a week, with increased exercise tolerance and ability to return to work, mirrored by a dramatic decrease in pulmonary vascular resistance of more than 50%. No significant adverse events were noted. There was a slight initial drop in blood pressure that reversed over time.

Comment

This paper is the first case report of the use of bosentan for treatment of portopulmonary hypertension. Although this paper presents only a single case report, the findings are striking and lend strong support to undertaking further trials in this rare but serious complication of cirrhosis.

Conclusion

The development of symptomatic portal hypertension remains an important marker in the evolution of the natural history of cirrhosis. Despite the implications of decompensation (developing ascites, encephalopathy, or variceal bleeding marks a rapid decline in life expectancy), progress has been slow to prevent each of these complications. The array of studies presented here represents a sample of this progress, including some of the advances in the basic sciences such as the recognition of another possible independent mediator of portal haemodynamics, H2S. The implications of this discovery have not been fully realized, but this advance will undoubtedly fuel the drive to discover more of the mechanism – and thereby, targets for intervention – or portal hypertension.

At the same time, clinical trials have also refined the management of complications using our current armamentarium. The development of non-invasive markers of liver fibrosis, and ultimately portal hypertension, may revolutionize the monitoring of patients with chronic liver disease. Direct measurement of the hepatic venous pressure gradient may stratify the risk of a patient's complications of portal hypertension, and thus allow newer therapies to be directed to high-risk patients, perhaps at the time of diagnosis, even before the initial development of varices, through an episode of bleeding, to prevention of recurrence. Other markers of disease severity, including estimates of renal function and its importance in disease scores such as the MELD score, continue to be highlighted.

The advances made in portal hypertension since the last publication of this text may lead to a shift in the paradigm of management, and thus to some optimism. Nonetheless, major questions and areas for discovery remain.

References

1. Lebrec D, Poynard T, Hillon P, Benhamou JP. Propranolol for prevention of recurrent gastrointestinal bleeding in patients with cirrhosis: a controlled study. *N Engl J Med* 1981; **305**: 1371–4.
2. Mukherjee S, Sorrell MF. Beta-blockers to prevent esophageal varices—an unfulfilled promise. *N Engl J Med* 2005; **353**: 2288–90.
3. Khuroo MS, Khuroo NS, Farahat KL, Khuroo YS, Sofi AA, Dahab ST. Meta-analysis: endoscopic variceal ligation for primary prophylaxis of oesophageal variceal bleeding. *Aliment Pharmacol Ther* 2005; **21**: 347–61.
4. Chalasani N, Boyer TD. Primary prophylaxis against variceal bleeding: beta-blockers, endoscopic ligation, or both? *Am J Gastroenterol* 2005; **100**: 805–7.
5. Stipanuk MH, Beck PW. Characterization of the enzymic capacity for cysteine desulphhydration in liver and kidney of the rat. *Biochem J* 1982; **206**(2): 267–77.
6. Feu F, Garcia-Pagan JC, Bosch J, Luca A, Teres J, Escorsell A, Rodes J. Relation between portal pressure response to pharmacotherapy and risk of recurrent variceal haemorrhage in patients with cirrhosis. *Lancet* 1995; **346**: 1056–9.
7. Patch D, Armonis A, Sabin C, Christopoulou K, Greenslade L, McCormick A, Dick R, Burroughs AK. Single portal pressure measurement predicts survival in cirrhotic patients with recent bleeding. *Gut* 1999; **44**: 264–9.
8. Boyer TD, Haskal ZJ. AASLD guidelines: the role of transjugular intrahepatic portosystemic shunt in the management of portal hypertension. *Hepatology* 2005; **41**: 386–400.

15

Hepatobiliary malignancies

BRENT LEMBERG, JAMILÉ WAKIM-FLEMING

Introduction

Hepatobiliary malignancies involve a spectrum of malignancies that are considered primary when they originate in the liver, such as in hepatocellular carcinoma (HCC) and cholangiocarcinoma, and secondary when they originate in other sites and metastasize into the liver. Resection and liver transplantation have been performed with the intention to cure. Liver transplantation offers the advantage of eradicating the primary liver tumour and treating the underlying liver disease, whereas liver resection may be curative for solitary liver metastasis.

Hepatocellular carcinoma is one of the most common malignant tumours worldwide, ranking fifth in men and eighth in women. The estimated number of HCC-related deaths approximates one million per year [1].

In the USA, the incidence of HCC has doubled since the 1980s, probably as a result of the rising rate of cirrhosis from viral hepatitis C. When liver transplantation is restricted to tumours meeting the Milan criteria (solitary tumour ≤5 cm or up to three tumours all ≤3 cm), the 5-year survival rate is 70% and the recurrence rate is less than 20% [2]. However, the demand for liver transplantation is increasing faster than the availability of donor organs, leading to a longer time on the waiting list. The consequences include tumour progression with a high recurrence rate following transplantation, and an increased number of patients dropping out from the waiting list.

Percutaneous interventional therapies for HCC have thus emerged. These include transarterial chemoembolization, radiofrequency ablation and percutaneous ethanol injection. These modalities are considered minimally invasive and constitute the best medical option for non-surgical HCC. Literature is scant on how these modalities compare with each other and which modality offers the best survival.

Cholangiocarcinomas arise from bile duct epithelial cells and are rare in the USA. These tumours are fatal because of their advanced stage at the time of diagnosis, which makes surgery not a good option. The incidence of cholangiocarcinoma is increasing globally. Established risk factors for cholangiocarcinoma relating to chronic biliary tract inflammation account for a small proportion of cases and additional risk factors are being recognized [3].

In this chapter we will discuss some of the progress made in this arena.

Mortality and hospital utilization for hepatocellular carcinoma in the United States

Kim WR, Gores GJ, Benson JT, Therneau TM, Melton LJ 3rd.
Gastroenterology 2005; **129**: 486–93

Background. The incidence of hepatocellular carcinoma continues to rise in the USA. Newer treatment options are now available but the prognosis remains poor. The authors of this review sought to determine whether mortality and hospital utilization from HCC has also increased over time. They used two nationally representative databases to assess mortality from HCC and to estimate hospital service utilization. They evaluated demographic and clinical characteristics that could explain any increase in HCC and the impact of various therapies on hospital utilization.

Interpretation. Two separate databases (the Multiple Cause of Death files and Nationwide Inpatient Sample) were used to analyse trends in mortality and hospital service utilization for HCC during the years 1988 to 2000. The authors showed that age, sex and race-specific mortality from HCC increased from 1.54 to 2.58 per 100 000 per year between 1980 and 1998. The proportion of HCC deaths in patients with viral hepatitis increased from <1% to 15% over the period evaluated. The estimated total hospital expenditure for HCC increased from $241 million in 1988 to $509 million in 2000 (adjusted for inflation). Hospitalizations for HCC increased by 76% from 1988 to 2000.

Comment

The Surveillance, Epidemiology, and End Results (SEER) Program of the National Cancer Institute has reported that the overall incidence of HCC increased by 114% between 1975 and 1998. This could imply that mortality and hospitalizations due to HCC may have increased accordingly. Indeed, the authors of this paper have shown that the number of deaths increased more than 2-fold from 1980 to 1998. A plausible explanation for the rise is the increasing number of people with long-standing HCV or non-alcoholic fatty liver disease, and the influx of immigrants from areas where hepatitis B is endemic, in whom the rate of mortality was the highest among the races studied. The economic burden also more than doubled, partly as a result of increased hospitalizations for diagnostic procedures, ablative and surgical therapies, including resection and liver transplantation. This study serves to highlight trends that will probably continue to increase in the foreseeable future.

Tumor size predicts vascular invasion and histologic grade: implications for selection of surgical treatment for hepatocellular carcinoma

Pawlik TM, Delman KA, Vauthey JN, *et al. Liver Transpl* 2005; **11**: 1086–92

Predictors of long-term survival after liver transplantation for hepatocellular carcinoma

Zavaglia C, De Carlis L, Alberti AB, *et al. Am J Gastroenterol* 2005; **100**: 2708–16

BACKGROUND. Hepatic resection and liver transplantation are two potentially curative modalities for patients with HCC. Currently, the size and number of tumours and the amount of underlying liver disease determine the feasibility of surgical therapy and the long-term survival rate. Prior to the establishment of strict selective criteria for transplantation, the recurrence rates were high and 5-year survival rates were poor. Studies have shown that both macroscopic and microscopic vascular invasion of the tumour are strong predictors of surgical outcome. The aim of the first study was to examine the relationship between tumour size, and microscopic (occult) vascular invasion and histological grade from data on a large number of patients who underwent resection of HCC. The aim of the second study was to identify predictors of both survival and tumour-free survival of patients with HCC who underwent liver transplantation for HCC.

INTERPRETATION. In the study by Pawlik *et al.*, the clinical data of 1073 patients, from five international hepatobiliary centres, who underwent resection of their HCC was evaluated. None of the patients had evidence of extrahepatic disease and all underwent an attempted curative resection. The incidence of microscopic vascular invasion increased with tumour size. Microscopic vascular invasion was present in 55% of the patients with tumours 5.1–6.5 cm and in 31% in patients with tumours smaller than 5 cm. Microscopic invasion was more common in solitary tumours measuring 5.1–6.5 cm (41%) compared with 27% of solitary tumours 5 cm or smaller. The size of the tumour also predicted histological grade. Fifty-four per cent of tumours 5.1–6.5 cm were high-grade compared with 36% of tumours smaller than 5 cm. Multivariate analysis revealed that histological grade, pre-operative alpha-feto-protein (AFP) level, number of tumour nodules and tumour size were independent predictors of microscopic vascular invasion (Table 15.1).

In the study by Zavaglia *et al.*, 549 patients received 603 liver transplants between 1989 and 2002. Median follow-up was 49 months. Overall 1-, 3-, 5- and 10-year survival was 84, 75, 72 and 62%, respectively. HCC was diagnosed in 116 patients before liver transplantation and in 39 on histological examination of liver explants. Eighty-four patients met Milan criteria on histological examination. A multivariate Cox model analysis was performed and five variables were found to affect survival (Fig. 15.1). These included histological grade of differentiation and micro- and macrovascular

Table 15.1 Factors predictive of microscopic vascular invasion in patients with tumours larger than 5 cm without evidence of major vascular invasion: multivariate analysis ($n = 502$)

Prognostic factor	Hazard ratio	95% CI	*P*-value
High-grade tumour	1.7	1.3–2.2	0.006
Large tumour size	1.5	1.3–1.8	0.001
AFP ≥1000 ng/ml	2.1	1.5–2.6	0.011
Multiple tumours	1.8	1.3–2.5	0.03
Tumour invasion into adjacent organ	1.1	0.70–1.5	0.22

CI, confidence interval; AFP, alpha-feto-protein.
Source: Pawlik *et al.* (2005).

invasion, AFP levels and encapsulation of the tumour. Histological grade and macrovascular invasion were strong and independent predictors of both survival and tumour recurrence in patients with cirrhosis who received liver transplantation.

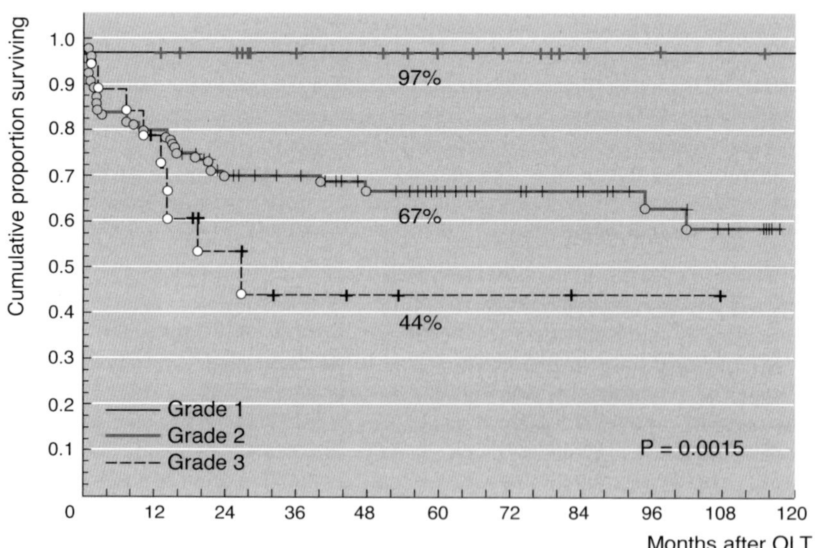

Patients at risk

Grade 1	33	32	30	22	22	18	15	12	11	10	8
Grade 2	85	68	54	47	39	31	26	20	16	13	7
Grade 3	19	13	7	4	3	2	2	1	1	0	

Fig. 15.1 Actuarial patient survival after liver transplantation for HCC according to the histological grade of differentiation (Grade 1 = well differentiated; Grade 2 = moderately differentiated; Grade 3 = poorly differentiated HCC). Source: Zavaglia *et al.* (2005).

Comment

These retrospective studies have shown that the size and number of tumours, even though they may correlate with histological grade and the degree of vascular invasion, are not sufficient to identify the patients who may benefit the most from resection or transplantation. This has major implications for how the scarce resource of donated livers should be best allocated. Selection criteria for such therapies may have to be modified to include the level of AFP, the degree of occult vascular invasion and the histological grade of the tumour. The task of diagnosing occult vascular invasion before making a decision regarding the management of such tumours is very challenging and new diagnostic modalities will be needed.

Critical appraisal of the clinical and pathologic predictors of survival after resection of large hepatocellular carcinoma

Pawlik TM, Poon RT, Abdalla EK, *et al.*; International Cooperative Study Group on Hepatocellular Carcinoma. *Arch Surg* 2005; **140**: 450–8

BACKGROUND. The incidence of HCC worldwide is increasing and the disease is predicted to afflict more than 500 000 persons in 2005. Tumours larger than 10 cm constitute about 15% of all cases of HCC and therapy is limited. Large tumours do not meet criteria for liver transplantation and ablative therapies are not curative. In this retrospective study, the authors attempted to assess the prognosis after resection of large liver tumours and to define factors that predict the best survival rate after resection.

INTERPRETATION. This was a retrospective study of a database from five major hepatobiliary centres. A total of 300 patients with an HCC 10 cm or larger and no evidence of extrahepatic disease underwent tumour resection. Perioperative mortality was 5%. At a median follow-up of 32 months, the median survival was 20.3 months. The 1-, 3-, 5- and 10-year overall survival rates were 65, 37, 27 and 18%, respectively (Fig. 15.2). Univariate analysis revealed that an AFP concentration of 1000 ng/ml or higher, multiple tumour nodules, the presence of vascular invasion and the presence of severe fibrosis were all significant predictors of poor survival. Multivariate analysis revealed that AFP level, vascular invasion, tumour number and the presence of severe fibrosis all remained independent predictors of poor survival. A clinical score was then devised using the four independent predictors in an attempt to stratify the patients with regard to prognosis. Patients with none of the independent predictors had the longest median survival (60 months). Patients with either one or two predictors had a survival of 19 months, and patients with three or four predictors had a survival of 10 months. There was no significant difference in survival between patients with one or two risk factors and those with three or four risk factors. The 5-year survival rates for patients with no risk factors, one or two risk factors, and three or four risk factors were 49, 19 and 14%, respectively.

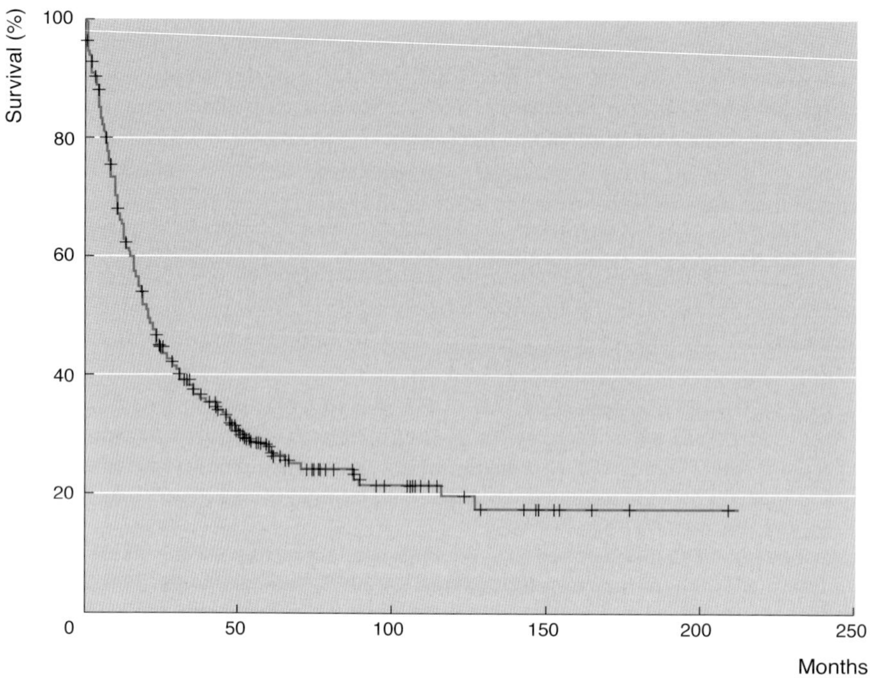

Fig. 15.2 At a median follow-up of 32 months (range, 0.2–208 months), the overall long-term median survival for patients with a hepatocellular carcinoma 10 cm in diameter or larger was 20.3 months. The 1-, 3-, 5-, and 10-year survival rates were 64.9%, 36.7%, 26.9%, and 17.8%, respectively. Source: Pawlik *et al.* (2005).

Comment

Worldwide, approximately 15% of hepatomas are larger than 10 cm. Therapeutic options are limited and ablative therapies are usually recommended. However, this study and others have shown that resection of large hepatomas can provide durable long-term survival. Like the previous two studies, this study underlines the importance of vascular invasion by the tumour as a poor predictor of survival but it also points out that the size of a hepatoma should not exclude patients from surgical resection. The good outcome could have been related to a lesser degree of fibrosis in the remainder of the liver.

Liver transplant results for hepatocellular carcinoma applying strict preoperative selection criteria

Santoyo J, Suarez MA, Fernandez-Aguilar JL, *et al.* *Transplant Proc* 2005; **37**: 1488–90

BACKGROUND. There is a range of treatments available for HCC. Liver transplantation is currently the best option for cure for a subset of cirrhotic patients who have a small HCC. Tumour recurrence rate and survival rate have improved dramatically owing to strict selection criteria based on the Milan criteria. The aim of this study was to analyse the results of a series of cirrhotic patients undergoing liver transplantation for small HCC when strict Milan criteria were applied.

INTERPRETATION. Fifty-three patients underwent liver transplantation for HCC. The distribution of Child–Pugh scores was as follows: A (32%), B (55%), C (13%). The Milan criteria were applied pre-operatively to all patients, but, despite this, 23 patients (43%) exceeded the Milan criteria when the explanted specimens were examined and 32% exceeded the University of California at San Francisco (UCSF) criteria when they were applied. The overall survival rate at 1, 3 and 5 years was 80, 70 and 70%, respectively. For those patients who exceeded the Milan criteria the survival rates at 1, 3 and 5 years were 72, 67, 67%, respectively and for those who exceeded the UCSF criteria the rates were 76, 69 and 69%, respectively,

Comment

Current methods of screening for HCC are imperfect. This study showed that 30–40% of the explanted livers had more disease than presumed when both the strict and extended criteria were applied to the explanted livers. Although this study does not address the survival at 1, 3 and 5 years in patients within the strict criteria, making the statistical significance between the group within the strict criteria and the group with the extended criteria hard to estimate, the survival in the latter group was lower than the overall survival. Given our current surveillance methods for HCC, extending the criteria for transplantation of cadaveric donors may not be recommendable at the moment in view of the lack of improved survival at a time when shortage of organ donors remains a major issue.

A randomized controlled trial of radiofrequency ablation with ethanol injection for small hepatocellular carcinoma

Shiina S, Teratani T, Obi S, *et al.* *Gastroenterology* 2005; **129**: 122–30

BACKGROUND. Therapeutic options for the treatment of HCC are multiple and consist of surgical and ablative therapies. When surgical therapy is not an option, ablative therapy with radiofrequency ablation, ethanol injection or chemoembolization

can be done. This randomized controlled trial aimed to assess the long-term outcomes of two therapies, radiofrequency ablation and percutaneous ethanol injection.

Interpretation. Two hundred and thirty-two patients with HCC were randomized to receive either radiofrequency ablation or ethanol injection. The patients were Child–Pugh class A or B; all had three or fewer tumours and all had tumours 3 cm or less. The 4-year survival rate for radiofrequency ablation was 74% and that for ethanol injection was 57% (Fig. 15.3). Radiofrequency ablation had a 46% lower risk of death, a 43% lower risk of overall recurrence and an 88% lower risk of local tumour progression than ethanol injection. The number of treatment sessions was smaller (2.1 vs 6.4) and the duration of hospitalization was shorter (11 vs 26 days) in the radiofrequency ablation group than in the ethanol injection group. The incidence of serious adverse events was not different between the two therapies.

Comment

Again in this well-designed randomized controlled trial, radiofrequency ablation proves to be superior to percutaneous ethanol injection in terms of survival rate, risk of death, recurrence and tumour progression when compared with ethanol injection.

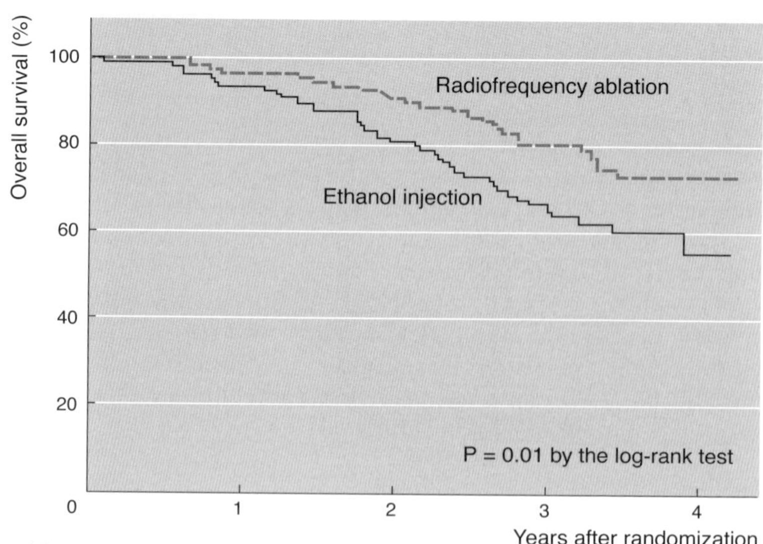

Number at risk	0	1	2	3	4
Radiofrequency ablation	118	114	108	72	13
Ethanol injection	114	107	93	51	8

Fig. 15.3 Survival in the 232 eligible patients, according to the treatment group. The actuarial 4-year survival rate was 74% in the radio frequency ablation group, whereas it was 57% in the ethanol injection group. Source: Shiina et al. (2005).

Percutaneous ethanol injection is the procedure of choice for tumours less than 3–4 cm in diameter, whereas radiofrequency ablation may ablate larger tumours; this could explain the difference in outcome when the number of sessions is controlled for.

Risk factors of intrahepatic cholangiocarcinoma in the United States: a case–control study

Shaib YH, El-Serag HB, Davila JA, Morgan R, McGlynn KA. *Gastroenterology* 2005; **128**: 620–6

BACKGROUND. The incidence of intrahepatic cholangiocarcinoma (ICC) and other biliary duct tumours has increased in the USA. The reason for the increased incidence remains unclear. Primary sclerosing cholangitis is known to be a major risk factor in the USA, but in other countries hepatitis B virus, hepatitis C virus (HCV) and/or diabetes mellitus have been described as potential risk factors. Using the SEER–Medicare database, this case–control study examined additional risk factors for ICC in the USA.

INTERPRETATION. The SEER–Medicare database is a linkage of SEER registry information with Medicare claims data. Since 1992, it has included population-based cancer registries in five US states and six metropolitan areas that represent approximately 14% of the US population. The Medicare database includes approximately 97% of individuals aged 65 years and older. Six hundred and twenty-five patients with ICC and 90 834 controls were included in the analysis. Twenty potential risk factors were examined. Several risk factors were significantly more prevalent. These included cirrhosis (adjusted odds ratio 27.2), alcoholic liver disease (adjusted odds ratio 7.4), HCV infection (adjusted odds ratio 6.1), HIV infection (adjusted odds ratio 5.9), diabetes (adjusted odds ratio 2.0) and inflammatory bowel disease (adjusted odds ratio 2.3), whereas for cholangitis the adjusted odds ratio was 8.8 and for chronic cholestasis it was 6.7.

Comment

This is a large study that examined risk factors for ICC in the US population. The authors confirm the validity of the previously known risk factors, such as inflammatory bowel disease, cholangitis and choledocholithiasis, in developing ICC, and suggest additional factors, such as chronic liver diseases (except haemochromatosis), especially in the setting of cirrhosis, HCV, HIV infection and diabetes mellitus. As the incidences of HCV infection and diabetes mellitus (and its comorbidities) continue to increase, unfortunately so could the incidence of ICC. The SEER registry has its own limitation and more studies are needed to confirm these findings.

Liver transplantation with neoadjuvant chemoradiation is more effective than resection for hilar cholangiocarcinoma

Rea DJ, Heimbach JK, Rosen CB, *et al. Ann Surg* 2005; **242**: 451–8

Surgical management of hilar cholangiocarcinoma

Hemming AW, Reed AI, Fujita S, Foley DP, Howard RJ. *Ann Surg* 2005; **241**: 693–9

BACKGROUND. Hilar cholangiocarcinoma is increasing in incidence. Radical resection offers a 5-year survival rate of 20–40% at best. Often patients are not candidates for surgical resection because of vascular involvement, bilateral lobe involvement and/or underlying primary sclerosing cholangitis. Liver transplantation for cholangiocarcinoma initially provided poor survival and high recurrence rates, and was for a long time considered a contraindication. In the study by Rea *et al.*, the authors compared survival after liver transplantation with neoadjuvant radiotherapy and chemosensitization ('the protocol') to survival after resection alone. The second study, by Hemming *et al.*, retrospectively looked at bile duct resection in addition to liver resection in patients with hilar cholangiocarcinoma.

INTERPRETATION. The study by Rea *et al.* included 71 patients from 1993 to 2004, 38 of whom underwent neoadjuvant radiotherapy, chemosensitization and liver transplantation. Fifty-four patients were explored for potential resection but 26 actually underwent resection for cure. Patient survival was significantly higher after the transplantation protocol plan than after resection. One-, 3- and 5-year survival rates were 92, 82 and 82%, respectively after the transplantation protocol and 82, 48 and 21%, respectively after resection ($P = 0.022$) (Fig. 15.4). In the study of Hemming *et al.*, patients who underwent curative resection had an operative mortality rate of 9% and a morbidity rate of 40%. Median overall survival was 40% and the 5-year survival was 35%. Negative margins were associated with improved 5-year survival (45%) (Fig. 15.5).

Comment

The results of this neoadjuvant-transplant protocol for the treatment of hilar cholangiocarcinoma in selected patients are significant in that the results showed that this management plan offer a better survival than resection. In addition, tumour resection and combined liver bile duct resection are potential surgical therapeutic options for patient with hilar cholangiocarcinoma.

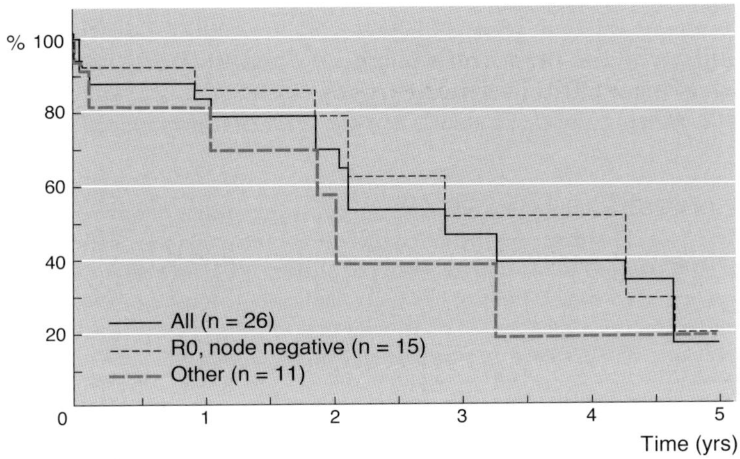

Fig. 15.4 Survival after operation for patients without PSC. Source: Rea *et al.* (2005).

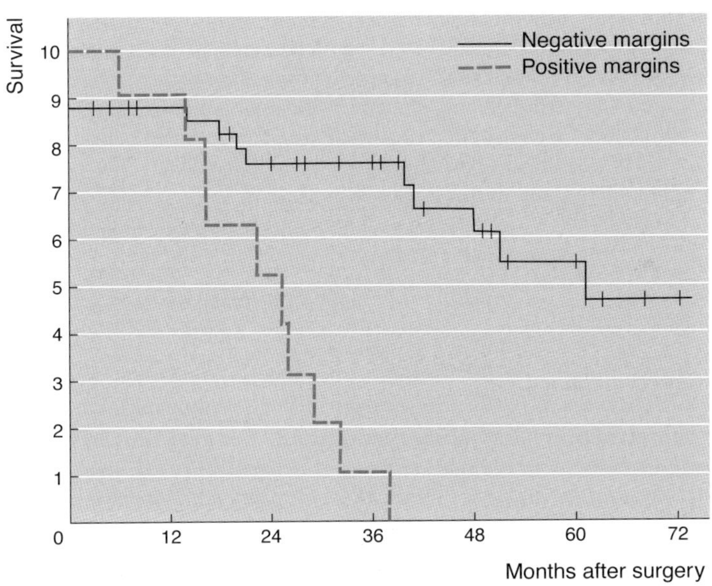

Fig. 15.5 Patient survival after resection. Source: Hemming *et al.* (2005).

Palliation of non-resectable bile duct cancer: improved survival after photodynamic therapy

Zoepf T, Jakobs R, Arnold JC, Apel D, Riemann JF. *Am J Gastroenterol* 2005; **100**: 2426–30

BACKGROUND. Surgical resection for bile duct cancer is potentially curative but only 33% of patients are candidates for resection. In unresectable bile duct cancer, palliative therapy with photodynamic therapy (PDT) or placement of an endoprosthesis for decompression has been suggested and has had some degree of success. In this study, the authors conducted a randomized controlled trial to compare PDT with endoprosthesis placement in patients with advanced non-resectable bile duct cancer.

INTERPRETATION. Thirty-two patients were randomized in this study; half of them underwent PDT and the other half had a prosthesis placed in the bile duct. The photosensitizing agent Photosan-3 was given intravenously prior to the laser irradiation. The agent concentrates in neoplastic tissue, and is then activated by non-thermal laser light, generating oxygen radicals that destroy malignant cells.

The goal of endoprosthetic treatment was bilateral hilar drainage. The primary outcomes were reduction in bile duct stenosis and survival. Secondary outcomes included acceptance of the treatment, quality of life, and a decrease in cholestasis. The median survival time after randomization was 7 months in the endoprosthesis group and 21 months in the PDT group (Fig. 15.6). Complications in the endoprosthesis group included one patient with bacterial cholangitis, which was responsive to antibiotic therapy. In the PDT group, three patients developed an infected biloma with cholangitis, again responsive to antibiotic therapy, and one patient underwent successful surgery for cholecystitis. There was no significant difference in cholestasis and quality of life. PDT was able to completely eliminate radiographic stenosis caused by the tumour.

Comment

For patients with unresectable bile duct cancer, the goal of treatment becomes essentially palliative. Patients will require relief from bile duct obstructions, either endoscopically or percutaneously. Radiation therapy and chemotherapy have had poor results. Although PDT was associated with a higher morbidity rate compared with endoprosthesis placement alone in this study, it improved survival and led to reduction in the size of malignant stenosis. PDT followed by prosthesis placement in the bile duct may become the treatment of choice in unresectable bile duct cancer.

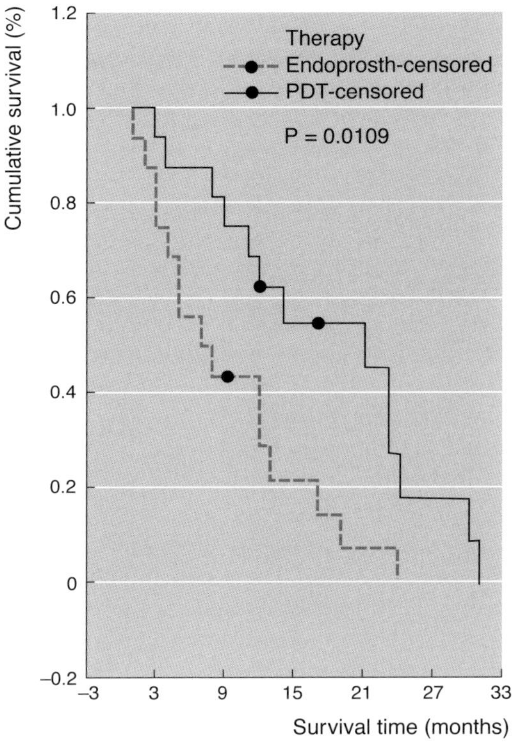

Fig. 15.6 Kaplan-Meier survival time. Source: Zoepf *et al.* (2005).

Biopsy of resectable colorectal liver metastases causes tumor dissemination and adversely affects survival after liver resection

Jones OM, Rees M, John TG, Bygrave S, Plant G. *Br J Surg* 2005; **92**: 1165–8

Background. The most common site of colorectal metastatic disease is the liver. Approximately 20% of patients are candidates for liver resection. Resection of colorectal liver metastases is associated with a median 5-year survival of 16–49%. Biopsy of liver metastases remains a controversial subject in the literature as some believe that it may cause tumour dissemination. This study involved a retrospective analysis of a database of patients who had undergone liver resection for colorectal metastases. The aim was to assess whether liver biopsy of colorectal metastases is necessary and whether it has any effect on long-term survival.

Interpretation. The end-points of the study were morbidity, operative mortality and long-term survival of the two groups. Ninety patients were in the biopsy group and 508 in the non-biopsy group. Operative morbidity and mortality were similar in the two groups. Seventeen patients (19%) in the biopsy group had evidence of needle-track deposits. The 4-year survival rate after liver resection was significantly different between the two groups: 33% in the biopsy group and 47% in the non-biopsy group. Pre-operative biopsy was an independent predictor of survival after resection of colorectal liver metastases. The inadvertent resection rate for patients with benign disease and no pre-operative histology was 1.2% (six out of a total of 514 patients).

Comment

This large study shows that almost one-fifth of all patients undergoing a liver biopsy to confirm colorectal–liver metastases will develop tumour seeding of the biopsy tract. These patients are potentially cured by their liver resection, but in reality they are left with remaining malignancy. The residual tumour seeding reduced their survival rate, with a 14% difference in survival between the two groups. Interestingly, 1.2% of the patients who did not undergo pre-operative biopsy were found to have benign disease and not metastatic disease. Unfortunately, these patients were subjected to unnecessary surgery and liver resection. These patients potentially could have been spared a liver resection if they had undergone a pre-operative

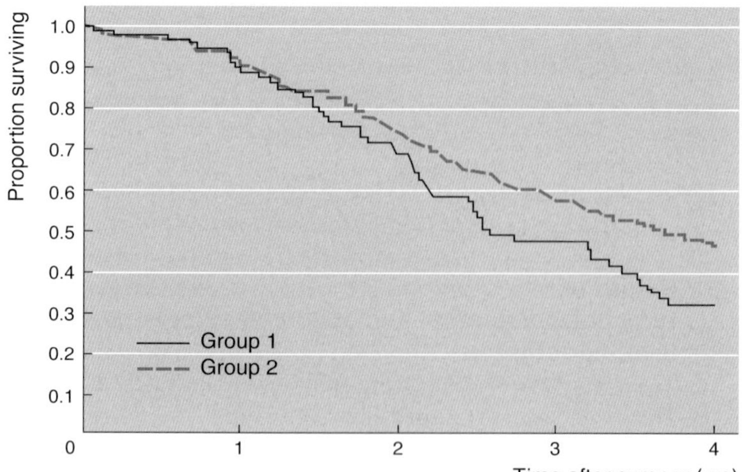

Number at risk

	0	1	2	3	4
Group 1	90	78	53	33	20
Group 2	508	407	273	165	104

Fig. 15.7 Kaplan–Meier survival curve comparing survival after liver resection in patients who had biopsy of suspected colorectal metastases (Group 1) and those who did not (Group 2). $P = 0{\cdot}008$ (log-rank test). Source: Jones *et al.* (2005).

biopsy; however, the 99% with malignant disease would then have had a 19% risk of seeding of the tract. This study highlights the fact that track seeding does occur at a high rate during biopsy of liver metastasis and reduces survival. However this study did not make note of the date of the biopsy in relation to the number of metastases, meaning that whether more metastases occurred as a result of seeding or as a result of the natural progression will therefore not be known. Imaging techniques have improved over time, and we hope to be able to rely on imaging modalities to enhance diagnostic accuracy, thus avoiding the need to biopsy potentially resectable metastatic liver disease.

Conclusion

It is likely that the incidence of hepatobiliary malignancies will continue to increase over the next several years. Mortality and the financial burden will increase accordingly.

Most common risk factors for HCC include viral hepatitis C and B and fatty liver disease [4,5]. Considerable effort has been devoted to establishing a prognostic model for HCC by using clinical and pathological information. Progress has been achieved and survival has improved, mainly pertinent to liver transplantation and to well-defined selection criteria.

Surgical and interventional modalities have been performed in recent years in combination or separately, with the intention of providing the best outcome for patients.

Although liver transplantation is considered the standard of care for most primary hepatobiliary malignancies, interventional modalities have emerged in the last few years as palliative therapies but also to reduce the tumour burden before transplantation, and as adjuvants to liver transplant. These modalities have been performed with increasing frequency because of the increased incidence of hepatobiliary tumours and the shortage of liver donors for transplantation. Results of randomized controlled trials for transarterial chemoembolization and radiofrequency ablation have shown beneficial effects on survival in specific situations. Several retrospective studies were performed last year attempting to analyse the outcome of the applied therapies. These studies have given us the kind of feedback that we need in order to assess whether a chosen modality has met its goal in terms of survival and recurrence of tumour. We learned that additional factors, such as those pertaining to tumour biology, have a great impact on survival. These factors include vascular invasion and the histological grade of the tumour. However, the greatest challenge remaining is the incorporation of these factors in selection criteria. As we continue to perfect our therapeutic armamentarium, enhanced diagnostic modalities for early detection will be needed. Genomics and imaging techniques are additional tools; progress in this area has been made in past years and will very likely continue. Such tools may become the future tools for the early diagnosis and therapy of hepatobiliary malignancies [6].

Interventional modalities for hepatobiliary malignancies as single therapies or in combination, along with transplantation, may also become the standard of care for such malignancies.

High-quality research related to cholangiocarcinoma has increased in the past few years. Primary sclerosing cholangitis may no longer be the sole risk factor for cholangiocarcinoma but cirrhosis, HCV, HIV infections and diabetes mellitus may continue to prove to be additional risk factors. Most cases of cholangiocarcinoma are discovered at an advanced stage; although surgery can be curative, few patients are candidates for surgery [**3**]. Palliative biliary decompression may be the only option for therapy because it can provide symptomatic relief. Photodynamic therapy can increase survival when the tumour burden shrinks, and may allow endobiliary prosthetic placement. In patients with hilar cholangiocarcinoma, combination neoadjuvant chemoradiation and liver transplantation in highly selected patients can offer a 5-year survival rate of 82%.

Finally, track seeding from biopsies of primary liver tumours or from metastatic lesions will continue to affect our diagnostic modalities, and whether or not to biopsy will remain a source of debate for years to come.

References

1. Bosch FX, Ribes J, Cleries R, Diaz M. Epidemiology of hepatocellular carcinoma. *Clin Liver Dis* 2005; **9**: 191–211, v.
2. Bruix J, Llovet JM. Prognostic prediction and treatment strategy in hepatocellular carcinoma. *Hepatology* 2002; **35**: 519–24.
3. Patel T. Cholangiocarcinoma. *Nat Clin Pract Gastroenterol Hepatol* 2006; **3**: 33–42.
4. Davila JA, Morgan RO, Shaib Y, McGlynn KA, El-Serag HB. Diabetes increases the risk of hepatocellular carcinoma in the United States: a population based case control study. *Gut* 2005; **54**: 533–9.
5. Zen Y, Katayanagi K, Tsuneyama K, Harada K, Araki I, Nakanuma Y. Hepatocellular carcinoma arising in non-alcoholic steatohepatitis. *Pathol Int* 2001; **51**: 127–31.
6. Parent R, Beretta L. Proteomics in the study of liver pathology. *J Hepatol* 2005; **43**: 177–83.

Further reading

1. Torok N, Gores GJ. Cholangiocarcinoma. *Semin Gastrointest Dis* 2001; **12**: 125–32.
2. Chamberlain RS, Blumgard LH. Hilar cholangiocarcinoma: a review and commentary. *Ann Surg Oncol* 2000; **7**: 55–66.
3. El-Serag HB. Hepatocellular carcinoma: an epidemiologic view. *J Clin Gastroenterol* 2002; **35**: S72–8.
4. Rocken C, Carl-McGrath S. Pathology and pathogenesis of hepatocellular carcinoma. *Dig Dis* 2001; **19**: 269–78.

16

Advances in paediatric hepatology

KADAKKAL RADHAKRISHNAN, ARIEL FELDSTEIN

Introduction

Many new and exciting advances have taken placed in paediatric hepatology in the last year that affect clinicians' ability to diagnose and treat many common causes of paediatric liver disease as well as our understanding of disease pathophysiology. In this chapter we will focus on new developments in four areas of paediatric hepatology because of their broad interest and potential impact. These topics are chronic hepatitis C infection, non-alcoholic fatty liver disease (NAFLD), paediatric liver transplantation and biliary atresia.

Hepatitis C infection

Hepatitis C virus (HCV) infection is one of the most common causes of chronic liver disease worldwide. The natural history of HCV in children remains incompletely defined. In general, it is thought to follow a benign clinical course, although, as in the adult population, HCV in children may progress to cirrhosis, liver failure and hepatocellular carcinoma [1]. The virus is transmitted parenterally and vertical transmission has become the most important route of transmission in children. There is currently no effective vaccination against this virus, and screening blood products and personal protection remain the mainstay of prevention [2]. In adults, addition of ribavirin to interferon has been extensively shown to improve virological responses [3], but until recently such data in children were lacking.

The exact timing of hepatitis C transmission during pregnancy or delivery remains unclear. This has been addressed recently in a study by Mok and colleagues from the European Paediatric Hepatitis C Virus Network [4]. This prospective cohort study included 54 HCV-infected children who had samples tested with the polymerase chain reaction (PCR) during the first 3 days of life. Seventeen of the 54 children tested positive for hepatitis C RNA (31%; 95% confidence interval 19–46%). Children with intrauterine infection were significantly more likely to be of lower birth weight and infected with HCV genotype 1. Mode of delivery was not associated with increased risk of vertical transmission. Although a higher proportion of infants born to HIV-co-infected women were PCR-positive in the first 3 days of life, this difference was not statistically significant. The results of this study show that at least a third to a half of children vertically infected with HCV acquired the infection *in utero*, and thus suggest that if effective maternal treatment were to become available it would probably need to be started early in pregnancy.

The European Paediatric Hepatitis C Virus Network this year also assessed the natural history of vertically acquired HCV infection in a large multicentre, prospective study of children born to HCV-infected women in Europe |**5**|. After reviewing follow-up data ranging up to 15 years (median 4.2 years) from 266 children, three broad modalities in the natural history of vertically acquired hepatitis C were detected. Approximately 20% of children appeared to clear the infection (i.e. they had two consecutive PCR test results negative for HCV RNA, normal alanine aminotransferase (ALT) values, and no clinical signs), 50% had evidence of chronic asymptomatic infections, characterized by intermittent viraemia and normal ALT levels, and 30% had evidence of chronic active infection, characterized by persistent viraemia, frequent abnormal ALT levels and, in some cases, hepatomegaly. In this study, clearance occurred by 3 years of age in most children, which is consistent with previous reports |**6**|. This is the largest longitudinal study of children with vertically acquired HCV infection described to date. Although the median follow-up was relatively short, the lack of any serious clinical manifestation or signs of progressive liver disease in this cohort confirms the relatively benign clinical course of HCV infection during childhood and the need to develop approaches for the long-term monitoring of outcomes in these patients.

A recent multicentre study by Gonzalez-Peralta *et al.* evaluated the efficacy of interferon α2b and ribavirin for the treatment of chronic hepatitis C in children |**7**|. The study consisted of Phase 1 and Phase 3 trials. The Phase 1 trial was conducted in two cohorts to establish the safety, efficacy and pharmacokinetics of interferon α2b (3 million IU/m^2 given subcutaneously three times weekly) plus ribavirin (8, 12 or 15 mg/kg/day). In Cohort 2 of Phase 1, 15 mg/kg/day of ribavirin was used. This dose was the optimal ribavirin dose determined from Cohort 1 of the Phase 1 study and comparable acceptable safety profile. In the Phase 3 trial, 3 million IU/m^2 of interferon α2b, given subcutaneously three times a week, and ribavirin 15 mg/kg/day were used. The authors were able to demonstrate a sustained virological response in 46% (54/118) of patients. The frequency of sustained virological response was 37% for HCV genotype 1 compared with 84% for genotype 2 or 3. These results are similar to those seen in adults. Dose modification was required in 31% of the study patients (37/118) and the most common reasons were anaemia and neutropenia. The study shows that combination therapy with interferon α2b and ribavirin is effective and reasonably safe in children. This therapy will probably become the treatment of choice for paediatric HCV, as it is currently in the adult population.

Non-alcoholic fatty liver disease

In both adults and children, NAFLD is an increasingly recognized form of chronic liver disease that can progress to end-stage liver disease [8,9]. NAFLD encompasses a spectrum of conditions associated with over-accumulation of fat in the liver. It ranges from steatosis (simple fatty liver), non-alcoholic steatohepatitis (NASH; fat with signs of hepatocellular injury with or without fibrosis) to advanced fibrosis and cirrhosis. Studies in the adult population suggest that, whereas simple fatty liver seems to be a benign condition, NASH may progress to fibrosis and cirrhosis [10]. NAFLD is strongly associated with obesity and insulin resistance and is currently considered by many as the hepatic component of the metabolic syndrome [11]. The importance of this observation is emphasized by the fact that in the USA and most of the Western world childhood obesity has reached epidemic proportions, which could potentially make NAFLD the most common liver condition in the paediatric population. In this chapter we will review two studies published in 2005 that may have a significant impact on our understanding of paediatric NAFLD.

In the first study, the prevalence of NAFLD in children with type 2 diabetes was examined. Nadeau and co-workers [12] reviewed retrospectively the clinical details of 118 children younger than 18 years of age diagnosed with type 2 diabetes at a paediatric diabetes clinic between 1996 and 2002. Children were excluded if they had a positive history of alcohol consumption, other liver disease (including viral, autoimmune and genetic/metabolic diseases) as well as a history of taking any potential hepatotoxic medications. Aminotransferase measurements were available in about half of the patients. Half of these latter patients were females, and the mean age of the patients was 15 years. Elevation of ALT was found in almost 50% of the patients, 29% (of the entire study group) having an elevation of ALT to more than twice the upper limit of normal. The mean ALT was 69 IU/l (range 8–357 IU/l) and mean aspartate aminotransferase (AST) was 44 IU/l (range 10–214 IU/l). The mean body mass index in these patients was 33 kg/m^2. The prevalence of elevated ALT in males was found to be higher than in females but the difference was not statistically significant. These numbers are significantly higher than those reported for the general paediatric population, in which the prevalence of elevated ALT ranges from 3 to 15% [12,13] and is higher than that in adults with type 2 diabetes [14], suggesting that children with type 2 diabetes may be at particular risk of having NAFLD. One limitation of this study was that liver biopsies were obtained in only three patients (in all three the result was consistent with NASH). Larger prospective studies are needed to validate these results.

The characteristic histological changes in NAFLD range from steatosis to steatohepatitis with or without fibrosis to cirrhosis. The histological features of NAFLD in adults are well described and include steatosis, lobular inflammation, hepatocellular injury, perisinusoidal or pericellular fibrosis, and Mallory hyaline. The pattern of macrovesicular steatosis with ballooning in hepatocytes and/or perisinusoidal fibrosis is considered diagnostic of NASH. In children, standard histological criteria for the diagnosis of NAFLD and NASH are not well established. A study by Schwimmer *et al.* |**15**| examined the liver biopsy findings in a large, well-characterized population of paediatric patients with NAFLD. One hundred children were included in the study. The median age was 12 years (range 2–18) and the median body mass index was 31 kg/m^2. Type 2 diabetes was present in 8% of the children. Almost two-thirds of the patients were male and the patients were predominantly of Hispanic ethnicity. Steatosis was mild in 19%, moderate in 28% and severe in 53%. Portal inflammation was mild in most of the children (70%); portal fibrosis was present in 60% of the patients, with moderate to severe fibrosis in half of these patients. Two histological patterns of steatohepatitis were characterized: type 1, with steatosis, ballooning degeneration and perisinusoidal fibrosis (similar to adult NASH); and type 2, with steatosis, portal inflammation and portal fibrosis. Type 2 NASH was more common (51/100) than type 1 (17/100), with overlap in the remaining cases. Boys were more likely to have type 2 NASH (P <0.01) and less likely than girls to have type 1 NASH. Patients with advanced fibrosis were more likely to have type 2 NASH. The results of this study suggest that NAFLD in children may present with histological characteristics different from those typically seen in adults. Although future studies are still needed, these findings may have significant implications for studies on the pathophysiology, natural history and response to therapy in paediatric NAFLD.

Liver transplantation

Liver transplantation has evolved into definitive treatment for fulminant and end-stage liver disease in children and adults. The development of newer immunosuppressive medications and advances in surgical techniques has made liver transplantation a viable form of treatment. With 5-year survival of paediatric liver transplant patients better than 85%, the long-term morbidity has become an important factor in the management of these children. The long-term issues include maintaining adequate growth and renal function as well as reducing the cardiovascular risks, which are some of the side effects of immunosuppressant medications. Moreover, a shortage of organs for transplantation has arisen as a result of the success of liver transplantation, the expanding indications and the lack of other effective therapeutic modalities. Developments in living related donor transplants may provide a means of reducing the wait for a liver transplant.

The Model for End-stage liver Disease (MELD) was developed for adults to ensure adequate allocation of organs to patients waiting for liver transplantation |**16**|. The Pediatric End-stage liver Disease (PELD) scoring system was created for the same purpose |**17**|. Data from the Studies of Pediatric Liver Transplantation (SPLIT) were used to develop the PELD scoring system. A variety of parameters were tested for their ability to predict either death while awaiting transplantation or the need for transfer to intensive care. The score includes total bilirubin, age

<1 year, international normalized ratio (INR), albumin and growth failure [17]. A recent study by Bourdeaux and colleagues [18] assessed the effect of the PELD score on post-transplant outcome. One hundred paediatric recipients of a primary liver transplant from living related donors ($n = 49$) and post-mortem donors ($n = 51$) were reviewed retrospectively. The PELD score was calculated for all patients at the time of pre-liver transplantation assessment and in the post-mortem donor group also at the time of liver transplantation, allowing the change in PELD score to be determined during the waiting period. There was no significant correlation between higher pre-transplant PELD score and worse patient or graft survival. Of the individual variables affecting the PELD score, a higher bilirubin and growth failure were associated with worse post-transplant patient survival. Also, a higher change in PELD score was found to be associated with poorer post-transplant patient survival, but this did not reach statistical significance. From this study, one could conclude that giving priority to patients with a high PELD score does not appear to result in a worse outcome after liver transplantation and may help to reduce pre-transplantation mortality. These findings will require further analysis in a larger group of patients followed in a prospective manner.

Concerns regarding the impact of the PELD score on organ allocation have recently been raised in the study by Shneider *et al.* [19]. In this study, the authors reviewed their experience with the PELD score from February 2002 to February 2004. They identified 48 patients who received a transplant for various reasons, the most common being biliary atresia ($n = 15$), followed by acute liver failure ($n = 12$). Twenty-five patients were excluded from analysis as the PELD score could not be applied. The reasons for this were several: four patients were above the age of 17 and the MELD score was used, ten had fulminant liver failure, two had a combined liver and kidney transplant, two had early re-transplantation for hepatic artery thrombosis and primary non-function, and one split liver was not allocated to the recipient. In three cases, the primary approach to transplantation was a living donor, and in three cases status 1 was granted by petition for concerns of hepatocellular carcinoma. After exclusion, 23 transplants were considered appropriate to assess the effectiveness of PELD scoring. Four patients were made status 1 because of life-threatening complications of their liver disease. Nineteen children (40% of the total cohort) underwent transplantation based on the PELD score, only two patients undergoing transplantation on the basis of their actual PELD score, while the rest required granting of a waiting list exception. This study brings out some potential major pitfalls of the PELD scoring system. The PELD score could be used in fewer than 10% of eligible candidates. Although these results could have been influenced in part by local variability and the small number of patients in the study, there is indeed an urgent need to further assess the effectiveness of PELD scoring in order to avoid potential unnecessary morbidity and mortality in children.

Renal dysfunction is an unfortunate side effect of calcineurin inhibitors cyclosporin A and tacrolimus in liver transplant recipients, and progression to end-stage renal failure with the requirement for renal replacement therapy may develop [20]. Evans *et al.* [21] looked at the effect of mycophenolate mofetil (MMF) on renal dysfunction in paediatric liver transplant patients being treated with calcineurin inhibitors. In this retrospective study, the authors assessed 48 children (23 males, median age 11) started on MMF for renal dysfunction and followed up for at least 1 year. They demonstrated a significant improvement from the baseline calculated glomerular filtration rate after 2 months on the MMF treatment. The dose of MMF used was 20 mg/kg/day in two divided doses and in a few selected patients the dose was increased to 40 mg/kg/day. Of the 48 patients, 36 were transferred to MMF monotherapy, four were on MMF and steroids and eight on MMF and low-dose cyclosporin A or tacrolimus. Children aged less than 3 years at the time of liver transplantation or who were started on MMF within 5 years of their liver transplant demonstrated the greatest increase in calculated glomerular filtration rate. Four patients did not respond to MMF and progressed to end-stage renal failure within 1 year of treatment. Mild side effects occurred in seven patients. Two patients showed typical features of acute rejection; one of these patients was non-adherent with the transplant medication. Both were treated with pulsed steroids and by increasing the dose of MMF to 40 mg/kg/day. Two patients developed chronic rejection and one of these responded to the reintroduction of low-dose tacrolimus. The other patient, who was reportedly non-adherent to therapy initially, had a more aggressive course and required re-transplantation. Renal dysfunction is an increasingly recognized morbidity in paediatric liver transplant recipients [22]. Paediatric liver transplant recipients receiving calcineurin inhibitor-based immunosuppression need to be monitored for renal dysfunction, preferably by estimating the glomerular filtration rate. Patients with renal dysfunction may be carefully moved to a non-calcineurin immunosuppressant such as MMF and should be monitored for rejection and side effects.

Biliary atresia

Biliary atresia is a progressive cholangiopathy in neonates and it is the most common cause of liver transplantation in children. The overall incidence is about 1 in 14 000 live births. Use of the Kasai portoenterostomy procedure in the first 8 weeks improves survival but liver transplantation before the age of 10 is still required in most patients [23].

Utterson and colleagues of the SPLIT Research Group reported on the clinical profiles, risk factors, and outcomes of a large population of patients with biliary atresia listed for liver transplantation [24]. A total of 755 patients were identified from the SPLIT registry between May 1995 and June 2003. More than 70% of patients were less than 1 year of age and 60% were females. Forty per cent of patients had growth failure, 16% receiving nasogastric feeding. The mean PELD score was 12; most scores were between 10 and 20.

At the time of the last follow-up, 24 (3%) patients had died while awaiting liver transplantation, 164 (22%) were alive without liver transplantation and 567 (75%) had undergone liver transplantation. A total of 81 patients died, one-third while awaiting transplantation, one-third after the first liver transplantation and one-third after re-transplantation. Of 65 patients who received a second transplant, 38% died. The survival rate after transplantation was 88% at 3 years. Multivariate analysis showed that significant risk factors for death on the waiting list included individual PELD components (bilirubin, INR and albumin) and the need for nasogastric/intravenous nutrition. Importantly, race, sex and year of listing were not significant. The most common cause of death after transplantation was infection, either viral or bacterial. Risk factors for death after transplantation included being an infant, lower height and weight *Z*-scores, the use of cyclosporin rather than tacrolimus, and re-transplantation. Significant factors predicting poor graft outcome included lower height and weight *Z*-scores, donor age equal to or lower than 5 months, cadaveric partial donors, the use of cyclosporin, and transplant rejection. The Kasai procedure did not affect post-transplantation mortality or graft survival. To date, this is the largest study describing the outcomes of children with biliary atresia following listing for liver transplantation. Improvement in the management of these children is still clearly needed, as evidenced by a mortality of 10% by 6 months after listing. The study identified several major predictors of poor outcome, both before and after liver transplantation, that may help in providing appropriate referral for liver transplantation and better care after liver transplantation. Future studies are needed to better address the outcomes of specific biliary atresia subtypes and the influence of the Kasai procedure and its timing on the outcome of patients with biliary atresia, as they were not examined in this study.

Conclusion

We have attempted to highlight some of the advances in the field of paediatric hepatology in 2005. The recent advances in our understanding of hepatitis C infection in children will open ways for newer and improved therapeutic strategies for the treatment of this disorder. Children can be at risk of metabolic syndrome, and its connection with NAFLD and NASH and the distinct histological changes of NASH in children are now becoming evident. These are areas that need further exploration. The controversial matter of PELD scoring, especially in the setting of a shortage of donor organs, will have to be evaluated critically. Also, with better survival after liver transplantation, the long-term effects of liver transplantation, such as renal dysfunction, will have to be monitored and studied prospectively. A large study on children with biliary atresia has provided us with a better understanding of the outcome of these patients. Further research in these areas will ensure better treatment and outcome and will help these children transition into a healthy adulthood.

References

1. Tovo PA, Lazier L, Versace A. Hepatitis B virus and hepatitis C virus infections in children. *Curr Opin Infect Dis* 2005; **18**: 261–6.
2. Hui AY, Sung JJ. Advances in chronic viral hepatitis. *Curr Opin Infect Dis* 2005; **18**: 400–6.
3. McHutchison JG, Bartenschlager R, Patel K, Pawlotsky JM. The face of future hepatitis C antiviral drug development: recent biological and virologic advances and their translation to drug development and clinical practice. *J Hepatol* 2006; **44**: 411–21.
4. Mok J, Pembrey L, Tovo PA, Newell ML. When does mother to child transmission of hepatitis C virus occur? *Arch Dis Child Fetal Neonatal Ed* 2005; **90**: F156–60.
5. European Paediatric Hepatitis C Virus Network. Three broad modalities in the natural history of vertically acquired hepatitis C virus infection. *Clin Infect Dis* 2005; **41**: 45–51.
6. Eyster ME, Sanders J, Goedert JJ. Viral clearance occurs very early during the natural resolution of hepatitis C virus infection in persons with haemophilia. *Haemophilia* 2004; **10**: 75–80.
7. Gonzalez-Peralta RP, Kelly DA, Haber B, Molleston J, Murray KF, Jonas MM, Shelton M, Mieli-Vergani G, Lurie Y, Martin S, Lang T, Baczkowski A, Geffner M, Gupta S, Laughlin M. Interferon alfa-2b in combination with ribavirin for the treatment of chronic hepatitis C in children: efficacy, safety, and pharmacokinetics. *Hepatology* 2005; **42**: 1010–18.
8. Angulo P. Non-alcoholic fatty liver disease. *N Engl J Med* 2002; **346**: 1221–31.
9. Wieckowska A, Feldstein AE. Non-alcoholic fatty liver disease in the pediatric population: a review. *Curr Opin Pediatr* 2005; **17**: 636–41.
10. Adams LA, Lymp JF, St Sauver J, Sanderson SO, Lindor KD, Feldstein A, Angulo P. The natural history of non-alcoholic fatty liver disease: a population-based cohort study. *Gastroenterology* 2005; **129**: 113–21.
11. Diehl AM, Clarke J, Brancati F. Insulin resistance syndrome and non-alcoholic fatty liver disease. *Endocr Pract* 2003; **9**(Suppl 2): 93–6.
12. Nadeau KJ, Klingensmith G, Zeitler P. Type 2 diabetes in children is frequently associated with elevated alanine aminotransferase. *J Pediatr Gastroenterol Nutr* 2005; **41**: 94–8.
13. Tominaga K, Kurata JH, Chen YK, Fujimoto E, Miyagawa S, Abe I, Kusano Y. Prevalence of fatty liver in Japanese children and relationship to obesity. An epidemiological ultrasonographic survey. *Dig Dis Sci* 1995; **40**: 2002–9.
14. Gupte P, Amarapurkar D, Agal S, Baijal R, Kulshrestha P, Pramanik S, Patel N, Madan A, Amarapurkar A, Hafeezunnisa. Non-alcoholic steatohepatitis in type 2 diabetes mellitus. *J Gastroenterol Hepatol* 2004; **19**: 854–8.
15. Schwimmer JB, Behling C, Newbury R, Deutsch R, Nievergelt C, Schork NJ, Lavine JE. Histopathology of pediatric non-alcoholic fatty liver disease. *Hepatology* 2005; **42**: 641–9.

16. Kamath PS, Wiesner RH, Malinchoc M, Kremers W, Therneau TM, Kosberg CL, D'Amico G, Dickson ER, Kim WR. A model to predict survival in patients with end-stage liver disease. *Hepatology* 2001; **33**: 464–70.

17. McDiarmid SV, Anand R, Lindblad AS. Development of a pediatric end-stage liver disease score to predict poor outcome in children awaiting liver transplantation. *Transplantation* 2002; **74**: 173–81.

18. Bourdeaux C, Tri TT, Gras J, Sokal E, Otte JB, de Ville de Goyet J, Reding R. PELD score and posttransplant outcome in pediatric liver transplantation: a retrospective study of 100 recipients. *Transplantation* 2005; **79**: 1273–6.

19. Shneider BL, Neimark E, Frankenberg T, Arnott L, Suchy FJ, Emre S. Critical analysis of the pediatric end-stage liver disease scoring system: a single center experience. *Liver Transpl* 2005; **11**: 788–95.

20. Falkenhain ME, Cosio FG, Sedmak DD. Progressive histologic injury in kidneys from heart and liver transplant recipients receiving cyclosporine. *Transplantation* 1996; **62**: 364–70.

21. Evans HM, McKiernan PJ, Kelly DA. Mycophenolate mofetil for renal dysfunction after pediatric liver transplantation. *Transplantation* 2005; **79**: 1575–80.

22. Alonso EM. Long-term renal function in pediatric liver and heart recipients. *Pediatr Transplant* 2004; **8**: 381–5.

23. Sokol RJ, Mack C, Narkewicz MR, Karrer FM. Pathogenesis and outcome of biliary atresia: current concepts. *J Pediatr Gastroenterol Nutr* 2003; **37**: 4–21.

24. Utterson EC, Shepherd RW, Sokol RJ, Bucuvalas J, Magee JC, McDiarmid SV, Anand R. Biliary atresia: clinical profiles, risk factors, and outcomes of 755 patients listed for liver transplantation. *J Pediatr* 2005; **147**: 180–5.

17

Liver transplantation

BIJAN EGHTESAD, JOHN FUNG

Introduction

Since the first successful orthotopic liver transplantation (OLT) reported in 1967 by Starzl [1] the procedure has passed many milestones. Better preservative solutions have improved the quality of organs and advances in immunosuppression have reduced the immune loss of livers. Refinements in surgical techniques in donors and recipients, increased expertise in intensive care, better understanding of the pathophysiology of metabolic disorders, acute liver failure, hepatocellular carcinoma (HCC) and more effective medical treatments for certain diseases, especially for hepatitis B, have shortened the list of contraindications of the procedure. Patient and graft survival have increased from weeks and months to years and decades. With longer survival, the fear of acute rejection has been replaced by worries about graft loss due to chronic rejection and recurrent disease. With more potent immunosuppressive agents, transplant recipients will survive longer to experience the complications associated with the use of these drugs.

Longer survival and better quality of life after OLT have caused more patients with end-stage liver disease to pursue the possibility of transplantation. In addition to the new patients, some survivors of OLT with graft failure are being added to lists for re-transplantation. Unfortunately, the number of candidates for OLT has increased at a much faster pace than the number of organs available, and the growing disparity has resulted in an increasing number of deaths while waiting for transplantation. In other words, liver transplantation has become the victim of its own success.

Today, the attention of the transplant community has changed from the problem of how to perform the transplant to how to better allocate transplantable organs, how to increase the number of organs available for transplantation, how to increase patient and graft survival, and how to prevent long-term complications. In this regard, most programmes have focused their efforts on preventing the recurrence of disease, particularly hepatitis C; on increasing the number of organs available by splitting single livers for two patients; on the use of livers from living donors; on the use of livers from donors selected on the basis of expanded criteria; on xenotransplantation; and on the prevention of the side effects of immunosuppressive drugs by using protective regimens and, more importantly, by extensive efforts to induce tolerance. At a US national level, changing the organ allocation policies from using the Child–Turcotte–Pugh (CTP) classification to a more objective system, the Model for End-stage Liver Disease (MELD), has improved prioritization policies |**2**|.

The number of publications in the field of liver transplantation is expanding rapidly. The articles discussed in this chapter cover a selection of highly popular related topics.

Model for End-stage Liver Disease

Addition of serum sodium into the MELD score predicts waiting list mortality better than MELD alone

Ruf AE, Kremers WK, Chavez LL, Descalzi VI, Podesta LG, Villamil FG. *Liver Transpl* 2005; **11**: 336–43

BACKGROUND. MELD, the new liver allocation system, was implemented in February 2002. The previous allocation system was based primarily on waiting time and subjective clinical parameters, such as ascites and encephalopathy. The new policy was developed using an evidence-driven model that provided more objective measures of mortality related to short-term liver disease. The system was found to be consistent and highly predictive of 3-month mortality. Since the implementation of the new system, fewer inappropriate patients have been placed on the waiting list, and there has been a trend towards reduced waiting list death rates and a statistically significant increase in transplantation rates. While the use of MELD has been a major advancement in liver allocation policy, like any other mathematical model it is not perfect. Recent reports have shown that certain patients, such as those with refractory ascites or a persistently low serum sodium concentration, may have a higher risk of death than predicted by their MELD score. These reports also argued that patients with ascites and encephalopathy have poor quality of life, and the MELD system does not reflect this.

INTERPRETATION. Of 262 patients consecutively listed for liver transplantation, 19 (7%) died, 175 (67%) survived and 68 (26%) underwent liver transplantation during 3 months of follow-up. Hyponatraemia (≤130 mEq/l) was present in 63% of the patients who died, compared with 13% of those who survived (P <0.001), whereas the proportion with elevated creatinine (≥1.4 mg/dl) was low and similar in the two groups. The risk of death across all MELD scores was higher for patients with hyponatraemia than for those without hyponatraemia. Cox regression considering data within 6 months of follow-up yielded quantitatively similar results, hyponatraemia being a significant predictor of a greater risk of death, with an odds ratio of 2.65 (P = 0.015). The authors concluded that hyponatraemia appears to be an earlier and more sensitive marker than creatinine to detect renal impairment and/or circulatory dysfunction in patients with advanced cirrhosis. They also concluded that the addition of serum sodium concentration to MELD can identify patients with a poor outcome in a more efficient way than the use of MELD alone, with a significant increase in the efficacy of the score in predicting waiting list mortality.

MELD fails to measure quality of life in liver transplant candidates

Saab S, Ibrahim AB, Spaner A, *et al. Liver Transpl* 2005; **11**: 218–23

BACKGROUND. The goal of this study was to evaluate the relationship between MELD score and quality of life and to compare MELD with CTP class and impaired quality of life. Quality of life questionnaires (Medical Outcome Short Form 36; SF-36) and the Chronic Liver Disease Questionnaire (CLDQ) were administered to 150 adult patients awaiting liver transplantation. Demographic data, laboratory results and recorded manifestations of hepatic decompensation in this cohort of patients were also collected.

INTERPRETATION. The scores found that both ascites and encephalopathy were predictive of quality of life when using the CLDQ. From these findings the authors concluded that, in liver transplant candidates, the severity of liver disease assessed by the MELD score was not predictive of quality of life. The presence of ascites and/or encephalopathy was significantly associated with a poor quality of life, and the CTP class correlated better with quality of life, probably because it includes ascites and encephalopathy.

Comment

The old liver allocation system was based primarily on waiting time, subjective clinical parameters such as ascites and encephalopathy, and the location of the patient (intensive care unit, hospital or home). This system had caused widespread dissatisfaction because it was not standardized and was subject to manipulation. The MELD model is based on three simple biochemical variables (creatinine and bilirubin concentrations and the international normalized ratio) which are readily available, highly reproducible, and inexpensive **|2|**. The system is consistent across diverse aetiologies of chronic liver disease and is fairly independent of the complications of end-stage liver disease, such as ascites, portosystemic encephalopathy, spontaneous bacterial peritonitis and variceal bleeding. It correlates well with other liver function tests and is a better predictor of short-term survival compared with the CTP score.

The presence of hyponatraemia in cirrhotic patients has always carried a poor prognosis, with difficulties in management, repeated episodes of hospitalization, neurological complications and increased mortality rates among this group of patients. In this study by Saab and colleagues, hyponatraemia showed the ability to identify a subgroup of high-risk patients who died with lower MELD scores. Thus, the incorporation of serum sodium concentration in the MELD formula can significantly increase the predictability of the short-term waiting list mortality rate.

Unlike other clinical parameters, serum sodium concentration is a laboratory value that is objective and readily available. If further prospective clinical studies confirm that hyponatraemia will improve the prediction of survival in patients with ascites, serum sodium could be added to the allocation system.

In liver transplantation, as in many other interventions in medicine, health-related quality of life has become an important parameter. Patients with end-stage liver disease have to endure a long time on the waiting list in the hope of transplantation. Many of these patients are suffering from major complications of cirrhosis and portal hypertension. Unlike the old CTP scoring system, the new MELD policy for liver allocation does not consider the complications of decompensated liver disease, such as ascites and encephalopathy, which are more or less subjective and amenable to diverse interpretations. On the basis of earlier studies, these parameters have not been shown to increase the predictive ability of the MELD system for the 3-month mortality end-point. The main matter of controversy in the transplant community has been the question of whether patients with intractable ascites and encephalopathy with poor quality of life but a low MELD score and a potentially lower risk of short-term mortality should be awarded a better chance to advance up the waiting list and receive earlier transplantation. Unfortunately, as long as the transplant community faces a severe organ shortage there is another legitimate question: should the chance to improve the quality of life take precedence over the chance to save life?

Hepatocellular carcinoma and liver transplantation

The impact of pre-operative loco-regional therapy on outcome after liver transplantation for hepatocellular carcinoma

Yao FY, Kinkhabwala M, LaBerge JM, *et al. Am J Transpl* 2005; **5**: 795–804

A prospective study on downstaging of hepatocellular carcinoma prior to liver transplantation

Yao FY, Hirose R, LaBerge JM, *et al. Liver Transpl* 2005; **11**: 1505–14

Background. While loco-regional therapies for HCC are associated with a significant risk of recurrence of tumour progression with longer follow-up, the effectiveness of these treatments in inducing tumour necrosis and providing temporary control of the spread of the tumour makes them ideal bridging procedures to OLT [3,4]. This is an important consideration as the waiting time for OLT has increased in recent years, leading to a greater risk of tumour progression, exceeding

the acceptable HCC criteria for OLT. This has prompted transplant centres to consider the same intervention to reduce the tumour to a size that would lie within conventional criteria for OLT or for facilitating resection.

INTERPRETATION. The first study is a subgroup analysis of 168 patients who underwent OLT for HCC to test the hypothesis that pre-operative loco-regional therapy confers a survival advantage in a subgroup of patients who are at intermediate risk of recurrence of HCC. Patients with pathological T3 HCC meeting the proposed University of California, San Francisco, expanded criteria (a single lesion not exceeding 6.5 cm or two or three lesions, none more than 4.5 cm, with total tumour diameter less than 8 cm) had a 5-year recurrence-free survival rate similar to that of patients with T2 HCC (88.5 vs 93.8%; $P = 0.56$). In the subgroup with pathological T2 or T3 HCC, the 5-year recurrence-free survival was 93.8% for the 85 patients who received pre-operative loco-regional therapy, versus 80.6% for the other 41 patients without treatment ($P = 0.049$). The treatment benefit, according to 5-year survival, appeared greater for pathological patients with T3 (85.9 vs 51.4%; $P = 0.05$) than for patients with T2 HCC (96.4 vs 87.1%; $P = 0.12$).

The second study is a prospective evaluation of the feasibility and outcome of loco-regional therapy intended for HCC downstaging to meet T2 criteria for OLT. Among 30 patients enrolled, 21 (70%) met criteria for successful downstaging, including 16 patients (53%) who subsequently received OLT, and nine patients (30%) were classified as treatment failures. In the explants of the 16 patients who underwent OLT, seven had complete tumour necrosis and seven met T2 criteria, but two exceeded T2 criteria. No recurrence of HCC was observed after a median follow-up of 16 months after OLT.

Comment

HCC is one of the most common solid organ cancers in the world. In the absence of effective chemotherapy or radiation therapy for HCC, surgery is considered the treatment of choice, and has the potential to cure. Because of the nature of the disease, and often the rapid growth of the tumour, most of the patients present in an advanced stage of the disease, so that fewer than 20% of them fulfil the criteria for resection |**5**|. Additionally, most cases of HCC occur in patients with underlying cirrhosis and there is a high chance of hepatic dysfunction after a major resection and a higher rate of tumour recurrence in the cirrhotic liver remnant. OLT offers the advantages of both eradication of the tumour and treating the underlying liver disease. In a study by Llovet *et al.* |**6**|, due to the limited donor organ availability, patients with HCC had to stay on the waiting list for a long time, with a yearly dropout rate of 30–40% because of the progress of the disease and no survival benefit after liver transplantation. With the new organ allocation rules under the MELD system and on the basis of the excellent results published by Mazzaferro *et al.* (Milan criteria: single tumour ≤5 cm or three nodules ≤3 cm each), patients with T2 HCC receive priority for organ allocation and expedited liver transplantation |**7**|.

Despite the adoption of the new rules and earlier transplantation, the continued shortage of organs means that many patients still do not get the chance of timely

OLT. It has been suggested that patients with untreated HCC may not benefit from OLT if their time on the waiting list is longer than 10 months [8].

With improved results gained from transplantation in patients with earlier stages of HCC, transplant programmes have focused on salvage protocols to prevent further growth of tumours in patients already on the waiting list, and to reduce the size of tumours in patients not fulfilling the criteria for listing in order to make them eligible for transplantation.

Loco-regional ablative therapies have been used as bridging modalities in patients with HCC, with the goals of minimizing the number of dropouts on the waiting list, reducing the post-transplant recurrence rate and reducing the size of some of the borderline tumours to make them eligible for transplantation [9]. The most frequently used modalities are transarterial chemoembolization (TACE) and percutaneous or laparoscopic ablation methods.

HCC is a highly vascularized tumour, receiving most of its blood supply from arterial neovascularization. Chemoembolization takes advantage of the arterial blood flow to the tumour and involves selective intra-arterial injection of the chemotherapeutic agent into the tumour region followed by embolization and occlusion of the arterial supply to the involved segment of the liver without jeopardizing the rest of the functional liver parenchyma. The effectiveness of the procedure was under question until a recently reported randomized, controlled trial from Barcelona showed improved patient survival [10].

The use of TACE in the pre-OLT period in patients with HCC has given relatively good results [7,11]. In a study by Sotriopoulos *et al.*, post-operative evaluation of liver explants from 21 patients showed regression in the size of tumours in 52% of patients and complete tumour necrosis in 24% of patients [11]. The procedure is well tolerated but has certain complications, including pain, fever, abscess formation and deterioration of liver function.

Ablative methods, such as percutaneous ethanol injection and percutaneous or laparoscopic radiofrequency ablation (RFA), are other ways to destroy tumour cells or reduce tumour size. Both procedures have their effect by inducing coagulative necrosis with alcohol or with heat generated by radiofrequency waves. In one study by Mazzaferro *et al.*, 50 patients with HCC underwent RFA before transplantation (mean interval 9 months). Evaluation of the explanted liver showed complete necrosis in 55% of the tumours. A tumour size of less than 3 cm was the most important factor in the achievement of complete ablation. Complications of the procedure include biliary injury and strictures, liver failure and peritonitis [12].

With increasing numbers of patients with HCC needing OLT in the MELD era, more efforts are being made to try to make these patients suitable for transplantation. Use of these loco-regional therapeutic measures alone or in combination has been promising, but because of controversial reports more randomized controlled trials to evaluate their benefits are needed.

HCV and liver transplantation

Liver transplantation and hepatitis C virus: systemic review of antiviral therapy

Triantos C, Samonakis D, Stigliano R, Thalheimer U, Patch D, Burroughs A. *Transplantation* 2005; **79**: 261–8

BACKGROUND. Post-transplantation recurrence of hepatitis C virus (HCV) infection is a universal phenomenon with a highly variable natural history. Approximately 40% of liver recipients may develop hepatic decompensation within 1 year, and 10–25% will develop cirrhosis within 5 years after transplantation [13,14]. Factors associated with recurrence include donor and recipient age, recipient gender and race, the use of strong antilymphocyte induction therapy, and high doses of corticosteroids. No single factor has been uniformly shown to be the strongest predictor of outcome. There is no consensus about the time to initiate antiviral therapy, the duration of therapy or the dosage. The current frequency of sustained virological response after treatment with a combination of pegylated interferon and ribavirin is approximately 25%.

INTERPRETATION. This review article presents both viral and histological responses to antiviral therapy in patients receiving liver transplantation for HCV infection. It covers the three areas of pre-transplantation therapy (five studies, 180 patients), pre-emptive therapy soon after transplantation (ten studies, 417 patients), and therapy for established disease (75 studies, 2027 patients). The authors found significant rates of dose reduction and drug stoppage in these patients. They also noted conflicting data on histological improvement and the risk of rejection with therapy. They concluded that the present antiviral therapy is neither easily used nor reasonably effective. The best treatment strategy could be pre-transplantation treatment, probably with newer drugs.

Comment

Recurrent HCV infection, as defined by detectable HCV RNA in serum, is an almost universal phenomenon. A recent study of post-transplant HCV kinetics showed that the first round of infection probably occurs during reperfusion of the new graft. The viral load then tends to increase over time and reaches 10- to 100-fold greater than pre-transplant levels at 1–3 months [**15–17**].

The course of the disease is highly variable after OLT. Histological progression of chronic hepatitis C is more aggressive and is associated with lower patient and graft survival when compared with non-HCV liver recipients [**15,18,19**]. In a study based on data from the United Network for Organ Sharing (UNOS), Forman *et al.* identified an increased rate of death (hazard ratio 1.23) and graft loss (hazard ratio 1.30) 1, 3 and 5 years after OLT for HCV-positive recipients compared with HCV-negative recipients [**20**]. The mechanism by which this injury is mediated is not well understood. Moreover, there are few data pertaining to the interrelation between the alloimmune response and the anti-HCV response in the state of immunosuppression. The lack of understanding of these associations makes it difficult to design guidelines for immunosuppression or the institution of antiviral therapy.

Based on the experience with OLT in hepatitis B infection and the use of pre-transplant antiviral treatment to lower the viral load and the use of hepatitis B immunoglobulin therapy at the time of transplantation, several groups have studied the possibility of using pooled serum from patients with demonstrated HCV clearance (hepatitis C immunoglobulin) |**21**|. Limited data are available regarding the efficacy of this treatment modality. Unfortunately, there are some limitations in the use of interferon and ribavirin in the pre-transplantation period. Patients with severe hypersplenism and low platelet and white blood cell counts and also patients with advanced liver disease (Child class C) cannot tolerate treatment. Most of the studies designed for pre-OLT antiviral therapy showed very high rates of adverse effects and patient dropout. Thus, interferon and ribavirin in the pre-OLT period may only be reliably used in cirrhotic patients with Child class A or B.

It has been shown that interferon is more effective in patients with lower viral loads. On this assumption, several programmes have used pre-emptive therapy protocols to prevent the recurrence of HCV after OLT. This is the time when the viral load is at its lowest. Unfortunately, interferon therapy in the first 14 days after OLT is difficult to start because of thrombocytopenia, leucopenia and the potential for bacterial infections, and renal dysfunction. There is also a theoretical risk of increasing cellular rejection. Several studies have shown some decrease in fibrosis and improvement in histology. However, it is not clear whether the responders were patients who might have had a less severe course of infection. Only randomized trials can address this issue and its cost-effectiveness.

Results of antiviral therapy in recurrent HCV after OLT have not been quite convincing either. There is a range of reports showing no response to histological improvement. Unfortunately, there is no standard time course for treatment, dosages, and modes of follow-up. It seems that only prolonged treatment and histological follow-up can evaluate whether fibrosis progression is halted after post-OLT treatment of recurrent HCV. Probably the most effective strategy will be to render patients negative for HCV RNA by PCR before transplantation, but better tolerated and more effective antiviral agents are needed to achieve this goal.

Fulminant hepatic failure

Cerebral hemodynamics and metabolic profiles in fulminant hepatic failure: Relationship to outcome

Aggarwal S, Obrist W, Yonas H, *et al. Liver Transpl* 2005; **11**: 1353–60

Blood lactate but not serum phosphate levels can predict outcome in fulminant hepatic failure

Macquillan GC, Seyam MS, Nightingale P, Neuberger JM, Murphy N. *Liver Transpl* 2005; **11**: 1073–9

BACKGROUND. Fulminant hepatic failure (FHF) is a rare disorder with devastating consequences. It is estimated that 2300–2800 cases occur each year in the USA. The mortality rate of the disorder is high and FHF accounts for 7% of liver transplants among adults |22|. Before the advent of liver transplantation, the reported mortality was more than 80%. With better understanding of the pathophysiology of the disease, advances in intensive care, better understanding of prognostic criteria and particularly the application of liver transplantation, the survival rate of these patients has improved significantly.

INTERPRETATION. These two articles focus on the use of additional clinical and biochemical parameters to identify patients with FHF who are at risk of dying without liver transplantation. The first article focuses on the correlations of (i) cerebral blood flow (CBF) and (ii) cerebral metabolic rate for oxygen and the adequacy of the oxygen supply to the brain. According to the authors' hypothesis, cerebral haemodynamic and metabolic changes undergo five sequential phases: phase 1, normal CBF and normal intracranial pressure (ICP); phase 2, high CBF and normal ICP; phase 3, high CBF and high ICP; phase 4, low CBF and high ICP; and phase 5, brain death. This model assumes that the changes in CBF precede and contribute to elevated ICP and brain swelling. Of the 26 patients studied, eight underwent OLT and all survived, including six with elevated ICPs. Of the 18 patients receiving medical treatment only, all seven with elevated ICP died, in contrast to nine survivors whose ICP remained normal. Of the six patients who died with brain death, all showed intracranial hypertension preceded by hyperaemia.

The second study is a retrospective analysis of 83 patients with FHF. Fifty-eight per cent survived with medical management, 23% underwent OLT and 19% died without a transplant. Survivors with medical management were younger, were more likely to have acetaminophen-induced hepatotoxicity, and had significantly lower serum bilirubin levels on admission. Although serum phosphate levels were significantly higher in non-survivors, this difference was mainly attributed to those who underwent transplantation. Arterial blood lactate levels were significantly lower among survivors compared with non-survivors. On multivariate analysis, the 12-h arterial blood lactate level was the only significant predictor of survival among patients with acetaminophen-induced hepatotoxicity and among patients without acetaminophen-induced hepatotoxicity after exclusion of patients who had undergone OLT.

Comment

The critical decision of when to perform OLT requires knowledge of accurate and sensitive prognostic factors for determining the likelihood of spontaneous recovery. Among the various prognostic criteria proposed, the King's College criteria have been widely accepted as a means of identifying patients with poor prognosis |**23**|.

However, the sensitivity of these criteria is limited because of their inability to identify a significant proportion of patients who will not survive without liver transplantation.

Timing is critical for successful transplantation; if OLT is performed too early it may not have been necessary, but if it is performed too late the patient with FHF may have already developed severe neurological damage or a life-threatening infection. Highly visible and professionally damaging error will lie in wait for the physician or surgeon who delays operation until a patient who might have been saved by transplantation has lost the chance. In contrast, the error of operating on patients who would have recovered spontaneously is seldom discovered and rarely proven.

It is crucial that an early decision is taken regarding liver transplantation in patients with FHF before the patient develops life-threatening complications of worsening cerebral oedema and multi-organ failure. The window for decision-making is thus short compared with the window for the majority of patients in need of a liver allograft. For the multidisciplinary team, faster evaluation of the patient and rapid decision-making based on a prognostic system of high diagnostic accuracy that can predict the outcome early in the clinical course is of prime importance. Such a system would not only help identify patients in need of emergency transplantation but would also ascertain spontaneous survivors, who would thus be spared a major procedure and lifelong immunosuppression.

Living donor liver transplantation

Outcomes of 385 adult-to-adult living donor liver transplant recipients: a report from A2ALL consortium

Olthoff KM, Merion RM, Ghobrial RM, *et al.*; A2ALL Study Group. *Ann Surg* 2005; **242**: 314–25

BACKGROUND. Adult living donor liver transplantation (ALDLT) has gained significant popularity during the last few years because the waiting list for deceased donor transplants has increased very rapidly. Unlike living donor transplantation for the paediatric population, a clear advantage of ALDLT over transplantation of the liver from a deceased donor has not been demonstrated. The liver transplantation procedure is a technically complex operation and the application of living donation to the adult recipient population has added more difficulty to the procedure. The operation requires a major hepatic resection in a healthy individual to obtain an adequate graft. Recent reports using national data from the Scientific Registry of Transplant Recipients (SRTR) demonstrate a worse outcome of right lobe grafts compared with whole grafts from deceased donors, but detailed data regarding many donor and recipient variables that may contribute to this outcome were not available [24,25]. Most of the reports were from single centres with different approaches to the presentation of the data,

which made it difficult to evaluate the real outcome. Therefore, the National Institutes of Health (NIH) organized a consortium of nine liver transplantation centres with experience in ALDLT in order to accrue and follow a sufficient number of patients undergoing right-lobe ALDLT to be able to collect adequate unified data for better outcome analysis.

INTERPRETATION. This report analyses detailed recipient outcomes of a US multicentre experience of 385 right-lobe ALDLT grafts between 1998 and 2003. The mean age of the recipients was 49 ± 11 years, and 59% were male. The most common diagnosis was hepatitis C (46%), followed by cholestatic liver disease (18%) and alcoholic cirrhosis (11%). HCC was the diagnosis in 16% and fulminant liver failure in another 4%. The mean MELD score at the time of transplantation was 15.6 ± 6.9 (range 6–40), 21% of patients having a MELD score of 6–10 and only 4% having a score greater than 30. Forty-one recipients (11%) were hospitalized at the time of transplantation. There were 42 deaths in the first year after transplantation and the patient survival rate was 94% at 90 days and 89% at 1 year. Survival with the original functioning graft was 87% at 90 days and 81% at 1 year. Infection and sepsis accounted for the largest numbers of deaths. There were 72 graft failures in the first year, of which 71% happened in the first 90 days. Hepatic artery and portal vein thrombosis were the major causes of graft failure ($n = 19$) and primary graft non-function was reported in twelve patients. Thirty-seven patients were re-transplanted (86% in the first 90 days), of whom seven died. Biliary complications were the most common technical problem; they were seen as biliary leaks in 30% and strictures in 8% of patients. Of 35 variables that were tested, three were associated with a significant independent risk of graft failure (re-transplantation or death): the recipient's age, cold ischaemia time, and the centre's experience.

Comment

Many studies have reported equivalent recipient results with living donor versus deceased donor liver transplantation in adult recipients. Short-term survival rates (90 days) are generally between 86 and 88% for both groups. In ALDLT, most centres in the USA and Europe use grafts from the right hepatic lobes because of their ability to fulfil the functional requirements of the adult recipient and avoid the negative impact of small-for-size syndrome (in consideration of donor safety, adequate graft size should correspond to 40–50% of the recipient's own liver volume).

The outcome of a segmental liver graft is influenced not only by its volume but also by technical complications |**26**|. The principal surgical challenges of this procedure, in addition to determining the graft size, include the optimization of vascular inflow, venous outflow and biliary drainage. This includes an appreciation of anatomical variations that may necessitate complex biliary or vascular reconstructions.

The analysis of patient and graft survival in this report is similar to that in reports from Europe and Asia. Broelsch *et al.* summarized the experience on 123 ALDLTs from eleven centres in Europe. Recipient and graft survival were 86 and

83% respectively [27]. Transplant programmes in Japan, Hong Kong and Korea and some other Asian programmes have reported survival rates of 85–90% in their patient populations [28,29].

This is the first report from the NIH-sponsored consortium of transplant programmes on ALDLT. The consortium is charged with addressing many issues by both retrospective data analysis from the centres that are involved and prospective cohort studies. Answering questions such as the impact of hepatitis C, HCC and optimal graft size in ALDLT and the standardization of reporting complications and outcomes are among the many tasks for this consortium to allow the successful and safe implementation of ALDLT in the future.

Renal function in liver transplantation

Renal histopathological lesions after orthotopic liver transplantation

Pillebout E, Nochy GH, Conti F, *et al. Am J Transpl* 2005; **5**: 1120–9

BACKGROUND. Renal dysfunction (acute or chronic) occurs in 17–95% of patients after OLT. The wide range of incidence reported may be due to the wide disparity in the criteria used to define renal failure as well as differences in the duration of follow-up. The commonly occurring aetiologies in this circumstance include acute tubular necrosis secondary to ischaemic or toxic insult to the kidneys, pre-existing hepatorenal syndrome (HRS) or renal insufficiency, diabetes mellitus, drug-induced interstitial nephritis and calcineurin inhibitor nephrotoxicity. The requirement for dialysis in the pre- and/or post-transplantation period, hepatitis C infection and age have also been variably shown to be associated with an increased risk of the development of chronic kidney disease [30–32].

INTERPRETATION. Kidney biopsies from 26 OLT recipients with chronic renal failure (CRF) were evaluated. Before transplantation, five patients had CRF, eight had diabetes and another nine were hypertensive. Renal biopsies were done at a mean of 5 years after liver transplantation. At this time twelve patients were diabetic and 25 hypertensive. Histological findings revealed significant renal destruction, with a mean of 45% interstitial fibrosis and 45% glomerular sclerosis. All biopsies showed severe arteriosclerosis. On the basis of these findings CRF was attributed to four associated primary lesions: (1) specific chronic cyclosporin A/tacrolimus (CyA/TAC) arteriopathy; (2) atypical diabetic nephropathy; (3) acute or chronic thrombotic microangiopathy attributed to CyA/TAC or α-interferon; and (4) tubular changes related to the administration of hydroxyethyl starch. At the end of the follow-up, after a mean of 6.4 years, twelve patients required dialysis and 13 had CRF; only one had normal renal function. The authors concluded that CRF in OLT recipients is more complex than originally thought and should not be classified as anti-calcineurin nephrotoxicity without further investigations, including renal histology. These investigations have therapeutic potential; that is, they may lead to more aggressive treatment of hypertension and/or diabetes.

Comment

The high incidence of CRF after liver transplantation and its multifactorial aetiology is not appreciated by the transplantation community. The cumulative incidence of severe CRF reaches 13.9% after a median follow-up of 36 months [33]. The incidence of less severe forms of renal dysfunction is probably many times higher than this estimate. The risk factors for the development of CRF after extrarenal transplantation include age, male sex, diabetes mellitus, hepatitis C infection and the presence of renal disease before transplantation. Patients with advanced liver disease can develop HRS, which is characterized by acute renal failure in the absence of pathological changes in the kidney. It has been more and more noticeable that these patients are also at increased risk of progressing to chronic renal failure after OLT.

Tacrolimus and cyclosporin A are the mainstay of immunosuppression in most transplant centres. It is customary to attribute post-transplant renal dysfunction to these agents. This study is important in that it highlights the multifactorial nature of renal dysfunction after OLT. Indeed, many patients with end-stage liver disease may have pre-existing renal problems. These problems can be overlooked because of a low serum creatinine level secondary to decreased muscle mass. Careful evaluation of these patients is important. If significant pre-existing renal dysfunction is found, the possibility of combined liver and kidney transplantation may need to be considered.

Renal function after orthotopic liver transplantation is predicted by duration of pre-transplantation creatinine elevation

Campbell MS, Kotlyar DS, Brensinger CM, *et al. Liver Transpl* 2005; **11**: 1048–55

BACKGROUND. Renal failure in patients with liver disease can be secondary to HRS, and other processes that can cause dysfunction in both liver and kidney, such as hepatitis C and B. The key to determining the need for renal replacement therapy following OLT, and thus the need for kidney transplantation, is the ability to predict the irreversibility of renal dysfunction or the progressive nature of the primary renal disease.

INTERPRETATION. A retrospective study of 69 OLT patients with a pre-transplant creatinine level of ≥1.5 mg/dl was performed. Fifty-three patients received liver transplantation alone and 13 combined kidney and liver transplantation. The authors evaluated the presence of HRS, the creatinine level, the MELD score, the albumin level, age, gender, the cause of liver disease, diabetes mellitus, hypertension, history of ascites, spontaneous bacterial peritonitis, variceal bleeding, hepatic encephalopathy, dialysis, and transjugular intrahepatic portosystemic shunting. After evaluation of all the potential variables in univariate and multivariable models, the authors concluded that the duration, but not the cause, of renal dysfunction predicts renal outcome in patients receiving only a liver transplant.

Comment

Patients with renal failure due to acute injury or the HRS have classically not been included as candidates for combined liver and kidney transplantation because of the reversibility of the renal dysfunction following OLT. However, the rate and duration of renal failure prior to OLT continues to be prolonged even with the new allocation system. Previous studies of HRS have emphasized its reversibility after OLT. However, most of these patients received their transplant after a short waiting period, and even then 5–9% progressed to end-stage renal disease over time [34]. The decision-making process for dual transplantation can be difficult and has been hampered by the lack of standardized evaluation and selection approach, the HRS, and the increasing illness severity of those undergoing OLT.

The findings of this study suggest that a prolonged period of HRS can have a large impact on kidney function and prevents full recovery. This gives the transplant programmes one more parameter to use in evaluating the need for combined transplantation. Unfortunately, there is no absolute cut-off time to use in selecting patients for combined transplantation.

Careful assessment of patients, knowledge of the cause of renal dysfunction and, if possible, obtaining a renal biopsy are helpful in decision-making, assessing the recoverability of the kidney and offering appropriate treatment to these patients. Caution should be used in selecting patients for these combined procedures to make certain that the available organs are used appropriately.

HIV and liver transplantation

Liver transplantation in patients with HIV infection

Fung J, Eghtesad B, Patel-Tom K, DeVera M, Chapman H, Ragni M. *Liver Transpl* 2004; **10**(Suppl 2): S39–S53

Pre-transplant survival is shorter in HIV-positive than HIV-negative subjects with end-stage liver disease

Ragni MV, Eghtesad B, Schlesinger KW, Dvorchik I, Fung JJ. *Liver Transpl* 2005; **11**: 1425–30

BACKGROUND. Human immunodeficiency virus (HIV) infection is associated with a spectrum of clinical conditions ranging from no symptoms to acquired immune deficiency syndrome (AIDS). Highly active antiretroviral therapy (HAART) has changed the course of the disease from an ultimately fatal illness to a more chronic disease in HIV-positive patients. Unfortunately, end-stage liver disease has become the leading cause of death in this group of patients. This is mainly due to the high rate of co-infection with chronic viral hepatitis B and hepatitis C. In several reports deaths due to end-stage liver disease have increased impressively from 11% in the early days to 50% in recent years [35]. Many transplant programmes around the world and also NIH have become interested in the analysis of outcomes of liver transplantation in this group of patients.

INTERPRETATION. In these two papers, the authors present the outcome of liver transplantation in HIV-positive patients from several large series, and discuss the criteria of eligibility for liver transplantation and the causes of morbidity and mortality in these patients while on the waiting list.

Comment

As a result of the increasing number of HIV-positive patients with liver failure, the increasing demand for liver transplantation in these patients and the better survival rate associated with HAART, a number of transplant programmes have proceeded with liver transplantation in selected patients with well-controlled HIV. Reported results of these programmes suggest that patient and graft survival rates are similar to those in HIV-negative recipients. In one report based on 19 patients receiving transplants in the HAART era, the overall patient survival rate was 79% with a median follow-up of 314 days; this was similar to the figure for non-HIV-positive liver transplant recipients, who had a 1-year survival rate of 88% [36]. The largest single-centre series comes from the University of Pittsburgh. A total of 29 HIV-positive patients with end-stage liver disease have received liver allografts and no other allografts since 1997. Overall, 89% were co-infected with HCV and 7% with hepatitis B virus, and the rest (4%) had fulminant liver failure. The 1-year survival rate of those who survived more than 30 days after transplantation was 89% and overall survival during 7 years of follow-up was 77%. The criteria for listing for liver transplantation in this group of patients were: (i) the demonstration of a good response to HAART with documentation of an undetectable viral load while on therapy; (ii) a CD4 count of more than 200; and (iii) the absence of opportunistic infections. Unfortunately, co-infected HIV-positive patients have shown much faster progression to end-stage liver disease and more rapid demise. Of 58 patients listed for liver transplantation, 15 (26%) received a transplant, whereas 21 (36%) died before transplantation, 57% of these dying from infection. This was in contrast to a waiting list mortality rate of only 15% in 1359 HIV-negative candidates. The cumulative survival period following initial evaluation was significantly shorter among HIV-positive than HIV-negative candidates (880 vs 1427 days; $P = 0.035$). Interestingly, these two groups of patients were in similar condition at the time of listing (similar MELD score, total bilirubin, creatinine and international normalized ratio).

These findings stress the importance of earlier referral of HIV-positive patients with end-stage liver disease to be evaluated for transplantation.

These reports and many smaller ones in the literature are indicative of the effectiveness of liver transplantation in HIV-positive patients with end-stage liver disease.

Conclusion

Thomas E Starzl, in an article entitled Evolution of Liver Transplantation, concluded with the following statement: '*what was inconceivable yesterday, and barely achievable today, often becomes routine tomorrow*' [37]. Liver transplantation has proved to be a prime example.

In the period reviewed, the field of liver transplantation has continued to advance. To overcome the impact of organ shortage, more attention was paid to the improvement of organ allocation, decreasing the death rate on the waiting list, and expanding the donor pool by innovative techniques such as the use of organs from live donors, better organ preservation and the use of organs from more marginal donors. Extensive effort in the prevention of disease recurrence in the transplanted livers continued. Newer immunosuppressive drugs and better protocols continued to change the pattern of rejection and to reduce the long-term complications of these agents, and, as a result, to increase patient and graft survival and improve quality of life. Xenotransplantation continued to progress and efforts to induce tolerance after organ transplantation had promising results.

References

1. Starzl TE, von Kaulla KN, Hermann G, Brittain RS, Waddel WR. Homotransplantation of the liver in humans. *Surg Gynecol Obstet* 1963; **117**: 659–76.

2. Weisner RH, McDiarmid SV, Kamath PS, Edwards EB, Malinchoc M, Kremer WK, Krom RAF, Kim WR. MELD and PELD: application of survival model to liver allocation. *Liver Transpl* 2001; **7**: 567–80.
3. Bruix J, Sherman M, Llovet JM. Clinical management of hepatocellular carcinoma; conclusions of the Barcelona-2000 EASL conference. *J Hepatol* 2001; **35**: 421–30.
4. Harnois DM, Steers J, Andrews JC. Pre-operative hepatic artery chemoembolization followed by orthotopic liver transplantation for hepatocellular carcinoma. *Liver Transpl Surg* 1999; **5**: 192–9.
5. Bismuth H, Majno PE, Adam R. Liver transplantation for hepatocellular carcinoma. *Semin Liver Dis* 1999; **19**: 311–22.
6. Llovet JM, Mas X, Apontte JJ. Cost-effectiveness of adjuvant therapy for hepatocellular carcinoma during the waiting time for liver transplantation. *Gut* 2002; **50**: 123–8.
7. Mazzaferro V, Regalia E, Doci R. Liver transplantation for the treatment of small hepatocellular carcinomas in patients with cirrhosis. *N Engl J Med* 1996; **334**: 693–9.
8. Sarasin FP, Majno PE, Llovet JM, Bruix J, Mentha G, Hadengue A. living donor liver transplantation for early hepatocellular carcinoma: a life-expectancy and cost-effectiveness perspective. *Hepatology* 2001; **33**: 1073–9.
9. Llovet JM, Fuster J, Bruix J. Intention-to-treat analysis of surgical treatment for early hepatocellular carcinoma: resection versus transplantation. *Hepatology* 1999; **30**: 1434–40.
10. Llovet J, Real MI, Montana X, Planas R, Coll S. Aponte J, Ayuso C, Sala M, Muchart J, Sola R, Rodes J, Bruix J; Barcelona Liver Cancer Group. Arterial embolisation or chemoembolisation versus symptomatic treatment in patients with unresectable hepatocellular carcinoma: a randomised controlled trial. *Lancet* 2002; **359**: 1734–9.
11. Sotiropoulos G, Malago M, Molmenti E, Paul A, Nadalin S, Brokalaki E. Efficacy of transarterial chemoembolization prior to liver transplantation for hepatocellular carcinoma as found in pathology. *Hepatogastroenterology* 2005; **62**: 329–32.
12. Mazzaferro V, Battiston C, Perrone S, Pulvirenti S, Regalia E, Romito R. Radiofrequency ablation of small hepatocellular carcinoma in cirrhotic patients awaiting liver transplantation: a prospective study. *Ann Surg* 2004; **240**: 900–9.
13. Everhart JE, Wei Y, Eng H, Charlton MR, Persing DH, Weisner RH. Recurrent and new hepatitis C virus infection after liver transplantation. *Hepatology* 1999; **29**: 1220–6.
14. Rosen HR, O'Reilly PM, Shackleton CR. Graft loss following liver transplantation in patients with chronic hepatitis C. *Transplantation* 1996; **62**: 1773–6.
15. Gane EJ, Naoumov NV, Qian KP, Mondelli MU, Maertens G, Portmann BC. A longitudinal analysis of hepatitis virus replication following liver transplantation. *Gastroenterology* 1996; **110**: 167–77.
16. Garcia-Retortillo M, Forns X, Feliu A, Moitinho E, Costa J, Navasa M. Hepatitis C virus kinetics during and immediately after liver transplantation. *Hepatology* 2002; **35**: 680–7.
17. Sreekumar R, Gonzales-Koch A, Maor-Kendler Y, Batts K, Moreno-Luna L, Poterucha J. Early identification of recipients with progressive histologic recurrence of hepatitis C after liver transplantation. *Hepatology* 2000; **32**: 1125–30.

18. Pelletier SJ, Lezzoni JC, Crabtree TD, Hahn YS, Sawyer RG, Pruett TL. Prediction of liver allograft fibrosis after transplantation for hepatitis C virus: persistent elevation of serum transaminase levels versus necroinflammatory activity. *Liver Transpl* 2000; **6**: 44–53.

19. Sanchez-Fueyo A, Restrepo JC, Quinto L, Bruguera M, Grande L, Sanchez-Tapia JM. Impact of the recurrent hepatitis C virus infection after liver transplantation on the long-term viability of the graft. *Transplantation* 2002; **73**: 56–63.

20. Forman LM, Lewis JD, Berlin JA, Feldman HI, Lucey MR. The association between hepatitis C infection and survival after liver transplantation. *Gastroenterology* 2002; **122**: 889–96.

21. Charlton M. Natural history of hepatitis C and outcomes following liver transplantation. *Clin Liver Dis* 2003; **7**: 585–602.

22. OPTN/SRTR 2003 Annual Report: Transplant data 1993–2002. HHS/HRSA/SPB/DOT; UNOS; URREA. Available at http://www.ustransplant.org. Accessed March 2005.

23. O'Grady JG, Alexander GJ, Hayllar KM, Williams R. Early indicators of prognosis in fulminant hepatic failure. *Gastroenterology* 1989; **97**: 439–45.

24. Abt PL, Mange KC, Olthoff KM, Markmann JF, Reddy KR, Shaked A. Allograft survival following adult-to-adult living donor liver transplantation. *Am J Transplant* 2004; **4**: 1302–7.

25. Thuluvath PJ, Yoo YH. Graft and patient survival after adult living donor liver transplantation compared to matched cohort who received a deceased donor transplantation. *Liver Transpl* 2004; **10**: 1263–8.

26. Brown SR Jr, Russo MW, Lai M, Shiffman ML, Richardson MC, Everhart JE, Hoofnagel JH. A survey of liver transplantation from living adult donors in the United States. *N Engl J Med* 2003; **348**: 818–25.

27. Broelsch CE, Malago M, Testa G, Gamazo CV. Living donor liver transplantation in adults: outcome in Europe. *Liver Transpl* 2000; **6**: S64–5.

28. Todo S, Furukawa H, Jin MB, Shimamura T. Living donor liver transplantation in adults: outcome in Japan. *Liver Transpl* 2000; **6**: S66–S72.

29. Chen CL, Fan ST, Lee SG, Makuuchi M, Tanaka K. Living-donor liver transplantation: 12 years of experience in Asia. *Transplantation* 2003; **75**(3 Suppl): S6–11.

30. Skluzacek PA, Szewc RG, Nolan CR, Riley DJ, Lee S, Pergola PE. Prediction of GFR in liver transplant candidates. *Am J Kidney Dis* 2003; **42**: 1169–76.

31. O'Grady JG, Forbes A, Rolles K, Calne RY, Williams R. An analysis of cyclosporine efficacy and toxicity after liver transplantation. *Transplantation* 1988; **45**: 575–9.

32. Zuber J, Martinez F, Droz D, Oksenhendler E, Legendre C; Groupe d'Étude des Nephrologues D'Île-de-France (GENIF). Alpha-interferon-associated thrombotic microangiopathy: a clinicopathologic study of 8 patients and review of the literature. *Medicine (Baltimore)* 2002; **81**: 321–31.

33. Ojo AO, Held PJ, Port FK. Chronic renal failure after transplantation of non-renal organ. *N Eng J Med* 2003; **349**: 931–40.

34. Gonwa TA, Morris CA, Goldstein RM, Husberg BS, Klintmalm GB. Long-term survival and renal function following liver transplantation in patients with and without hepatorenal syndrome—experience in 300 patients. *Transplantation* 1991; **51**: 428–30.

35. Bica I, McGovern B, Dhar R, Stone D, McGowan K, Scheib R, Snydman DR. Increasing mortality due to end-stage liver disease in patients with human immunodeficiency virus infection. *Clin Infect Dis* 2001; **32**: 492–7.

36. Roland M, Stock PG. Review of solid-organ transplantation in HIV-infected patients. *Transplantation* 2003; **75**: 425–9.

37. Starzl TE, Iwatsuki S, Van Thiel DH, Gartner JC, Zitelli BJ, Malatack JJ, Schade RR, Shaw BW Jr, Hakala TR, Rosenthal JT, Porter KA. Evolution of liver transplantation. *Hepatology* 1982; **2**: 614–36.

Abbreviations

5-ASA	5-aminosalicylic acid
AAP	American Academy of Pediatrics
AASLD	American Association for the Study of Liver Diseases
AC-1	Amsterdam-1 criteria
ACBE	air-contrast barium enema
ACT 1, ACT 2	Active Ulcerative Colitis Trials 1 and 2
AFP	alpha-feto-protein
AIDS	acquired immune deficiency syndrome
AIH	autoimmune hepatitis
ALDLT	adult living donor liver transplantation
ALT	alanine aminotransferase
ALT	alanine transaminase
ANA	antinuclear antibodies
ANCA	antineutrophil cytoplasmic antibodies
anti-HB	anti-hepatitis B surface antigen
ASCA	anti-Saccharonyces cervesiae antibodies
AST	aspartate aminotransferase
AST	aspartate transaminase Bb-12 bifidobacteria
BMD	bone mineral density
BMI	body mass index
BNP	B type natriuretic peptide
CAM	complementary and alternative medicine
CARD	caspase activation and recruitment domain
CBF	cerebral blood flow
CBS	cystathionine β-synthase
CC	collagenous colitis
CCFA	Crohn's and Colitis Foundation of America
CD	Crohn's disease
CDAI	Crohn's disease activity index
CDC	Centers for Disease Control
CDEIS	Crohn's Disease Endoscopic Index of Severity
CEA	carcinoembryonic antigen
CGQL	Cleveland Global Quality of Life score
CH	compensatory hyperinsulinaemia
CHS	Clalit Health Services
CI	confidence interval
CLDQ	Chronic Liver Disease Questionnaire
COX 2	cyclooxygenase 2
CRF	chronic renal failure
CSA	cross-sectional area
CSE	cystathionine γ-lyase
CTC	computed tomographic colonography
CTC	computed tomographic colonoscopy
CTP	Child–Turcotte–Pugh

CyA/TAC cylosporin A/tacrolimus
DDW Digestive Disease Week
DES diffuse oesophageal spasm
EBUS-TBNA endobronchial ultrasound-guided transbronchial needle aspiration
EGD oesophagogastroduodenoscopy
EIM oesophageal impedance monitoring
ELH electrohydraulic lithotripsy
EMD oesophageal motility disorders
EMR endoscopic mucosal resection
EOTR end-of-treatment response
EPS Endoscopic Plication System
ERCP endoscopic retrograde cholangiopancreatography
EUS endoscopic ultrasonography
EUS-FNA endoscopic ultrasound fine-needle aspiration
EV oesophageal varices
EVL endoscopic variceal ligation
FAP familial adenomatous polyposis
FDA Food and Drugs Administration (USA)
FGF fibroblast growth factor
FHF fulminant hepatic failure
FNA fine-needle aspiration
FOBT faecal occult blood testing
FPI fasting plasma insulin
FS flexible sigmoidoscopy
FSS Fatigue Severity Score
GER gastro-oesophageal reflux
GERD gastro-oesophageal reflux disease
GETAID Groupe d'Étude Thérapeutique des Affections Inflammatoires Digestives
GGT gamma-glutamyltransferase
GGT gamma-glutamyl-transpeptidase
GM-CSF granulocyte–macrophage colony stimulating factor
HAART highly active antiretroviral therapy
HAV hepatitis A virus
HBeAg hepatitis B envelope antigen
HBsAg hepatitis B surface antigen
HBV hepatitis B virus
HCC hepatocellular carcinoma
HCIG hepatitis C-enriched immune globulin
HCIG hepatitis C immunoglobulin
HCV hepatitis C virus
HE hepatic encephalopathy
HIV human immunodeficiency virus
HMG-CoA 3-hydroxy-3methyl-glutaryl coenzyme A

HNPCC	hereditary non-polyposis colorectal cancer
HOMA	homeostasis model assessment
HRM	high-resolution manometry
HRS	hepatorenal syndrome
H2S	hydrogen sulphide
HVPG	hepatic venous pressure gradient
IBD	inflammatory bowel disease
IBDQ	inflammatory bowel disease questionnaire
IBS	irritable bowel syndrome
IBS-QOL	Irritable Bowel Syndrome Quality of Life score
ICC	intrahepatic cholangiocarcinoma
ICP	intracranial pressure
ICP	intrahepatic cholestasis of pregnancy
IEM	ineffective oesophageal motility
IFN-α	interferon α
IgG4	immunoglobulin G4
IL	interleukin
IMPDH	inosine monophosphate dehydrogenase
INR	international normalized ratio
IPAA	ileal pouch–anal anastomosis
IPMN	intraductal papillary mucinous neoplasm
IPS	irritable pouch syndrome
IQR	interquartile range
IR	insulin resistance
KGF	kerationocyte growth factor
KGFR	KGF receptor
La-5	lactobacilli
LADR	low accelerating dose regimen
LES	lower oesophageal sphincter
LESP	lower oesophageal sphincter pressure
LOH	loss of heterozygosity
MELD	Model for End-stage Liver Disease
mIU	million international units
MMF	mycophenolate mofetil
MMPD	merimepodib
MMR	mismatch repair
MRI	magnetic resonance imaging
MSI	microsatellite instability
MSI-H	MSI-high
MSI-L	MSI-low
MSS	microsatellite stable
mU	million units
NAFLD	non-alcoholic fatty liver disease
NASH	non-alcoholic steatohepatitis
NBD	nasobiliary drainage
NF-κB	nuclear factor κB
NHANES	National Health and Nutrition Examination Survey
NIH	National Institutes of Health
NNC	number needed to encounter one complication
NNS	number needed to screen
NO	nitric oxide

NOD2	nucleotide oligermization domain 2	PSC	primary sclerosing cholangitis
NPS	National Polyp Study	RFA	radiofrequency ablation
NSAID	non-steroidal anti-inflammatory drug	rFVIIa	recombinant factor VIIa
NTx	amino telopeptide of type I collagen of organic bone matrix	ROC	receiver operating characteristic
OLT	orthotopic liver transplantation	SBP	spontaneous bacterial peritonitis
OmpC	outer membrane porin C	SEER	Surveillance, Epidemiologic, and End Results
OR	odds ratio	SF36	Medical Outcome Short Form 36
PAB	Performance Assessment Battery	SIBO	small intestinal bacterial overgrowth
pANCA	perinuclear antineutrophil cytoplasmic antibodies	SIR	standardized incidence ratio
PBC	primary biliary cirrhosis	SNP	single-nucleotide polymorphism
PCDAI	Pediatric Crohn's Disease Activity Index	SOM	sphincter of Oddi manometry
PCR	polymerase chain reaction	SPECT	single photon emission computed tomography
PDAI	Pouchitis Disease Activity Index	SPLIT	Studies of Pediatric Liver Transplantation
PDT	photodynamic therapy	SRTR	Scientific Registry of Transplant Recipients
PELD	Pediatric End-stage Liver Disease	STP	spatiotemporal plot
PELD	Pediatric End-stage Liver Transplantation	SVR	sustained viral response
S-PIIINP	serum pamino-terminal propeptide of type III procallagen	SVR	sustained virological response
ppb	parts per billion	TACE	transarterial chemoembolization
PPI	proton pump inhibitor	TGF-β1	transforming growth factor β1
ppm	parts per million	TIPS	transjugular intrahepatic portosystemic shunt
PSA	prostate specific antigen		

TLESR	transient lower oesophageal sphincter relaxation
TLR	toll-like receptor
TNF	tumour necrosis factor
UC	ulcerative colitis
UCDAI	ulcerative colitis disease activity index
UCSF	University of California at San Francisco
UDCA	ursodeoxycholic acid
UNOS	United Network for Organ Sharing
VAS	visual analogue score
WCE	wireless capsule endoscopy

Index of papers reviewed

General index

KEEPING UP TO DATE IN ONE SERIES

"THE YEAR IN ..."

EXISTING AND FUTURE VOLUMES

The Year in Allergy 2003	ISBN 1 904392 05 9
The Year in Allergy 2004	ISBN 1 904392 25 3
The Year in Allergy Volume 3	ISBN 1 904392 60 1
The Year in Anaesthesia and Critical Care Volume 1	ISBN 1 904392 47 4
The Year in Diabetes 2004	ISBN 1 904392 20 2
The Year in Gastroenterology and Hepatology Volume 1	ISBN 1 904392 48 2
The Year in Gastroenterology and Hepatology Volume 2	ISBN 1 904392 81 4
The Year in Gynaecology 2003	ISBN 1 904392 10 5
The Year in Heart Failure Volume 1	ISBN 1 904392 38 5
The Year in Hypertension 2004	ISBN 1 904392 28 8
The Year in Hypertension Volume 6	ISBN 1 904392 56 3
The Year in Infection Volume 2	ISBN 1 904392 32 6
The Year in Infection Volume 3	ISBN 1 904392 72 5
The Year in Interventional Cardiology 2003	ISBN 1 904392 14 8
The Year in Interventional Cardiology Volume 3	ISBN 1 904392 33 4
The Year in Lipid Disorders Volume 1	ISBN 1 904392 96 2
The Year in Neurology 2004	ISBN 1 904392 22 9
The Year in Osteoporosis Volume 1	ISBN 1 904392 27 X
The Year in Osteoporosis Volume 2	ISBN 1 904392 62 8
The Year in Post-Menopausal Health 2004	ISBN 1 904392 23 7
The Year in Renal Medicine Volume 1	ISBN 1 904392 39 3
The Year in Respiratory Medicine 2004	ISBN 1 904392 31 8
The Year in Respiratory Medicine Volume 3	ISBN 1 904392 53 9
The Year in Rheumatic Disorders Volume 4	ISBN 1 904392 29 6
The Year in Rheumatic Disorders Volume 5	ISBN 1 904392 57 1
The Year in Schizophrenia Volume 1	ISBN 1 904392 04 0
The Year in Therapeutics Volume 1	ISBN 1 904392 50 4
The Year in Urology Volume 2	ISBN 1 904392 30 X
The Year in Urology Volume 3	ISBN 1 904392 82 2

KEEPING UP TO DATE IN ONE VOLUME
THE YEAR IN GASTROENTEROLOGY AND HEPATOLOGY
VOLUME 2

SUBJECT MATTERS DEALT WITH IN PREVIOUS VOLUME
THE YEAR IN GASTROENTEROLOGY AND HEPATOLOGY VOLUME 1

ISBN 1 904392 48 2

Diseases of the upper gastrointestinal tract
- Acid-related diseases
- Upper gastrointestinal motility
- Advances in gastro-oesophageal reflux disease
- Nutrition

Disease of the lower gastrointestinal tract
- Colorectal neoplasia
- Therapy for Crohn's disease
- Epidemiological studies in inflammatory bowel disease
- Inflammatory bowel disease genetics
- Risk factors and treatment for pouchitis
- Overview of irritable bowel syndrome

Gastrointestinal endoscopy and pancreatic diseases
- Endoscopic ultrasonography
- Biliary endoscopy
- Non-steroidal anti-inflammatory drugs—cyclooxygenase-2 inhibition
- Pancreatic disease

Hepatology and liver transplantation
- Chronic viral hepatitis
- Cholestatic liver diseases
- Non-alcoholic fatty liver disease and portal hypertension
- Hepatobiliary malignancies
- Overview of liver transplantation

Clinical Publishing
Oxford Centre for Innovation
Mill Street
Oxford OX2 0JX, UK
T: +44 1865 811116
F: +44 1865 251550
E: info@clinicalpublishing.co.uk
W: www.clinicalpublishing.co.uk